Textbook on
Nutrition and Dietetics
for Post Basic BSc Nursing Students

Textbook on
Nutrition and Dietetics
for Post Basic BSc Nursing Students

I Clement
MA (Sociology) MA (Child Care and Education) MSc (Nursing)
PG Diploma in Hospital Administration

Principal
VSS College of Nursing, Nagadevanahalli
Bengaluru, Karnataka, India

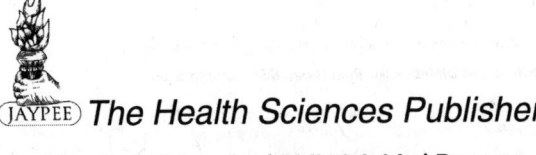

JAYPEE The Health Sciences Publishers

New Delhi | London | Philadelphia | Panama

Jaypee Brothers Medical Publishers (P) Ltd

Headquarters

Jaypee Brothers Medical Publishers (P) Ltd
4838/24, Ansari Road, Daryaganj
New Delhi 110 002, India
Phone: +91-11-43574357
Fax: +91-11-43574314
Email: jaypee@jaypeebrothers.com

Overseas Offices

J.P. Medical Ltd
83 Victoria Street, London
SW1H 0HW (UK)
Phone: +44 20 3170 8910
Fax: ++44 (0)20 3008 6180
Email: info@jpmedpub.com

Jaypee Medical Inc
The Bourse
111 South Independence Mall East
Suite 835, Philadelphia, PA 19106, USA
Phone: +1 267-519-9789
Email: jpmed.us@gamil.com

Jaypee Brothers Medical Publishers (P) Ltd
Bhotahity, Kathmandu, Nepal
Phone: +977-9741283608
Email: kathmandu@jaypeebrothers.com

Jaypee-Highlights Medical Publishers Inc
City of Knowledge, Bld. 237, Clayton
Panama City, Panama
Phone: +1 507-301-0496
Fax: +1 507-301-0499
Email: cservice@jphmedical.com

Jaypee Brothers Medical Publishers (P) Ltd
17/1-B Babar Road, Block-B, Shaymali
Mohammadpur, Dhaka-1207
Bangladesh
Mobile: +08801912003485
Email: jaypeedhaka@gmail.com

Website: www.jaypeebrothers.com
Website: www.jaypeedigital.com

© 2015, Jaypee Brothers Medical Publishers

The views and opinions expressed in this book are solely those of the original contributor(s)/author(s) and do not necessarily represent those of editor(s) of the book.

All rights reserved. No part of this publication may be reproduced, stored or transmitted in any form or by any means, electronic, mechanical, photocopying, recording or otherwise, without the prior permission in writing of the publishers.

All brand names and product names used in this book are trade names, service marks, trademarks or registered trademarks of their respective owners. The publisher is not associated with any product or vendor mentioned in this book.

Medical knowledge and practice change constantly. This book is designed to provide accurate, authoritative information about the subject matter in question. However, readers are advised to check the most current information available on procedures included and check information from the manufacturer of each product to be administered, to verify the recommended dose, formula, method and duration of administration, adverse effects and contraindications. It is the responsibility of the practitioner to take all appropriate safety precautions. Neither the publisher nor the author(s)/editor(s) assume any liability for any injury and/or damage to persons or property arising from or related to use of material in this book.

This book is sold on the understanding that the publisher is not engaged in providing professional medical services. If such advice or services are required, the services of a competent medical professional should be sought.

Every effort has been made where necessary to contact holders of copyright to obtain permission to reproduce copyright material. If any have been inadvertently overlooked, the publisher will be pleased to make the necessary arrangements at the first opportunity.

Inquiries for bulk sales may be solicited at: jaypee@jaypeebrothers.com

Textbook on Nutrition and Dietetics for Post Basic BSc Nursing Students

First Edition: **2015**

ISBN 978-93-5152-299-7

Printed at Sanat Printers, Kundli

Dedicated to

Professor (Mrs) Jessie Sudarsanam
Former President
Trained Nurses' Association of India (TNAI)
Tamil Nadu Branch

Head
Department of Medical Surgical Nursing
Annai JKK Sampoorani Ammal College of Nursing
Namakkal, Tamil Nadu, India

Preface

Nursing is a challenging profession where the nurses play dynamic roles in day-to-day life. One of such roles is becoming a 'talented nutritionist'. Learning of nutrition and dietetics has become a vital part of nursing care since the therapeutic nutrition forms an important part of treatment for all age-groups, though the medications will treat the pathological causes. But stability of a patient's health depends upon providing the right kind of nutrition as per the patient's disease condition. Therefore, imparting, updating and inculcating knowledge about nutrition in relation to the disease condition became an important need for each nurse. This is the reason why in the Post Basic BSc Nursing curriculum, nutrition and dietetics have been added as their subject in the first year.

Keeping all these aims in mind, this textbook on nutrition and Dietetics is prepared to meet the requirement as per the Indian Nursing Council recommendations. This book is divided into four sections: first—nutrition, second—dietetics, third—infant and child nutrition, and fourth—community nutrition, and contains 32 chapters.

For better understanding of the content, each chapter has the glossary, illustrations done with simple lucid language, and with adequate tables and diagrams wherever needed. For students' betterment, previous years' question papers (six in number) have also been provided. Be it the students or teachers, whosoever goes through this book, is sure to get clear-cut knowledge about the concept of nutrition and dietetics. For students, contents in this book will be adequate, apt to the point, and also helpful for them to score well in the examinations.

I wish the students all the best!

I Clement

Acknowledgments

I am thankful to the Lord Almighty who strengthens me with his abundant blessings through innumerable means, helping me in all my accomplishments.

My heartfelt thanks to Shri Sommana, Former Minister of Karnataka, and Chairman of VSS Group of Institutions, for his constant support and encouragement.

My sincere thanks to my guru Dr BT Basavanthappa, Principal, Rajarajeswari College of Nursing, Bengaluru, Karnataka, India, and PV Ramachandran, Chairman, College of Nursing, Sri Ramachandra University, Chennai, Tamil Nadu, India, a great philosopher and an internationally renowned teacher of nursing, who helped me in discovering the world of knowledge. I am thankful to Ms Shylaja Sommana, Managing Director, Dr BS Arun, Dr BS Naveen and Ms Divya from VSS Group of Institutions, Bengaluru, Karnataka, India, for their support and encouragement.

I am also grateful to Dr BC Bhagavan, Professor, Department of Surgery, Kempegowda Institute of Medical Sciences, Bengaluru, Karnataka, India, and Dr Ashwathnarayan, MLA, Chairman, Padmashree Group of Institutions, Bengaluru, Karnataka, India.

Special thanks to Dr TV Ramakrishnan, Professor of Anesthesiology and Head of Clinical Services, Department of Accident and Emergency Medicine, Sri Ramachandra University, Chennai, Tamil Nadu, India. Dr Jeyaseelan Manickam Devadasan, Dean, Dr Tamilmani, Principal, Professor (Mrs) Jessie Sudarsanam, Head, Department of Medical Surgical Nursing, Annai JKK Sampoorani Ammal College of Nursing, Namakkal, Tamil Nadu, India, and all my teachers and students.

I convey my sincere thanks to my beloved parents, brothers and sisters, and my wife Nisha Clement for her continuous support and constant encouragement in each step of my life. I take this opportunity to thank my little ones, Cabin, Cynthia and Cavin. I extend thanks to my beloved friend and brother Mr Regi T Kurien.

Special thanks to Shri Jitendar P Vij (Group Chairman), Mr Ankit Vij (Group President), Mr Tarun Duneja (Director–Publishing), Mr KK Raman (Production Manager) of M/s Jaypee Brothers Medical Publishers (P) Ltd, New Delhi, and Mr Venugopal V (Regional Manager, Bengaluru), Mr Santhosh Kumar (Author Coordinator), Ms Sajini SV (Team Head) and all other staff members of M/s Jaypee Brothers Medical Publishers (P) Ltd, Bengaluru Branch.

Contents

SECTION 1: NUTRITION

Chapter 1: Introduction to Nutrition   3
    Nutrition   4
    History of Nutrition   4
    Concept of Nutrition   8
    Nutrition and Health   9
    Nutrition—A Basic Human Need   12
    Physiology of Nutrition   14
    Importance of Nutrition in Health   17
    Relation of Nutrition to Health   18
    Nutrition-related Health Problems   19
    Food   21
    Functions of Food   21
    Classification of Foods   24
    Food Groups   26
    Nutritive Value of Common Foods   26
    Healthy Food Substances   29
    Calorie   31
    Body Mass Index (Quetelet's Index)   32
    Basal Metabolic Rate   32
    Energy   33

Chapter 2: Review of Macro- and Micro-nutrition   39
    Macro- and Micro-nutrients   39
    Carbohydrates   40
    Fiber   48
    Proteins   49
    Lipids   62
    Vitamins   72
    Fat-soluble Vitamins   73
    Vitamin D   78
    Vitamin E   84

Vitamin K   86
Thiamine   88
Riboflavin   92
Niacin   95
Pyridoxine   98
Pantothenic Acid   101
Folic Acid   101
Cyanocobalamin   103
Vitamin C   105
Vitamin Deficiencies   109
Mineral Elements   111
Calcium   112
Phosphorus   118
Microminerals   120
Trace Elements   132

Chapter 3: Balanced Diet   134
Importance   134
Meaning   135
Elements   135
Components of Healthy Balanced Diet   138
Factors Influencing   140
Calculation   143
Effects of Unbalanced Diets   145
Specific Nutritional Deficiencies   146
Conditions with Specific Dietary Requirement   147
Nurses' Health Promotion Role   151

Chapter 4: Meal Planning   152
Importance   152
Objectives   153
Goals   153
Factors Affecting   154
Steps in Meal Planning   158
Meal Planning for Different Meals in a Day   159
Budget for Food   163

Chapter 5: Food Hygiene/Sanitation   168
Hygiene   168
Principles of Food Sanitation   170
Sources of Food Contamination   171

Food Poisoning 172
Practical Rules for Food Sanitation 175
Hygiene Control 176
Effects of Unsafe Practices 178
Legislation, Regulations and Codes of Practice 179
Hazard Analysis and Critical Control Point 180

Chapter 6: Food Adulteration 182
Concept of Adulteration 183
Meaning of Food Adulteration 184
Food Adulteration and Health 185
Adulterants 186
Packaging Materials and Hazards 190
Food Laws and Standards 192
Consumer Protection 194
Sale of Certain Admixtures is Prohibited 195
Procedures for Sampling and Analysis 195
Penalties 196
Important Miscellaneous Provisions 196

Chapter 7: Cooking Methods 198
Objectives of Cooking 198
Different Methods of Cooking 199
Combination of Cooking Methods 209

Chapter 8: Food Preservation 212
Food Spoilage 212
Principles of Food Preservation 213
Methods of Food Preservation 213

SECTION 2: DIETETICS

Chapter 9: Introduction to Dietetics 229
Diet as a Therapeutic Agent 230
General Objectives of Diet Therapy 231
Meaning of Diet Therapy 231
Principles of Diet Therapy 231
Factors to Consider in Planning Therapeutic Diets 232
Modification of Nutrients in Therapeutic Diets 232
Team Approach 232

Chapter 10: Diet in Sickness — 236
Purposes 236
General Rules of Treatment 236
Problems During Sickness 237
Diet 238
Special Feeding Methods (Management of Special Diets) 246

Chapter 11: Dietary Modifications — 249
Important Factors Involved 249
Kilocalorie Modifications 251
Nurse's Responsibilities in Food Serving 263

Chapter 12: Diet Therapy for Perioperative Conditions — 267
Preoperative Diet 267
Postoperative Diet 269
Diet Plan for Pre- and Post-operative Surgery 271

Chapter 13: Diet Therapy in Fevers — 274
Diet for Common Fevers 274
Diet Therapy in Different Types of Fever 275
Causes of Fever 276
General Dietary Management 278
Typhoid Fever 279

Chapter 14: Diet Therapy for Gastrointestinal Disorders — 284
Diarrhea 285
Constipation 286
Peptic Ulcer 290

Chapter 15: Diet Therapy for Liver Diseases — 294
Infective Hepatitis (Jaundice) 295
Cirrhosis of Liver 297
Hepatic Coma 299
Cholelithiasis 301
Dietary Restriction for Liver Diseases 302

Chapter 16: Diet Therapy for Endocrine and Metabolic Disorders — 306
Diabetes Mellitus 306
Various Metabolic Disorders 314

Chapter 17: Diet Therapy for Urinary Disorders — 320
Glomerulonephritis 320
Nephrosis (Degenerative Bright's Disease) 321
Acute Renal Failure 322
Chronic Renal Failure 323
Urolithiasis or Urinary Calculi 326

Chapter 18: Diet Therapy for Cardiovascular Disorders — 329
Types 329
Dietary Management in Cardiovascular Disorders 330
Hypertension 331

Chapter 19: Diet Therapy for Allergy — 334
Food as Allergens 334
Immediate versus Delayed Hypersensitivity 336
Diagnosis of Food Allergy 337
Treatment 339
Food Intolerance 340

Chapter 20: Diet Therapy for Respiratory Disorder — 343
Tuberculosis 343

Chapter 21: Nurse's Role in Diet Therapy — 346
Factors Affecting the Risk of Malnutrition 347
Assistance with Meals 350
Feeding Adults 351
Feeding the Helpless Patient 353
Nasogastric Tube Insertion 356
Gastric Gavage 359
Gastrojejunostomy Feeding 362

Chapter 22: Fluid and Electrolytes — 366
Importance of Water 366
Functions of Water 367
Requirements 368
Dehydration 369
Electrolyte 370
Hyponatremia 372
Hypernatremia 374

Hypokalemia 377
Hyperkalemia 379
Hypocalcemia 380
Hypercalcemia 383
Hypomagnesemia 385
Hypermagnesemia 387
Hypophosphatemia 389
Hyperphosphatemia 391

SECTION 3: INFANT AND CHILD NUTRITION

Chapter 23: Nutritional Needs of Infants 397
Need of Infant Nutrition 397
Dietary Requirements 398
Infancy 399
Childhood 400
Exclusive Breastfeeding 400
Artificial Feeding 414
Complementary Feeding 422

Chapter 24: Premature Infant Feeding 427
Importance of Preterm Nutrition 427
Nutritional Requirements 431
Goals of Nutrition 433
Feeding Protocol 434
Intolerance to Feedings 436

Chapter 25: Weaning and Supplementary Feeding 440
Weaning 440
Baby-friendly Hospital Initiative 449
Supplementary Feeding 452

Chapter 26: Nutritional Assessment 456
Concept 456
Assessment of Nutritional Status 457
Anthropometric Approach 462
Nutritional Assessment Guidelines 463
Road-to-Health Chart 467

Chapter 27: Nutrition for a Sick Child — 470
Effects of Illness on Food   470
Special Feeding Methods   471
Emergency Nutrition for Sick   476
Nutritional Problems of the Child   478
Malnutrition   480

Chapter 28: Child Nutrition Programs — 484
Special Nutrition Program   484
Applied Nutrition Program   487
Integrated Child Development Services   490
Minimum Need Program   492
Twenty Point Program   492
Child Survival and Safe Motherhood Program   493

SECTION 4: COMMUNITY NUTRITION

Chapter 29: Community Nutrition — 499
Nutritional Needs of Individuals   499

Chapter 30: Nutritional Problems and Policies — 526
Factors Affecting Nutritional Status   526
Steps to Solve Nutritional Problems   527
Nutritional Deficiency   528
National Nutritional Policy   544
Obesity   549

Chapter 31: Community Nutrition Programs — 551
Nutrition Programs   551
Current Nutritional Deficiency Status   556
Five Year Plans on Nutritional Aspects   557
Integrated Child Development Service   558
Mid-day Meal Program   561
National Nutritional Anemia Program   563
Special Nutrition Program   566
National Goiter Control Program   567
National Program for Prophylaxis against Blindness due to Vitamin A Deficiency   568
Balwadi Nutrition Program   569
Applied Nutrition Program   569
World Food Program   570

Chapter 32: Community Nutritional Rehabilitation — 574
Rehabilitation for Protein-Energy Malnutrition Children 574
Community Nutrition Training 576
Nutrition Education 581
Food and Nutrition Board 586
Activities of Food and Nutrition Board 586
Nutrition Society of India 587
Food and Agriculture Organization 587
Cooperative for Assistance and Relief Everywhere 589
National Institute of Nutrition, Hyderabad 589
Central Food Technological Research Institute, Mysore 591
National Institute of Public Cooperation and Child Development 593

Previous Years' Question Papers — 597
Nutrition and Dietetics—September 2012 599
Nutrition and Dietetics—March 2012 599
Nutrition and Dietetics—August 2011 600
Nutrition and Dietetics—February 2011 601
Nutrition and Dietetics—August 2010 601
Nutrition and Dietetics—February 2010 602

Glossary — 603
Nutrition 605
Dietetics 607
Infant and Child Nutrition 609
Community Nutrition 612

Index — 615

SECTION 1

Nutrition

Chapter 1

Introduction to Nutrition

▶ INTRODUCTION

Food is prime necessity of life. The food we eat is digested and assimilated in the body, and used for its maintenance and growth. Food also provides energy for doing work. Man has exhibited much thought and foresight in cultivating a variety of grains, fruits, vegetables, nuts and oil seeds, and in rearing birds and animals for use as food. Nutrition deals with the way in which the human body receives, and uses all the substance or materials necessary for its growth and development and for keeping it in good condition. This begins in eating food. The food swallowed then digested as it is passed through the stomach and small intestines. During digestion, the food is broken up into simple substances. These are absorbed into bloodstream and carried to the liver, where they are either stored, or changed further or sent out to other parts of the body for use as required.

▶ DEFINITIONS

1. **Food:** It is defined as anything solid, liquid or semisolid, which when ingested putting into the mouth, digested and assimilated, nourishes the body. The edible stuff that provides us with nutrients is termed as food. It is broadly classified as cereals, pulses, vegetables, fruits, milk, eggs, flesh foods, fats and sugar.
2. **Nutrients:** These are defined as those chemical substances, which are supplied by food, and are needed as a source of energy and as a structural material for every cell of the body. These are constituents in food that must be supplied

to the body in suitable amounts. They include proteins, fats, carbohydrates, minerals, water and vitamins.
3. **Nutrition status:** It is defined as the extent to which a customary diet meets the body's requirement. In other words, it signifies the condition of the body after the consumption of food. The condition of individual's health is influenced by the utilization of nutrients. It can be assessed by dietary survey, anthropometry, clinical and laboratory investigations.

NUTRITION

Nutrition is the combination of processes by which the living organism receives and utilizes the materials necessary for the maintenance of its function, and for the growth and renewal of its components.

Nutrition is that condition, which permits the development and maintenance of the highest state of fitness. And also it involves is processes or activities by which the human body receives and uses all the food necessary for its growth, development, regulation and repair. It is the science of food, the nutrients and other substances therein, their action, interaction and balance in relationship to health and disease.

▶ HISTORY OF NUTRITION

Nutritional discoveries from the earliest days of history have had a positive effect on our health and well-being (Table 1.1). The word nutrition itself means "the process of nourishing or being nourished, especially the process by which a living organism assimilates food, and uses it for growth and replacement of tissues." Nutrients are substances that are essential to life, which must be supplied by food. Today more than ever, obtaining nutritional knowledge can make a big difference in lives. Air, soil and water pollution in addition to modern farming techniques, have depleted soils of vital minerals. The widespread use of food additives, chemicals, sugar and unhealthy fats in the diets contributes to many of the degenerative diseases such as cancer, heart disease, arthritis and osteoporosis.

CHAPTER 1: Introduction to Nutrition

Here is a brief history of the science that offers the hope of improving health naturally.

The first recorded nutritional experiment is recorded in the book of Daniel in the Bible. Daniel was among the finest young men captured by the King of Babylon when the Babylonians over ran Israel and was to serve in the King's court. He was to be fed from the King's table of fine foods and wine. Daniel objected and preferred his own choices, which included vegetables (pulses) and water. The chief steward was afraid for his head, but agreed to a trial. Daniel and his friends received his own diet for 10 days and then were compared to the King's men, as they appeared fitter and healthier. They were allowed to continue with their own foods, not defiling themselves with those of the King. The 20th century became the era of the Golden Age of Nutrition, when most of the discoveries of the nutrients took place. Stephen Babcock was instrumental in helping to open the age. Babcock, better known for the Babcock test for milk fat that bears his name and conceived the idea to feed dairy cattle feed from just one source, all corn plant or all wheat plant.

Table 1.1: Highlights of history of nutrition

Sl No	Year	Description
1.	400 BC	Hippocrates, the 'Father of Medicine', said to his students, "Let food be thy medicine and medicine be thy food". He also said, "wise man should consider that health is the greatest of human blessings". Foods were often used as cosmetics or as medicines in the treatment of wounds. In some of the early Far Eastern Biblical writings, there were references to food and health. One story describes the treatment of eye disease, now known to be due to vitamin A deficiency, by squeezing the juice of liver onto the eye. Large amounts of vitamin A is stored in the liver.
2.	1447	James Lind, a physician in the British Navy, performed the first scientific experiment in nutrition. At that time, sailors were sent on long voyages for years and they developed scurvy (a painful, deadly bleeding disorder). Only non-perishable foods such

Contd...

SECTION 1: Nutrition

Contd...

Sl No	Year	Description
		as dried meat and breads were taken on the voyages, as fresh foods would not last. In his experiment, Lind gave some of the sailors seawater, others vinegar and the rest lime. Those given the lime were saved from scurvy. As vitamin C was not discovered until the 1930s, Lind did not know it was the vital nutrient. As a note, British sailors became known as 'Limey'.
3.	1500	Scientist and artist Leonardo da Vinci compared the process of metabolism in the body to the burning of a candle.
4.	1770	Antoine Lavoisier, the 'Father of Nutrition and Chemistry' discovered the actual process by which food is metabolized. He also demonstrated where animal heat comes from. In his equation, he describes the combination of food and oxygen in the body, and the resulting giving off heat and water.
5.	1800	It was discovered that foods are composed primarily of four elements such as carbon, nitrogen, hydrogen and oxygen, and methods were developed for determining the amounts of these elements.
6.	1840	Justus Liebig of Germany, a pioneer in early plant growth studies, was the first to point out the chemical make up of carbohydrates, fats and proteins. Carbohydrates were made up of sugars, fats were made up of fatty acids and proteins were made up of amino acids.
7.	1897	Christiaan Eijkman, a Dutchman working with natives in Java, observed that some of the natives developed a disease called beriberi, which cause heart problems and paralysis. He observed that when chickens were fed the native diet of white rice, they developed the symptoms of beriberi. When he fed the chickens, unprocessed brown rice (with the outer bran intact), they did not develop the disease. Eijkman then fed the brown rice to his patients and they were cured. He discovered that food could cure disease. Nutritionists later learned that the outer rice bran contains vitamin B_1, also known as thiamine.

Contd...

CHAPTER 1: Introduction to Nutrition

Contd...

Sl No	Year	Description
8.	1912	a. McCollum EV, while working for the US Department of Agriculture at the University of Wisconsin, developed an approach that opened the way to the widespread discovery of nutrients. He decided to work with rats rather than large farm animals such as cows and sheep. Using this procedure, he discovered the first fat-soluble vitamin (vitamin A). He found that rats fed butter were healthier than those fed lard, as butter contains more vitamin A. b. Casimir Funk was the first to coin the term 'vitamins' as vital factors in the diet. He wrote about these unidentified substances present in food, which could prevent the diseases of scurvy, beriberi and pellagra (a disease caused by a deficiency of niacin or vitamin B_3). The term vitamin is derived from the words vital and amine, because vitamins are required for life and they were originally thought to be amines—compounds derived from ammonia.
9.	1930	William Rose discovered the essential amino acids, the building blocks of protein.
10.	1940	a. The water soluble B and C vitamins were identified. b. Russell Marker perfected a method of synthesizing the female hormone progesterone from a component of wild yams called diosgenin.
11.	1950 to the present	The roles of essential nutrients as a part of bodily processes have been brought to light. For example, more came to known about the role of vitamins and minerals as components of enzymes and hormones that work within the body.
12.	1968	Linus Pauling, a Nobel Prize winner in chemistry, created the term 'orthomolecular nutrition'. Orthomolecular is literally 'pertaining to the right molecule'. Pauling proposed that by giving the right molecules to the body in the right concentration (optimum nutrition), nutrients could be used by people to achieve better health and prolong life. Studies in the 1970s and 1980s conducted by Pauling and colleagues suggested that very large doses of vitamin C given intravenously could be

Contd...

Contd...

Sl No	Year	Description
		helpful in increasing the survival time and improving the quality of life of terminal cancer patients.
13.	1994–2000	Have you ever wondered, why vitamin bottle labels and nutritional websites include a phrase saying that their products and information are not intended to diagnose, cure or prevent any disease? They usually state that their health claims have not been evaluated by the Food and Drug Administration (FDA). Here is why: The Dietary Supplement Health and Education Act was approved by Congress in October of 1994 and updated in January 2000. It sets forth, what can and cannot be said about nutritional supplements without prior FDA review.

▶ CONCEPT OF NUTRITION

Nutrition is also known as nourishment or aliment in the form of food in order to support life. The diet of an organism refers to what they eat. Many common health problems can be prevented by having a healthy diet. Dietitians are professionals who specializes human nutrition, meal planning, preparation and so on. They are trained people to provide dietary advice for every individual in health and disease. There are seven major classifications of nutrients, they are, carbohydrates, fibers, fats, proteins, minerals, water and vitamins. These classes of nutrients are categorized as macronutrients are needed in relatively large amounts. Micronutrients are needed in smaller quantities. Macronutrients are carbohydrates, fats, fibers, water and proteins, while micronutrients are vitamins and minerals.

The macronutrients provide energy, which is measured in Joules or kilocalories and written with a capital 'C' to distinguish them from gram calories. Carbohydrates and proteins provide 17 kJ (4 kcal) of energy per gram, while fats provide 37 kJ (9 kcal) of energy per gram. Vitamins, minerals, fiber and water do not provide energy, but are necessary for other reasons. Other nutrients include antioxidants and photochemicals. These substances were recently discovered, which have

CHAPTER 1: Introduction to Nutrition

been not yet recognized as vitamins or contribute to health, but they are necessary to the bodies. Photochemical may act as antioxidant, but not all of them are antioxidants.

▶ NUTRITION AND HEALTH

Health is defined by the World Health Organization (WHO) as the "state of complete physical, mental and social well-being and not merely the absence of disease or infirmity." To maintain good health and nutritional status, one must eat a balanced food, which contains all the nutrients in the correct proportion. The essential requisites of health would include the following:

1. Achievement of optimal growth and development, reflecting the full expression of one's genetic potential.
2. Maintenance of the structural integrity and functional efficiency of body tissues necessary for an active and productive use.
3. Mental well-being.
4. Ability to withstand the inevitable process of aging with minimal disability and functional impairment.
5. Ability to combat diseases such as:
   a. Resisting infections (immunocompetence).
   b. Preventing the onset of degenerative diseases.
   c. Resisting the effect of environmental toxins/pollutants.

Till 3 decades, the role of nutrition in growth and development, and tissue integrity alone was clear, but now the persuasive role nutrition plays in the other dimensions of health is implicit. Hence an optimal nutritional status is an indication of good health. This recent advance has brought about a large-scale change in dietary habits and practices of the population.

Facts About Basic Nutrition and Health

1. The amount and kinds of food taken affect his/her health and well-being.
2. Eating the recommended servings of food 'from the food guide pyramid' will provide key nutrients and enable a

person to meet the dietary recommendations outlined in this concept.
3. Counting food servings is important to assuring that adequate choices are made from the pyramid.
4. New dietary guidelines are available to help a person to plan for sound nutrition.

The number of calories needed per day depends upon the basal metabolic rate (BMR), which in turn, depends upon factors such as age, sex, size, muscle mass, glandular function, emotional state, climate and exercise.
5. Eating well can reduce risk of various health problems and increase quality of life.

Fat Dietary Recommendations

For Fats

1. Excess fat in the diet, particularly saturated fat, is associated with an increased risk of disease and is inversely related to optimal health.
2. Modified fats and fat substitutes in the diet can have varying health consequences.
3. There are some recommendations that can be followed to assure healthy amounts of fat in the diet.

For Carbohydrates

1. For optimal health, carbohydrates, especially complex carbohydrates, should be the principle source of calories in the diet.
2. There are some recommendations that can be followed to assure healthy amounts of carbohydrate in the diet.

For Proteins

1. Protein is the basic building block for the body, but dietary protein constitutes a relatively small amount of daily calorie intake.

CHAPTER 1: Introduction to Nutrition

2. There are some recommendations that can be followed to assure healthy amounts of protein in the diet.

For Vitamins

1. Adequate vitamin intake is necessary to good health and wellness, but excessive vitamin intake is not necessary and can be harmful.
2. There are some recommendations that can be followed to assure healthy amounts of vitamins in the diet.

For Minerals

1. Adequate mineral intake is necessary for good health and wellness, but excessive mineral intake is not necessary and can be harmful.
2. There are some recommendations that can be followed to assure healthy amounts of minerals in the diet.

For Water and Other Fluids

1. Water is a critical component in the healthy diet. Beverages other than water are a part of many diets. Some beverages can have an adverse effect on good health.
2. There are some recommendations that can be followed to assure healthy amounts of water and fluids in the diet.

Facts About Sound Eating Practices

1. Healthy snacks can be an important part of good nutrition.
2. Consistency (with variety) is a good general rule of nutrition.
3. Moderation is a good general rule of nutrition.
4. Careful selection of food choices is important for those who rely on fast foods as a significant part of their diet.
5. There are some recommendations that can be followed concerning fast foods.

SECTION 1: Nutrition

Facts About Nutrition and Physical Performance

1. Carbohydrate loading and carbohydrate replacement during exercise can enhance sustained aerobic performances exceeding 1 hour in length.
2. The timing may be more important than the make up of the pre-event meal.
3. High-protein diets advocated for active people and athletes have been questioned by leading organizations in the areas of health, physical activity and nutrition.
4. People who are interested in enhancing physical performance are especially subject to nutrition quackery.

▶ NUTRITION—A BASIC HUMAN NEED

Nutrition is a basic human need that changes throughout the life cycle and along the health-illness continuum. The body requires food to provide energy for organ functions, body movement and work, maintain body temperature, and to provide raw materials for enzymes function, growth replacement of cells and repair. Food provides nutrition for both the body and mind. Eating has evolved from being simply a necessity; is an integral component of medical treatment. The science of nutrition encompasses the study of nutrients and how they are handled by the body, as well as the impact of human behavior and environment on the process of nourishment. Nutrients alter specific substances used by the body for growth and development, activity, reproduction, lactation, health maintenance and recovery from illness or injury. Good nutrition is a basic component of health, growth and development for maintaining health throughout the life. Proper nutrition of the nation is necessary for the nation's growth and economic development.

Nurses must understand the functions of the basic nutrients and metabolism. An understanding of the guidelines for adequate diet is essential so that nurses can teach about nutrients and answer for the questions related to diet. Nurses must be able to assist the nutrients of the diet. They must also recognize that many divergent factors influence food intake and consider

CHAPTER 1: Introduction to Nutrition

the factors when attempting to modify food intake. The factors that influence nutrient requirements are developmental consideration, i.e. age, sex, health status, culture and religion, socioeconomic status, personal preference, medications, alcohol and drugs, etc. Nurse also must be able to identify clients at risk for nutritional problems and be aware of common nutritional conditions (Table 1.2).

The term 'food' refers to anything, which nourishes the body. It would obviously include solids, semisolids and liquids, which can be consumed. The food helps to sustain the body to keep it healthy. The terms 'food' and 'nutrition' are sometimes used synonymously, but it is not strictly correct. Food is defined as "what one feeds on and is a composite mixture of many nutrient substances ranging from a fraction of a gram in some cases to hundred of gram in others. The foodstuff is defined as anything, which can be used as food. Therefore, the word 'nutrition' is derived from the word 'nutricus', which means 'to suckle at the breast'. Nutrition is defined as combination of dynamic process by which the consumed food is utilized for nourishment, structural and functional efficiency of every cell of the body.

Metabolism refers to all the biochemical reactions within the body. It consists of anabolic reactions that build substances, body tissues and catabolic reactions those breakdown substances. Food is ingested, digested and absorbed to produce the energy needed for these reactions. The energy requirement of an awake person at rest is called the 'basal metabolic rate'. BMR is the energy needed at a person's lowest level of cellular functions. Age, body size, temperature, growth, sex, nutritional status, emotional status and good intake affect individual energy requirements beyond the BMR. When energy requirements are completely met by caloric intake in food, people maintain that activity levels without weight change. If the number of calories ingested exceeds energy needs, people gain weight. When the calories ingested fail to meet energy requirements, people lose weight.

Nutrition encompasses all of the processes involved in consuming and utilizing food for energy, maintenance and growth.

SECTION 1: Nutrition

The processes include ingestion, digestion, absorption, metabolism and excretion. Much of the discussion throughout this chapter focuses on ingestion. Because this is the process that the indicial can control and with which the nurse can assist the client. Basic information is presented about proper nutrition and the role of the nurse in assisting clients to meet their nutritional needs. Topics covered include, specific nutrients and their functions in the body; photochemicals; promoting proper nutrition factors influencing nutrition; nutritional needs during the life cycle; nutrition and health; weight management; food labeling; quality and safety; food allergies and nutrition and the nursing process.

▶ PHYSIOLOGY OF NUTRITION

Five processes are involved in the body's use of nutrients:
1. Ingestion.
2. Digestion.
3. Absorption.
4. Metabolism.
5. Excretion.

Ingestion

Nutrition begins with ingestion, taking food into the digestive tract, generally through the mouth. In special circumstances, ingestion occurs directly into the stomach, through a feeding tube.

Digestion

Digestion refers to the mechanical and chemical processes that convert nutrients into a physically absorbable state. Mechanical digestion includes mastication (chewing), breaking food into fine particles and mixing it with enzymes in saliva and deglutition (swallowing food), the peristaltic waves and mucus secretions that move the food down the esophagus. Chemical digestion includes the digestive juices changes food into the individual nutrients that can be used by the body.

CHAPTER 1: Introduction to Nutrition

Digestion begins in the stomach (except in the case of some starches for which digestion begins in the mouth) and is completed in the intestines. Peristalsis [rhythmic, coordinated, serial contractions of the smooth muscles of the gastrointestinal tract (GIT) forces], chyme (an acidic, semifluid paste) pass through the small and large intestines. Only carbohydrates, proteins and fats require chemical digestion to make the nutrients available or absorption.

Absorption

Absorption is the process, whereby the end products of digestion (i.e. individual nutrients) pass through the epithelial membranes in the small and large intestines, and into the blood or lymph systems. The nutrients are absorbed and taken to the parts of the body that need them. Most nutrients are water soluble, and can be absorbed directly through the villi (finger-like projections that line the small intestine) and into the blood. Fats, which are not water soluble are absorbed first into the lymph system and eventually enter the circulatory system (Fig. 1.1).

Metabolism

The conversion of nutrients into energy by the body is called metabolism. This process is the sum total of all the biological and chemical processes in the body as they relate to the use of nutrients in every body cell. Metabolism involves two processes:
1. Anabolism.
2. Catabolism.

Anabolism

Anabolism is the constructive process of metabolism, wherein new molecules are synthesized and new tissues are formed, as in growth and repair. This process requires energy.

Catabolism

Catabolism is the destructive process of metabolism, wherein tissues or substances are broken into their component parts.

SECTION 1: Nutrition

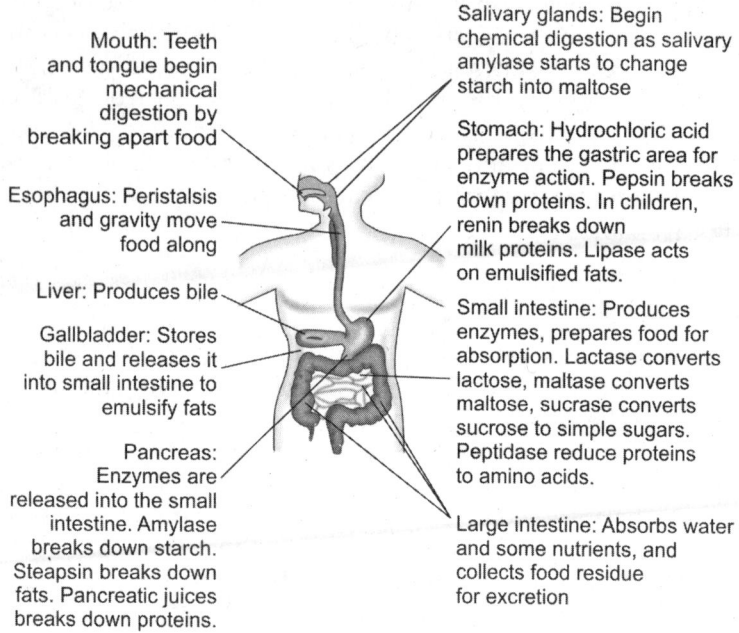

Fig. 1.1: Digestion and absorption of food at various parts of gastrointestinal tract (GIT)

Labels in figure:

- **Mouth:** Teeth and tongue begin mechanical digestion by breaking apart food
- **Esophagus:** Peristalsis and gravity move food along
- **Liver:** Produces bile
- **Gallbladder:** Stores bile and releases it into small intestine to emulsify fats
- **Pancreas:** Enzymes are released into the small intestine. Amylase breaks down starch. Steapsin breaks down fats. Pancreatic juices breaks down proteins.
- **Salivary glands:** Begin chemical digestion as salivary amylase starts to change starch into maltose
- **Stomach:** Hydrochloric acid prepares the gastric area for enzyme action. Pepsin breaks down proteins. In children, renin breaks down milk proteins. Lipase acts on emulsified fats.
- **Small intestine:** Produces enzymes, prepares food for absorption. Lactase converts lactose, maltase converts maltose, sucrase converts sucrose to simple sugars. Peptidase reduce proteins to amino acids.
- **Large intestine:** Absorbs water and some nutrients, and collects food residue for excretion

This process releases energy. During metabolism, energy is also produced by the process of oxidation, which is the chemical process of combining nutrients with oxygen. The energy produced by the body is used in a number of ways such as electrical energy for brain and nerve activities, chemical energy for metabolism, mechanical energy for muscle contractions and thermal energy to keep the body warm.

Metabolic rate: It is the rate of energy utilization in the body; it is expressed in units called calories. One calorie is the amount of heat required to raise the temperature of 1 g of water by 1°C. Because of the large quantity of energy released during metabolism, the energy is expressed in kilocalories (kcal), each of which is equal to 1,000 calories.

Basal metabolism: It is the amount of energy needed to maintain essential physiologic functions, when a person is at complete rest, i.e. the lowest level of energy expenditure. The major factor affecting basal metabolism is body composition. Lean muscle tissue has a higher metabolic rate and thus produces more energy than fat tissue. Generally, women have a lower metabolism than men, because they have a higher percentage of fat tissue; however, metabolism increases during menstruation, pregnancy and lactation. Age has also an influence, because growth periods increase metabolism. Glandular activity, especially of the thyroid gland, affects metabolism. The rate of metabolism is governed primarily by the hormones triiodothyronine (T3) and thyroxine (T4). Hypothyroid activity, a decrease in the secretion of thyroid hormones, causes a lower rate of metabolism, whereas hyperthyroid activity, an increase in the secretion of thyroid hormones, causes a higher rate of metabolism.

Excretion

Excretion is the process of eliminating or removing waste products from the body. Dietary fiber, indigestible materials, salts and other products such as bile and water are converted into feces, and excreted from the body as solid waste. Other excretory organs that aid the digestive system in the elimination of wastes include the kidneys, bladder, sweat glands, skin and lungs. Most liquid waste is sent through the kidneys and bladder to be excreted as urine. Some liquid waste is removed through the sweat glands of the skin as perspiration. Gaseous waste is eliminated through the lungs.

▶ IMPORTANCE OF NUTRITION IN HEALTH

Nutrition may be defined as the science of food and its relationship to health. It is concerned primarily with the part played by nutrients in body growth, development and maintenance. The word nutrient or 'food factor' is used for specific dietary constituents such as proteins, vitamins and minerals. Dietetics is the practical application of the principles of nutrition; it includes the planning of meals for the well and the sick. Good nutrition means "maintaining a nutritional status that enables us to grow well and enjoy good health."

Nutrition deals with the way in which the human body receives, and uses all the substance or materials necessary for its growth and development, and for keeping it in good condition. This begins in eating food. The food is swallowed and then digested as it is passed through the stomach and small intestines. During digestion, the food is broken up into simple substances. These are absorbed into bloodstream and carried to the liver, where they are either stored or changed further or sent out to other parts of the body for use as required.

Some are used to supply the body with heat and energy, and others for the building and repair of the tissues, and yet others are used to control the chemical changes taking place in the body or to protect the body from diseases, finally the waste products, which cannot be used are excreted.

▶ RELATION OF NUTRITION TO HEALTH

Good nutrition is a basic component of health. The relation of nutrition to health may be seen from the following view points.

Growth and Development

Good nutrition is essential for the attainment of normal growth and development. Not only physical growth and development but also the intellectual development, learning and behavior are affected by malnutrition. Malnutrition during pregnancy may affect the fetus resulting in stillbirth, premature birth and 'small-for-dates' babies. Malnutrition during early childhood delays physical and mental growth; such children are slow in passing their milestones and are slow learners in school. Good nutrition is also essential in adult life for the maintenance of optimum health and efficiency. In short, nutrition affects human health from birth till death.

Specific Deficiency

Malnutrition is directly responsible for certain specific nutritional deficiency diseases. The commonly reported ones in India are kwashiorkor, marasmus, blindness due to vitamin A deficiency, anemia, beriberi, goiter, etc. Good nutrition therefore is essential for the prevention of specific nutritional deficiency diseases and promotion of health.

Resistance to Infection

Malnutrition predisposes to infections like tuberculosis. It also influences the course and outcome of many of the clinical disorders. Infection, in turn, may aggravate malnutrition by affecting the food intake, absorption and metabolism.

Mortality and Morbidity

The indirect effects of malnutrition on the community are even more striking; a high general death rate, high-infant mortality rate, high-sickness rate and a lower expectation of life. Overnutrition, which is another form of malnutrition, is responsible for obesity, diabetes, hypertension, cardiovascular and renal disease, disorders of the liver and gallbladder. More recent reports suggest that diet perhaps plays an important role in certain types of gastrointestinal cancers. It is now quite well-accepted that diet and certain diseases are inter-related.

▶ NUTRITION RELATED HEALTH PROBLEMS

Diet and Nutrition

A balanced dietary intake promotes nutritional health. Genetic predisposition seems to play subsidiary role in dietary intake. Malnutrition in developing countries is essentially because of the nature of undernutrition. Inadequate dietary intake causes health problem in pregnant women, lactating mothers and growing children.

Diet and Chronic Diseases

Modern epidemics of nutrition-related chronic diseases have appeared in developed countries of the world, which is attributed to the intake of 'affluent diet'. The disease includes hypertension, coronary heart diseases, diabetes, etc. Chronic liver diseases include cirrhosis of liver, which are also prevalent in the affluent classes, are related to excessive intake of alcohol.

Diet and Cancer

Epidemiological studies carried out all over the world have established that nearly one third of all cancers types are directly related to one or the other dietary component. Diet rich in saturated fats is particularly linked to colon cancer and prostate cancer. Breast cancer and rectum cancer are also related to high-fat intake. Epidemiological studies have revealed that regular intake of fruits and vegetables, high in fiber content, low in saturated fats and rich in several antioxidants, vitamins namely, retinol, carotene, vitamin C and vitamin E act are potential carcinogenic agents.

Diet and Dental Diseases

Diet rich in sugar content predispose to dental caries. Sugar has casual association with dental caries; the association is particularly strong during childhood years with sugars that are consumed in between meals rather than with meals. High-starch diet is not cacogenic obviously because it contains complex sugars.

Diet and Skeletal Diseases

Consumption of diet, poor in calcium may predispose to osteoporosis. Alcohol intake and smoking habit are also related to osteoporosis. Osteoporosis predisposes to fracture especially in elderly people.

CHAPTER 1: Introduction to Nutrition

Diet and Mental Health

Inadequate dietary intake deficient in nutrients likes iodine, nicotinic acid and iron can retard mental development or impair mental performance. Iodine deficiency can cause an extreme degree of mental impairment as seen in cretinism. Nicotinic acid deficiency can lead to dementias in extreme cases of pellagra.

Diet and Diet Therapy

Dietetics is the word used to describe the practical application of the principles of nutrition to the human body in health and disease. Diet therapy is the science dealing with prescription of appropriate diet to patients, which constitutes an important component of their treatment.

FOOD

▶ FUNCTIONS OF FOOD

Food is the basic necessity of man. It is a mixture of different nutrients such as carbohydrate, protein, fat, vitamins and minerals. These nutrients are essential for growth, development and maintenance of good health throughout the life. They also play a vital role in meeting the special needs of pregnant and lactating women, and patients recovering from illness.

Physiological Functions

Energy-yielding Foods

Foods rich in carbohydrates and fats are called energy-yielding foods. They provide energy to sustain the involuntary processes essential for continuance of life, to carry out various professional, household and recreational activities, and to convert food ingested into usable nutrients in the body. The energy needed is supplied by the oxidation of foods consumed. Cereals, roots and tubers, dried fruits, oil, butter and ghee are all good sources of energy.

SECTION 1: Nutrition

Bodybuilding Foods

Foods rich in protein are called bodybuilding foods. Milk, meat, eggs and fish are rich in proteins of high quality. Pulses and nuts are good sources of protein, but the protein is not of high quality. These foods help to maintain life, promote growth and also supply energy.

Protective and Regulatory Foods

Food rich in protein, minerals and vitamins are known as protective and regulatory foods. They are essential for health and regulate activities such as maintenance of body temperature, muscle contraction, control of water balance, clotting of blood, removal of waste products from the body and maintaining heartbeat. Milk, egg, liver, fruits and vegetables are protective foods.

Social Function

Food has always been the central part of our community, social, cultural and religious life (Table 1.2). It has been an expression of love, friendship and happiness at religious, social and family get-togethers. Food is served at many social events such as teas, breakfasts, banquets, athletic award dinners, dances and meeting of all sorts. On all these occasions, food indirectly serves as an instrument to develop social support.

Psychological Function

Besides other functions, food satisfies certain emotional needs also. People often find it difficult to get adjusted to unfamiliar food, although it may be nutritionally sound. Traditional habits are characterized by certain foods, which are pleasing to people of one culture and distasteful for those of another. In addition to satisfying physical and social needs, foods also satisfy certain emotional needs of human beings. These include a sense of security, love and acceptance. For example, preparation of delicious foods for family members is a token of love and affection.

CHAPTER 1: Introduction to Nutrition

Table 1.2: Factors affecting food and nutrition

Sl No	Factors	Description
1.	Social factors	Food habits are handed over from generation to generation in the society, particularly in the developing countries. Though these factors have very little or no scientific basis, people rigidly adhere to them in many parts of India; pregnant women are not allowed to consume papayas as it is believed that papayas produce a lot of heat in the body, which in turn induce abortion.
2.	Religious factors	Many Hindus are vegetarians; Jains do not eat curd and do not eat after sunset. To eat meat, is to destroy the seed of compassion. Islamic food laws prohibit the consumption of unclean foods such as swine and animals killed in a manner that prevents their blood from being fully drained from their bodies. Jews do not eat pork and shellfish.
3.	Cultural factors	It is a custom in most of the communities in India that women and girls eat only after men and boys finish their eating. Curd and citrus fruit should not be taken by a person suffering from cold or cough.
4.	Traditional factors	The traditional cooking practices also act as a barrier in achieving a balanced diet, e.g. using polished rice, draining away the rice water and prolonged boiling of vegetables add to the great loss of nutrients. Women should take only bread and coffee for 2 days after the delivery of a child and a very small quantity of water should be given.
5.	Economical factors	Financial resources determine the type of food, depending on the availability one selects the food. People in lower income groups in India consume a combination of cereals and cheaply available green leafy vegetables, roots and tubers.

Relationship of Food to Main Functions

Nutrition is the process or an activity by which the human body receives and uses all the food necessary for its growth, development and functions or activities:

SECTION 1: Nutrition

1. Food supplies heat and energy for work and play.
2. Food supplies materials for growth and repair of the body.
3. Food supplies materials for regulation or control of body process and for protection of the body. People are familiar with food, but in order to understand the different types of nutrients that are used in the body, it is necessary to know what substances or materials present in food. These substances are called nutrients. The nutrients present in food are proteins, fats, minerals, elements and vitamins.

An adequate diet should contain liberal amounts of protein rich and protective foods, and it should supply all the dietary essentials in the required amounts.

▶ CLASSIFICATION OF FOODS

Classification by Origin

1. Foods of animal origin.
2. Foods of vegetable origin.

Classification by Chemical Composition

1. Carbohydrates.
2. Proteins.
3. Fats.
4. Vitamins.
5. Minerals.

Classification by Predominant Function

1. Bodybuilding foods, e.g. milk, meat, poultry, fish, eggs, pulses, groundnuts, etc.
2. Energy-giving foods, e.g. cereals, sugars, roots and tubers, fats and oil.
3. Protective foods, e.g. vegetables, fruits, milk.

Classification by Nutritive Value

1. Cereals and millets.
2. Pulses (legumes).

CHAPTER 1: Introduction to Nutrition

3. Vegetables.
4. Nuts and oil seeds.
5. Fruits.
6. Animal foods.
7. Fats and oil.
8. Sugar and jaggery.
9. Condiments and spices.
10. Miscellaneous foods.

Since the foods vary in their contents of various nutrients, they have been broadly grouped under three categories from the nutritional point of view:

1. Energy-yielding foods.
2. Bodybuilding foods.
3. Protective foods.

These are briefly discussed below.

Energy-yielding Foods

Food rich in carbohydrates and fats are called energy-yielding foods. Cereals, roots and tubers, dried fruits, sugars and fats are included in this group. Cereals contain fair amounts of proteins, minerals and certain vitamins, and form the important sources of the above nutrients.

Bodybuilding Foods

Food rich in proteins are called bodybuilding foods. Milk, meat, fish, eggs, pulses, oil seeds and nuts, and low-fat oil seed flours are included in the group of bodybuilding foods.

Protective Foods

Food rich in proteins, vitamins and minerals are termed protective foods. Milk, eggs, liver, green leafy vegetables and fruits are included in this group. Protective foods are broadly classified into two groups:

1. Food rich in vitamins, minerals and proteins of high biological value, e.g. milk, eggs and liver.

2. Foods rich in certain vitamins and minerals only, e.g. green leafy vegetables and fruits.

▶ FOOD GROUPS

Five Food Group Plans

The nutritional expert group of Indian Council of Medical Research, India suggested a five food group plan and the nutrients supplied by each food group are given in Table 1.3.

Basic Seven Food Groups

The seven food group plan was developed by US Department of Agriculture (USDA) in 1943. The seven groups with their nutrient contribution are given in Table 1.4.

▶ NUTRITIVE VALUE OF COMMON FOODS

Food contains nutrients in different proposition and different organoleptic properties. Hormonal substance enzymatic substance and antioxidants are present in various propositions in addition, micro and macronutrients.

Cereals

Cereals are rich in carbohydrate, low protein (6%–12%) low fat, poor in iron and calcium. Rice, barley, ragi, millets and wheat are some of the examples of cereals. Insulin stimulants are present in ragi and millet, firstly rich in calcium and latter they are sources of fiber. Except yellow maize and sorghum cereals are free of vitamin A (ascorbic acid). Wheat has acarbose, a chemical helpful to maintain normal blood sugar level. Richest source of iron are bajra and samai (*Panicum miliare*). 100 g of staple food, cereals yield 346 kcal of energy.

Pulses and Legumes

Pulses and legumes are generally called protein foods. They contain 22% of protein soluble and insoluble fibers. They are

CHAPTER 1: Introduction to Nutrition

Table 1.3: Five food group plans

Sl No	Food groups	Description
1.	Group I	Cereals, roots and tubers: All these foods primarily supply energy. This group includes foods such as wheat, jowar, bajra, ragi and other cereals. Tapioca, potato, sweet potato, arbi and yam come under roots and tubers. This group provides calories, proteins, iron and vitamins. These foods are cheap and are taken in large amounts by the low-income groups. This also provides thiamine and niacin.
2.	Group II	Protein giving foods: The foodstuffs in this group are primary sources of protein; though cereals also furnish proteins. Dals, grains, peas, beans, groundnuts, cashew nuts, almonds, coconut, milk, curd, buttermilk, paneer (cottage cheese), khoa, eggs, fish, mutton, chicken, pork and other flesh foods come under this group. It provides protein both from the vegetables and animal kingdom. Milk and dairy products also provide calcium and riboflavin. Meat, fish and eggs are good sources of protein, iron and niacin.
3.	Group III	Fats/oils, sugar/jaggery: All these foodstuffs supply energy. These include—vegetable oils, vanaspati oil, ghee, butter, cream, sugar and jaggery. This group constitutes about one sixth of the energy value of the diet, but does not add appreciably to the protein, mineral or vitamin levels. Butter is a good source of vitamin A.
4.	Group IV	Protective vegetables and fruits: These are rich sources of minerals and vitamins. These include green leafy vegetables, yellow or orange fruits and vegetables, and citrus fruits.
5.	Group V	Other vegetables: They provide variety in taste and texture, and furnish roughage in the diet. These include fruits stems, leaves and flowers of plants, lady's finger, brinjals, bitter gourds, cauliflower and others. They are fair sources of certain vitamins and minerals.

SECTION 1: Nutrition

Table 1.4: Basic seven food groups

Sl No	Food groups	Description
1.	Group I	Green and yellow vegetables—provide carotene, ascorbic acid and iron.
2.	Group II	Oranges, grapes, tomatoes or raw cabbage or salad greens. These give ascorbic acid (vitamin C).
3.	Group III	Potatoes, other vegetables and fruits. They are good sources of vitamins and minerals in general and fibers.
4.	Group IV	Milk and milk products are sources of calcium, phosphorus, proteins and vitamins.
5.	Group V	Meat, poultry, fish and eggs provide proteins, phosphorus, iron and vitamin B.
6.	Group VI	Bread flour and cereals provide thiamine, niacin, riboflavin, iron, carbohydrates and fiber.
7.	Group VII	Butter or fortified margarine are rich sources of fat and vitamin A.

rich in potassium and vitamin B, deficient in methionine, but rich in lysine. More than 40% of protein is present in soybean. It is richest source of protein among plant foods. Calorific value of pulses and legumes are ranging from 315 to 372 kcal for every 100 g. But green peas and soybean provide 93–432 kcal respectively. Source of pulses and legumes are Bengal gram, black gram, red gram, lentil, rajma, horse gram, cowpea and field bean.

Green Leafy Vegetables

Green leafy vegetables are low-calorie foods, having 90% moisture, high fiber, low protein, rich vitamins and minerals particularly, beta carotene and calcium. In general greens do not have protein in sufficient amount, but agathi greens contain 8% protein. Low-cost nutritious food like curry leaves have 800 mg calcium for every 100 g. Arai keerai is richest source of iron. Familiar greens like *Amaranthus gangeticus* are good for normal cardiac function, as it provides potassium. *A. tristis* and *A. viridis* green are excellent source of iron and ascorbic acid respectively. Commonly used green leafy vegetables are coriander leaves, drumstick leaves, mint, amaranth, celery, spinach and curry leaves.

Other Vegetables

Vegetables are known as low-caloric foods, which contain potassium, soluble fiber, vitamin B and ascorbic acid. Some types of vegetable are good source of calcium, e.g. sundakkai and field beans. Folic acid present in lady's finger and chow chow helps in malnutrition of red blood cell (RBC). Choline of pumpkin and cauliflower is vital and regulates fat metabolism.

Roots and Tubers

Roots and tubers are poor source of protein, but good source of carbohydrate. The beta carotene in carrot and yam, ascorbic acid in potato, magnesium in pink radish and phosphorus in *Colocasia* are particularly helpful to meet normal requirements of recommended dietary allowances for an individual.

▶ HEALTHY FOOD SUBSTANCES

1. Tomato: It has lycopene, which is anticancer carotenoid.
2. Bitter gourd: It is an insulin stimulant.
3. Cruciferous vegetables: Brussels sprouts and broccoli, which has indole resists cancer of womb.
4. Cucumber: It is diuretic and has arginine.
5. Green tea: It contains catechins—an antioxidant.

Fruits

Fruits are roughage, provide bulk to the stools. Most of the fruits are good sources of vitamins and minerals. Ascorbic acid in amla is richer than fruits such as orange, lime and grapes. 100 g of Indian gooseberry yields 600 mg vitamin C. The beta carotene a precursor of vitamin A found in mango and papaya helps to maintain good vision because of an action similar to pepsin.

Papain relieves the symptoms of episiotomy (surgical incision of vulva during delivery). Watermelon is very meager energy yielder, whereas dried fruits provide high calories. A report by national academy of sciences found that resveratrol, a chemical known to be highly concentrated in grapes skin, acts like estrogen, a hormone known to protect against heart diseases.

Nuts and Oil Seeds

Nuts and oil seeds are rich in saturated fat; contain tocopherol thiamine and niacin. Almond, cashew nut, groundnut, walnut, sesame seed, linseed are some sources of nuts and oil seeds. Groundnuts contain monounsaturated fatty acid, 25% protein and 40% fat. Nutritious ball made from groundnut and jaggery in healthy food for children. Coconut meals raises hemoglobin content, as it provides approximately 70 mg iron. Most of the nuts and oil seeds are energy yielder and rich in phosphorus. Short-and medium-chain fatty acid of coconut oil is good for infant intestine.

Eggs

Eggs are good mixture of all nutrients except carbohydrate and fiber; supplies essential amino acids and termed as good quality proteins. Raw egg white contains antinutritional factor avidin, which is binding with biotin and makes it unavailable. Ovalbumin, ovomucoid, flavoprotein are egg white proteins. One egg yolk contains 200 g cholesterol and proteins such as lipovitellin and phosvitin. 13% fat, 170 kcal energy, 2 mg iron, 60 mg calcium, 220 mg phosphorus can be obtained from 100 g of egg. Cooked egg is better than raw egg.

Meat, Poultry and Fish

Beef meal is richest source of iron among meat products. Protein in the meat and meat products are superior compared to vegetable proteins. Essential amino acids and biological value are responsible to upgrade the quality. Protein value of mutton

CHAPTER 1: Introduction to Nutrition

is less than that of chicken, but fat percentage is higher than fish and chicken. They all are moderate source of phosphorus Common fish varieties rohu and katla have 1.4% and 2.4% of fat respectively. Cat fish is free from fat. Fatty fish are hilsa, tapsee and dried chela. Omega-3 fatty acid content of fish is helpful in preventing cardiac diseases. Consumption of cod-liver oil protects eyes from night blindness.

Milk and Milk Products

Milk is ideal food since infant to aged. Skimmed milk, cheese, tinned milk powder, khoa and supplementary foods are made from milk. Cow milk, buffalo milk and processed milk are widely consumed. Protein content of cow milk is higher than human milk, but buffalo milk is rich in fat. High protein and calcium content among milk products is in skimmed milk powder. This group of foods have sufficient phosphorus, thiamine, niacin, but deficit in iron and vitamins. Energy value of 100 g cow milk, buffalo milk, goat milk, human milk is 67, 117, 72 and 65 calories respectively.

▶ CALORIE

The scientific definition of a calorie is a unit of energy for heat in particular. One calorie is the amount of heat that increases the temperature of 1 kg of water by 1°C; any food may contain one or more nutrients, but carbohydrates, fats and proteins are the nutrients, which gives calories to the body. The caloric value of these nutrients and of any common foods has been determined by burning a known weight of the nutrient or food in an atmosphere of oxygen in what is known as a bomb calorimeter. The caloric values of the nutrients are given in Table 1.5.

The following examples of calorie intake are based on USDA guidelines.

Table 1.5: Caloric values of the nutrients

Sl No	Nutrients	Caloric values (kcal/g)
1.	Carbohydrates	4
2.	Fats	9
3.	Proteins	4

SECTION 1: Nutrition

A person's daily calorie intake should be based on age, gender and physical activity level. Men generally need more calories than women and active people need more calories than sedentary (inactive) people:
1. Children aged 2 and 8: 1,000–1,400.
2. Active women aged 14 and 30: 2,400.
3. Sedentary women aged 14 and 30: 1,800–2,000.
4. Active men aged 14 and 30: 2,800–3,000.
5. Sedentary men aged 14 and 30: 2,000–2,600.
6. Active men and women above 30: 2,200–3,000.
7. Sedentary men and women 30: 1,800–2,200.

▶ BODY MASS INDEX (QUETELET'S INDEX)

The body mass index (BMI) is used as a reference standard for assessing the prevalence of obesity in the community:

$$\text{Body mass index} = \frac{\text{Weight in kg}}{\text{Height in square meter}}$$

Ideal body mass index:
1. Ideal body mass index for Indian women: 19–24.
2. Ideal body mass index for Indian man: 20–26.

Once the BMI exceeds the normal limit; the person can be termed as overweight or obese.

▶ BASAL METABOLIC RATE

Basal metabolic rate is the minimum number of calories needed to maintain vital functions, such as breathing and keeping the heart beating. It is the energy expenditure necessary to maintain basic physiologic conditions such as respiration, cardiac contraction, conduction of nerve impulses, metabolic activity such as synthesis of macromolecules under standard conditions, reabsorption of kidney, iron transport across impulse. This function occurs continuously with one's own conscious or awareness. Basal metabolic needs are surprisingly large person whose total energy expenditure amounts to 2,000 calories/day, spends as much as 1,200–1,400 calories to support usual metabolism.

Definitions

1. Basal metabolism is the minimum amount of energy needed by the body for maintenance of life when the person is at postabsorptive state, physical and emotional rest.
2. Basal metabolic rate is a measure of the energy required by the activities of resting tissue can be measured directly from the heat produced (using a respiration calorimeter and metabolic chamber) or indirectly from O_2 intake and CO_2 expenditure when the subject is at rest.

Normal Values

1. Basal metabolic rate values are expressed as kcal or kJ square meter of body surface per hour.
2. In adults, BMR for healthy males 40 kcal/h (168 kJ) and in healthy females is 37 kcal/h (155 kJ).

Factors Affecting BMR

There are many factors, which affect the BMR; the most common factors are given in Table 1.6.

▶ ENERGY

Energy is defined as the capacity for doing work. It is the heat produced in the body, which is utilized for performing the involuntary and voluntary activities, to maintain body temperature to synthesize new body constituents.

Basal Metabolic Rate

A number of processes go on in the body without any conscious effort, even when subject is at complete rest and no physical work is done. These include involuntary processes,

Table 1.6: Factors affecting basal metabolic rate (BMR)

Sl No	Factors	Description
1.	Surface area of the body	The larger the surface area of the body in relation to its bulk, the greater is the heat lost by radiation.
2.	Sex	The basal metabolic rate is higher per square meter of body surface area in men than in women. According to western standards the requirements are: a. 40 cal/m²/h for men. b. 37 cal/m²/h for women.
3.	Age	Growing children and adolescent have high BMRs in relation to their weight than adults.
4.	Diseases	Some diseases, especially of thyroid gland, may raise or lower the BMRs. A rise of body temperature of 1°F is found to increase BMRs by about 7%.
5.	Nutritional status	The BMR is lower in starvation and undernourishment, as compared to well-fed state. Under prolonged or chronic undernutrition, the BMR is decreased.
6.	Stress	Psychological stress and tension caused by worry or stress will increase the BMR.
7.	Environmental factors	In cold climate, the BMR is increased and in tropical climate, the BMR proportionally low.
8.	Drugs	Smoking (nicotine), coffee (caffeine) increases the BMR, whereas, beta blockers tend to decrease energy expenditure.

such as the beating of heart, the circulation of blood, etc. These activities are called basal metabolic processes. The energy used for carrying out these activities is known as the BMR. The basal energy need constitute more than half of the total energy need, for most of the people.

Unit of Energy

The energy value of food is expressed in terms of kilocalories (kcal or C). A kilocalorie is defined as the amount of heat required to raise the temperature of 1 kg of water by 10°C. In

the metric system, the international unit, which is kilojoules, is used instead of kilocalories. One kilojoule energy is expended when 1 kg of mass is moved by 1 meter using a force of a Newton:
- 1 Calorie = 4.184 Joule (J)
- 1 kcal or C = 4.184 kilojoules (kJ)
- 1,000 kcal or C = 4.184 Megajoule (MJ)
- 1 kJ = 0.239 kcal
- 1 MJ = 239 kcal.

Factors Influencing the Total Energy Requirement

Among factors, which influences energy needs are age, sex, body size, climate, secretion of endocrine glands, status of health, altered physiological activity.

Age

During the growth period, the BMR is high. Therefore during infancy, the energy need per kilogram of body weight is higher than during adulthood. Energy requirement also decline progressively after early adulthood due to steady decline in BMR thereafter. The basal metabolism during rapid growth is at a high level. The younger the individuals the higher, the basal metabolism since, much energy are stored for growth. The period at which the basal metabolism reaches its highest level is between the ages of 1 and 2 years. A gradual decline occurs between the age of 2 and 5 years, with a more rapid decline until adult age is reached.

Sex

The BMR is higher in adolescent boys and adult males as compared to adolescent girls and adult females though it is not due to direct influence of sex differences, but are due to the differences in body composition. Males have a greater amount of muscles and glandular tissues, which is metabolically more active whereas, females have greater adipose tissues, which is metabolically less active. Hence, energy requirement of males is higher than of females.

Body Size

Body size will have an important effect on energy needs, because a larger body has a greater amount of muscles and glandular tissue to maintain, thus requiring higher energy allowances. Heat is continuously lost through the skin by radiation. Since the heat loss is proportional to the skin surface, the basal heat production is directly proportional to the surface area. A tall thin individual has a greater surface area than an individual of the same weight who is short and fat, and the former will therefore, have a higher BMR.

Climate

Climate is known that the BMR is lower in tropics then in temperate zones. Hence the energy cost of work is slightly higher when the temperature falls below 140°C. However, it is felt that there is no need to make any adjustment for temperature in India.

Secretion of Endocrine Glands

The thyroid gland, in particular, exerts a marked influence on the energy requirement. If it is overactive (hyperthyroidism), the BMR will increase; if the activity of the gland decreases (hypothyroidism), the BMR will be reduced. Thereby, increasing or decreasing energy requirement accordingly.

Status of Health

During the periods of fever as well as malnutrition, the BMR of an individual is affected. Illness involving an elevation of body temperature markedly increases the basal heat production thus increasing the BMR, hence increased energy requirement.

Altered Physiological States

During pregnancy and lactation, the energy needs are increased because of an elevated BMR. In pregnancy this additional energy is needed to support the growth of fetus and maternal tissues. During lactation energy is required for synthesis of milk.

Effect of Food

A certain amount of work is expended in the digestion of food, its absorption, transfer to the tissues and utilization. The increased heat production as a result of the ingestion of food is known as the specific dynamic action of the food. Protein, when eaten alone has been shown to increase the metabolic rate by 30%. On the basis of the mixed diets, which are usually consumed, the specific dynamic action of food is approximately 10% of the energy requirement.

Extent of Physical Activity

Any kind of physical activity increases the energy expenditure above the basal energy need. Energy for the performance of all types of physical activities ranks next to basal metabolism in amount of energy expended. Sleep causes a reduction of about 10% in the BMR depending on the number of hours spent in sleeping and its manner, i.e. restless/peaceful.

The energy need is determined by the nature and duration of physical activity. Sedentary work such as includes office work, bookkeeping, typing, teaching, etc. calls for lesser energy than moderate work (more active and strenuous occupations) such as nursing, homemaking or gardening. A still greater amount of energy is required by those individuals who are involved in heavy work (hard manual laborer) such as ditch digging, shifting freight, etc. Energy needs vary with age, occupation and physiological state.

▶ CONCLUSION

Nutrition is essential for growth and development, health and well-being. Eating a healthy diet contribute to preventing future illness and improves quality and length of life. Nutritional status is the state of health as determined by the dietary habits. There are several ways of assessing nutritional status, including anthropometric (i.e. physical body measurement), food intake and biochemical measurement. Proper nutrition is a powerful good: people who are well-nourished are more likely to be healthy, productive and able to learn. Good nutrition benefits families, their communities and the world as a whole. Undernutrition is by the same logic, devastating. It blunts the intellect, saps the productivity of everyone it touches and perpetuates poverty.

Chapter 2

Review of Macro- and Micro-nutrition

▶ INTRODUCTION

Nutrients, which are needed by the body for good nutritional status, are provided by food. An individual nutritional status is dependent on the provision of sufficient nutrients and the good utilization of these nutrients. Power status of nutrition may be caused by eating that is inadequate in amount and kind or it may be caused by failure in digestion and utilization of these nutrients. The nutrients present in foods fall into three major categories, i.e. proximate, vitamins and minerals. The proximate usually referred to as proximate principles include only those nutrients that yield energy on oxidation, i.e. carbohydrates, proteins and fats. Nutrients are organic and inorganic complexes contained in food.

▶ MACRO- AND MICRO-NUTRIENTS

Macronutrients

Carbohydrates, proteins and fats are macronutrients, which are often called 'proximate principles' because they form a main bulk of the food as given below:

- Carbohydrate: 65%–80%
- Protein: 7%–15%
- Fats: 10%–30%.

Micronutrients

Vitamins and minerals are called micronutrients because they are required in small amounts. A vitamin is an organic compound that cannot be manufactured by the body and is needed in small quantities to catalyze metabolic process. When this vitamins are lacking in the diet, metabolic deficits results. Minerals are found in organic compounds and inorganic compounds as free ions. On oxidation, minerals leave an ash, which can be acid or alkaline.

▶ CARBOHYDRATES

Carbohydrates are macronutrients containing carbon, hydrogen and oxygen. They are primary energy yielder, present in plant foods as well as animal foods. Polyhydroxy aldehyde or ketone group occurs in some sugar units. Glucose is physiologically significant among carbohydrate.

Carbohydrates are the chief, cheapest and main source of energy. Carbohydrate normally should provide 50%–60% of total caloric requirements. All the carbohydrates contain carbon, hydrogen and oxygen. All the carbohydrates are changed in the body to simple form called glucose (Table 2.1).

Composition

Carbohydrates are organic compounds composed of carbon, hydrogen and oxygen with the later elements in the ratio of 2:1. The general formula is $C_n H_{2n} O_n$. They are viewed as hydrated carbon atoms.

Classification

Carbohydrates are chemically known as saccharides. They are classified according to number of sugar units present in the molecular structure. The classifications of carbohydrate are shown in the Figure 2.1.

Monosaccharides

Monosaccharides are simple form of carbohydrates, which yields only one molecule of sugar on hydrolysis, e.g. glucose, fructose and galactose:

CHAPTER 2: Review of Macro- and Micro-nutrition

1. Trioses—glyceraldehyde and dihydroxyacetone.
2. Tetroses—erythrose, threose.
3. Pentoses—arabinose, xylose, ribose and deoxyribose.

Table 2.1: Sources of carbohydrate

Sl No	Source	Percentage
1.	Arrowroot powder	83%
2.	Sago	87%
3.	Syrup, jelly, jam	65%–85%
4.	Rice	79%
5.	Barley, dried dates	75%
6.	Mango powder	64%
7.	Ragi	72%
8.	Tapioca	38%
9.	Jaggery	90%
10.	Bread	55%
11.	Honey	79%

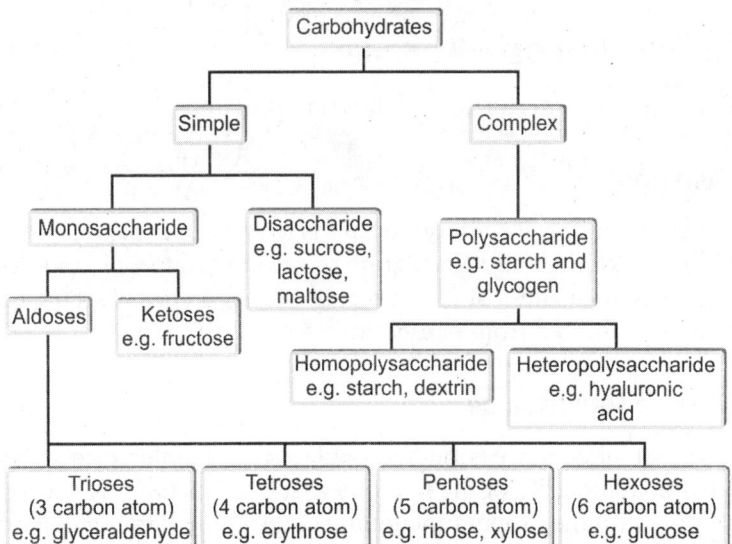

Fig. 2.1: Classification of carbohydrates

Disaccharides

1. Boise—glycolic bald headed.

Oligosaccharides

Oligosaccharides yield 2–10 molecules of monosaccharides on hydrolysis, e.g. disaccharides (maltose, lactose and sucrose), trisaccharides (raffinose) and tetrasaccharides (stachyose).

Polysaccharides

Polysaccharides yield more than ten molecules of monosaccharide on hydrolysis such as given below:
1. Pentosans: For example, araban, xylan.
2. Hexosans:
    a. Starch, dextrin and glycogen.
    b. Cellulose, inulin, mannan.

Complex polysaccharides: They are not digested by human enzymes, e.g. hemicelluloses, gums, mucilages and pectins.

Functions of Carbohydrate

Carbohydrates perform the following functions.

Yield Energy

Principle function of carbohydrates is to serve as a major source of energy for the body. Each gram of carbohydrate yields 4 kcal of energy regardless of its source. In Indian diets, 60%–80% of energy is derived from carbohydrate.

Glucose Maintenance

Glucose maintenance is indispensable for the maintenance of the functional integrity of the nervous tissue and is the sole source of energy for the proper functioning of the brain. Prolonged lack of glucose may cause irreversible damage to the brain.

CHAPTER 2: Review of Macro- and Micro-nutrition

Protein Sparing Action

Carbohydrates exert a protein sparing action. If sufficient amounts of carbohydrates are not available in the diet, the body will convert protein to glucose in order to supply energy. Hence, to spare proteins for tissue building, carbohydrates must be supplied in optimum amounts in the diet. This is called the protein sparing action of carbohydrates.

Fat Metabolism

Carbohydrates are essential to maintain normal fat metabolism. Insufficient carbohydrates in the diet results in larger amounts of fat being used for energy than the body are equipped to handle. This leads to accumulation of acidic intermediate products called ketone bodies.

Synthesis of Body Substances

Carbohydrates aid in the synthesis of non-essential amino acids, glycoproteins (which function as antibodies) and glycolipids (which form a part of cell membrane in body tissues especially brain and nervous system). Lactose remains in the intestine longer than other disaccharides and thus, encourages growth of beneficial bacteria.

Precursors of Nucleic Acid

Carbohydrates and products derived from them, serve as precursors of compounds like nucleic acids, connective tissue matrix and galactosidase of nervous tissue.

Detoxification Function

Glucuronic acid, a metabolite of glucose serves as a detoxifying agent. It combines with harmful substances containing alcohol or phenolic group converting them to harmless compounds, which are later excreted.

Roughage of the Diet

Insoluble fibers known as composite carbohydrates can absorb water and give bulk to the intestinal contents, which aids in the elimination of waste products by stimulating peristaltic movements of the gastrointestinal tract (GIT).

Other Roles

Carbohydrate has a variety of functions in the animal and human body. It plays crucial role in biological system they are:

1. Carbohydrate of 1 g provides 4 kcal on oxidation.
2. Protein sparing action helps to regulate protein metabolism. When carbohydrate and fat is in adequate amount in the diet, major protein is used for tissue building.
3. Ketone body from fat metabolism is prevented when carbohydrate is sufficient.
4. Pentose (five-carbon sugar) is utilized in the formation of deoxyribonucleic acid (DNA) and ribonucleic acid (RNA).
5. It supplies fuel to brain tissues, otherwise irreversible damage occurs.
6. If carbohydrate exceeds the normal requirement, fat synthesis in adipose tissue.
7. Lactose in gastrointestinal tract promotes the growth of bacteria, which is responsible for the synthesis of B complex vitamins.
8. Complex polysaccharides cellulose and hemicellulose contribute bulk to the stool.
9. Carbohydrate in well-balanced diet keeps the blood sugar level within normal limits.

Digestion and Absorption of Carbohydrates

Digestion

The first stage of digestion of carbohydrate takes place in the mouth. Chewing breaks up food, and exposes starch and sugars to the action of enzymes. Saliva contains salivary amylase

CHAPTER 2: Review of Macro- and Micro-nutrition

(ptyalin). It converts starch to maltose, but time limits the action of salivary amylase, because as food enters the stomach, the acid present in the stomach blocks the action of salivary amylase.

In the stomach, the acid causes hydrolysis of sucrose. In the small intestine, pancreatic amylase and intestinal amylase digest starch up to the stage of maltose:

$$\text{Starch} \xrightarrow[\text{Salivary amylase}]{\text{Pancreatic amylase}} \text{Maltose + Isomaltose}$$

Glycogen is also broken by these enzymes to disaccharides. Enzymes maltase, sucrase and lactase present in the brush borders of the columnar cells of small intestine convert disaccharides to monosaccharides:

$$\text{Maltose} \xrightarrow{\text{Maltase}} \text{Glucose + Glucose}$$

$$\text{Lactose} \xrightarrow{\text{Lactase}} \text{Glucose + Galactose}$$

$$\text{Sucrose} \xrightarrow{\text{Sucrase}} \text{Glucose + Fructose}$$

Cellulose and other polysaccharides are not digested by enzymes, so undigested material passes to large intestine forming bulk, which contributes to feces.

The end products of carbohydrate digestion are monosaccharides—glucose, galactose and fructose. They are absorbed by process of active absorption by the mucosa of the small intestine.

Metabolism

Metabolism occurs inside the various cells of the body.

There are two types of metabolism: Anabolism (building up) and catabolism (breaking down):

1. The major carbohydrate anabolic pathways are conversion of glucose into glycogen (glycogenesis), which takes place in the liver and muscles.

SECTION 1: Nutrition

2. The conversion of glucose into fat (lipogenesis) takes place in the liver and adipose tissue.
3. Carbohydrates follow two major catabolic pathways:
   a. The breakdown of glucose releasing energy (glycolysis) and converting it into usable energy adenosine triphosphate (ATP) and which in turn gets converted to glycogen glucose (glycogenolysis).
   b. After digestion and absorption of glucose into the bloodstream, it is utilized directly by the tissues for energy. When the absorbed glucose exceeds the body's need for energy, it is stored as glycogen in the liver and muscle, and excess glucose is converted to triglycerides and stored as fat in adipose tissue.

Glucose Formation from Non-carbohydrate Sources

1. Glucose can be formed by the metabolism of protein and from the glycerol of fat. It has been estimated that the glycerol present in 100 g of fat can give rise to 50–60 g glucose.
2. Lactate, which is formed from glucose, can be reconverted into glucose in the liver.

Regulation of Blood Sugar

1. Blood circulates glucose continuously to each and every cell of the body as a source of energy, and for the synthesis of a number of substances.
2. In fasting state, blood sugar level is 60–85 mg/100 mL of blood. Soon after a meal, it raises to 140–150 mg/100 mL.
3. If the body is in a good carbohydrate metabolic pathway, the concentration will fall down to a normal blood sugar level of 60–85 mg/100 mL.
4. The liver very efficiently maintains the normal blood sugar level. The liver is the only organ in our body, which can either supply glucose to the circulation or to remove the excess sugar from blood.
5. If the blood sugar concentration is high, the condition is known as hyperglycemia. Hypoglycemia occurs when the

blood sugar level is below normal level. This occurs in certain abnormalities of liver function or when insulin is produced in excessive amount by the pancreas.

Carbohydrate Requirements

As carbohydrate is utilized as main source of energy, at least 40% of the total energy in the food should come from carbohydrates. In our country, 60%–80% of a day's energy needs are met from carbohydrates in the form of starch furnished by cereals and pulses. In developed countries, only 30%–40% of days energy needs are met from carbohydrates:

1. The body has a specific need for carbohydrates as a source of energy for the brain and other tissue cells, for synthesis of lactose of milk (lactating women) and galactose, and other sugars present in the cerebrosides, mucopolysaccharides, etc.
2. Carbohydrate is essential for the oxidation of fat and for the synthesis of certain non-essential amino acids.
3. The carbohydrate calories should be at least 40% in well-balanced diets. The level of carbohydrates calories in the diet will also depend on the availability of fat and the economic conditions of the people as fat is about twice as costly as cereals on equicalorie basis in the developing countries and per capita production of fat per day is low (10–15 g).
4. The optimal levels of carbohydrates in the diet, taking into physiological needs for proteins and fats are given in Table 2.2.

Table 2.2: Carbohydrate requirements of various age groups

Sl No	Age group	Optimal level of carbohydrate calories as % of total calories
1.	Adults	50%–70%
2.	Expectant and nursing mothers	40%–60%
3.	Infants (1–12 month)	40%–50%
4.	Preschool children (1–5 year)	40%–60%
5.	Older children and adolescents	50%–70%

SECTION 1: Nutrition

Deficiencies

1. Low level of glucose (40 mg% or below) in the blood is called hypoglycemia. This is not common in healthy individual. Diabetic people may get this condition on poor or irregular treatment.
2. The signs and symptoms of diabetes are tiredness, convulsions, dizziness, tingling, faintness, headache, firmness, tachycardia, palpation, confusion, slurred speech, staggering gait, lack of coordination and coma.
3. Low carbohydrate with high-protein and high-fat foods are dangerous, leads to weight loss, ketosis, dehydration, electrolyte deficits, retention of uric acid and some symptoms of gout.

Diabetes Mellitus

1. Diabetes mellitus is a chronic disease in which blood glucose level is raised above 180 mg/dL of blood and glucose is excreted in urine.
2. The disease is primarily due to the insufficient production of the hormone, insulin by the β-cells of the islets of Langerhans of the pancreas.

▶ FIBER

Fiber or roughage consists of cellulose and hemicellulose. These parts of carbohydrates are not digested by digestive juice. They are left unchanged after digestion. Dietary fiber is defined as that portion of plant material ingested in the diet that is resistant to digestion by gastrointestinal secretions. It consists of hemicellulose, cellulose, lignins, oligosaccharides, pectins, gums and waxes.

Some bacteria in the large intestine can degrade some components of fiber releasing products that can be absorbed into the body and used as energy source. Two categories of fiber are found in food. Crude fiber (CF) is defined as the residue remaining after the treatment with hot sulfuric acid, alkali and alcohol.

CHAPTER 2: Review of Macro- and Micro-nutrition

The major component of CF is a polysaccharide called cellulose. CF is a component of dietary fiber. Several other carbohydrate and related compounds are called pectins; hemicellulose and lignins are the second category found in plant foods and are also resistant to digestion. These together with cellulose are collectively known as dietary fiber.

Role

Fibers are indigestible substance of plant foods, roughage not digested by human enzyme contribute bulk to the stool. For example, fibrous foods contain whole cereals, fenugreek, cabbage and greens. Fiber part of the foods is cellulose hemicellulose and lignin.

Functions

1. Fiber absorbs water and this increases the bulk of the stool and helps to reduce the tendency of constipation by encouraging bowel movements.
2. The cholesterol-lowering effect of certain types of dietary fiber appears firmly established.
3. Fiber may also have a role in weight reduction; people who eat well-balanced diets obtain enough roughage.
4. Prevents constipation and reduce the effects of carcinogens.
5. Increases the motility of small intestine, colon and decreases the transit time.

▶ PROTEINS

In Greek, proteins mean the first importance. They are nitrogenous constituents made up of chain of amino acids present in both plant and animal foods.

The name 'protein' was suggested by Mulder in 1838 to the complex organic nitrogenous substances found in animal and plant tissues. Protein constitute about one fifth (20%) of animal body on the fresh weight basis. They are essential for life processes. They plan an important role in many biochemicals, biophysical processes in the body.

SECTION 1: Nutrition

Proteins differ from carbohydrates and fats in that they contain nitrogen in addition to carbon, hydrogen and oxygen and a few contain sulfur. Most of the proteins also contain phosphorus and some specialized proteins contain iron, iodine, copper and other organic elements. Contribution made by proteins to the energy value of most well-balanced diets is usually between 10% and 15% of the total. But they are most important because every cell in the body is composed of proteins, which are subjected to continuous wear and replacement.

Chemical Composition

Proteins contain carbon, hydrogen, oxygen and nitrogen. They are distinguished from carbohydrates and fats by the presence of nitrogen.

Protein is synthesized from basic units called amino acids. Protein molecules, which contain up to hundred amino acids, are much larger than carbohydrates or lipid molecule. Chemically amino acids are composed of a carbon atom to which is attached a carboxyl (COOH) group, a hydrogen atom (H), an amino group (NH_2) and an amino acid radical (R) as shown below.

The carboxyl group, the amino group and the hydrogen atom are the same for all amino acids. The R group however distinguishes one amino acid from another. R varies from a single hydrogen atom as found in glycine to longer chain of up to 7 carbon atoms. A protein molecule is made up of chains of amino acids joined to each other by a peptide linkage. The amino group of one amino acid is linked to the carboxyl group of another amino acid by removal of water.

Thus, two amino acids form dipeptide and three forms a tripeptide. Proteins consist of hundreds of such linkages, hence called polypeptides:

1. Proteins contain carbon, hydrogen, nitrogen and sulfur and also some contain phosphorus.
2. Proteins are large molecules formed from the combination of a number of simpler substances known as amino acids.

3. Proteins are larger than carbohydrates and fat molecules; its molecular weight is 13,000.
4. They are colloids, which are large particles and do not pass through semi-permeable membrane.
5. The nitrogen content of proteins varies from about 14% to 20% and in most of the proteins; the value is near about 16%.
6. This average figure of 16% is used commonly for converting nitrogen content of foodstuffs or tissues into proteins by multiplying by the factor 6.25 (100/16).

Structure

Proteins are large molecules formed by the combination of a number of amino acids. About 23 amino acids have been found to occur in proteins:

1. **Monoamine monocarboxylic acids:** These include glycine, alanine, valine, isoleucine, norleucine, serine and threonine.
2. **Monoamino dicarboxylic acid:** These are aspartic acid and glutamic acid.
3. **Diamino monocarboxylic acid:** Arginine and lysine belong to this group.
4. **Sulfur-containing amino acids:** These are cystine, cysteine and methionine.
5. **Aromatic and heterocyclic amino acids:** These include phenylalanine, tyrosine, histidine, tryptophan, proline and hydroxyproline.

Properties

1. Proteins are colloids; they act both as weak acids and bases.
2. Proteins are soluble in sodium hydroxide and when the alkaline solutions of proteins are acidified, the proteins are precipitated.
3. When proteins are heated, a decrease in their solubility is observed, this is known as denaturation.

Classification

Proteins are classified into three types they are:
1. **Simple proteins:** These include albumins, globulins, glutelins, prolamins, fibrous proteins, histones and protamins.
2. **Conjugated proteins:** These include nucleoprotein, glycoprotein, phosphoproteins, hemoglobin and lipoproteins.
3. **Derived proteins:** These include proteins, metaproteins, coagulated proteins, peptones and peptides.

The main functions of proteins are to replace the daily loss of body protein, to provide amino acids for the formation of tissue proteins during growth, to provide the amino acids necessary for the formation of enzymes, blood, proteins and certain hormones of protein nature, and to provide amino acids for the growth of fetus in pregnancy and for the production of milk proteins during lactation.

Amino Acids

Amino acids are simplest molecule derived from large molecule of protein. Animal foods have good quality amino acids compare to plant containing amino acid. There are 23 amino acids.

Classification

Amino acids are classified into two groups:
1. **Essential (indispensable):** This is one that cannot be synthesized by the body to meet the physiological needs and hence, should be supplied by the diet. The essential amino acids are histidine, isoleucine, leucine, lysine, methionine, phenylalanine, threonine, tryptophan and valine.
2. **Non-essential (dispensable):** They are those that the body can synthesize. They are alanine, arginine, asparagine, aspartic acid, cysteine, glutamic acid, glutamine, glycine, proline, serine and tyrosine.

CHAPTER 2: Review of Macro- and Micro-nutrition

Other Classifications

Essential amino acids (EAA) 8: It can be defined as body cannot synthesis certain amino acids, which must be supplied by the diet, e.g. methionine, tryptophan, valine, isoleucine, lysine and phenylalanine.

Semiessential amino acids (SEAA)—2: Methionine essential amino acids can be converted to cystine, but cystine cannot be converted to methionine. Likewise phenylalanine is converted to tyrosine, but tyrosine cannot be converted to phenylalanine. When cystine and tyrosine are present in the diet, the requirement for methionine and phenylalanine.

Non-essential amino acids (NEAA)—13: They are synthesized in the body, i.e. they are derived from other amino acids, e.g. alanine, aspartic acid, cystine, glutamine, glutamic acid, glycine, hydroxylysine, proline, serine, tyrosine and cysteine.

Classification of Proteins Based on Content of Amino Acids

1. **Complete proteins:** It contains enough essential amino acids to maintain the growth and the development of cells and it has high biological value, e.g. milk and meat. These foods are referred to be having a high-biological value (Table 2.3).
2. **Partially complete proteins:** It will maintain life, but they lack some of the amino acids, which are necessary for growth and development, e.g. gliadin of wheat.
3. **Incomplete proteins:** They are incapable of replacing or building new tissues and hence cannot support life, e.g. zein in corn.

Biological Value of Protein

Biological value of protein is the percentage of protein nitrogen that is absorbed and available for use by the body for growth and maintenance:

1. Proteins are functionally divided into complete, partially complete and incomplete proteins.
2. A complete protein contains all essential amino acids in relatively the same amounts as human beings require promoting and maintaining normal growth, e.g. protein derived from animal foods.
3. A partially complete protein contains sufficient amounts of amino acids to maintain life, but fail to promote growth, e.g. gliadin in wheat.
4. Incomplete proteins are incapable of replacing or building new tissue and cannot support life or growth, e.g. protein in wheat germ.
5. The quality of a protein is determined by the kind and proportion of amino acid it contains. Proteins that contain all essential amino acids in proportions capable of promoting growth are described as complete protein, good quality protein or proteins of high biological value.

Table 2.3: Sources of amino acids

Amino acids	Sources
Valine	Rice, jackfruit, agathi, cheese, Brewer's yeast, egg, apple, sweet potato, cauliflower, pumpkin, radish, horse gram, potato, bitter gourd.
Leucine	Thinai (millet), cholam (jowar), kambu (bajra), rice, Bengal gram dal, black gram dal, whole green gram, agathi, knol khol, greens, potato, yam, brinjal, cashew nut, apple, beef, pork, curd, buffalo milk, wheat, egg.
Isoleucine	Ragi, rice, kesari dal, black gram dal, agathi, radish, potato, tomato, pork, cheese, banana, egg.
Methionine	Ragi, celery, leaves, yam, ladies finger, dried coconut, grapes, egg.
Phenylalanine	Dairy products, egg, pork, banana, almond, groundnut, yam, colocasia, spinach, agathi, rice, barley, red gram dal, horse gram, Bengal gram dal.
Tryptophan	Kambu (bajra), rice, potato, cauliflower, egg, papaya, mango, milk, radish, carrot, beetroot.

CHAPTER 2: Review of Macro- and Micro-nutrition

6. A good quality protein is digested and utilized well. Egg protein is a complete protein and is considered as a reference protein with the highest biological value. The quality of other proteins is determined based on their comparison with egg protein.
7. The protein of animal foods like milk, meat and fish generally compare well with egg in the essential amino acid composition and are categorized as good quality proteins. Plant proteins are of poor quality, since the essential amino acid composition is not well-balanced. The amino acid, which is not present in sufficient amount in food protein, is called the limiting amino acid of that food, e.g. lysine in cereal protein, tryptophan in wheat germ.

Functions of Proteins

1. **Building block:** The most important function is to supply amino acids to cells for the continuous replacement of cells throughout life. It is the most abundant organic compound in our body. It is the building blocks of our body.
2. **Regulatory functions:** Different proteins perform highly specialized regulatory function in the body. Hemoglobin, which is the chief constituent of the red blood cells, carries oxygen to the tissues. Oxyhemoglobin and their alkaline salts permit oxygen to entire into tissues and receive carbonic acid from the cells.
3. **Formation of enzymes, hormones and other secretions:** Proteins supply raw materials for the body to synthesis enzymes like trypsin and pepsin. Hormones like insulin and thyroxine are protein in nature. Antibodies, which give resistance power to the body, are protein in nature. They are known as immune proteins.
4. **Sources of energy:** Protein is generally considered as the building material of our body. But when the diet contains insufficient carbohydrate and fat for fuel, proteins are used as a fuel in the body. Energy value of protein is 4 cal/g, which is as same as carbohydrate.

5. **Proteins from part of vital compounds in body:** Nitrogenous compounds are present in certain substances of immunological antigenic reactions; examples of these are globulin of blood serum and chromatin in nucleus.
6. **Body protection:** There is a protein called γ-globulin, which has a capacity to fight against invading organism. The body's resistance to disease is maintained in part by antibodies, which are protein in nature.
7. **Energy yielding:** The energy needs of the body take priority over other needs and if the diet does not furnish sufficient energy from carbohydrates and fats. The proteins of the diet as well as tissue protein will be used up for giving energy. 1 g of protein gives 4 calories.
8. **Maintenance of body temperature:** During the metabolism of proteins extra heat is liberated, which is used for maintaining the body temperature.

Factors Affecting the Protein Requirement

1. Sufficient amount of protein is required to recover the daily losses of nitrogen in the urine, feces, sweat, etc.
2. Essential amino acids in sufficient amount should be supplied to meet the daily needs.
3. Energy requirement should be met through other sources (carbohydrates and fats), so the proteins are spared for its own function and not for supplying energy.
4. Infants and children demand more protein per kg of body weight for the normal growth and development.
5. The need for protein is increased tremendously during pregnancy to maintain the development of maternal tissues as well as fetus.
6. During lactation, the production of milk increases the protein requirement.
7. Additional amounts of proteins are needed during conditions, such as kwashiorkor and marasmus.

CHAPTER 2: Review of Macro- and Micro-nutrition

8. The protein needs are greatly increased during infections, in burns, surgery and injuries because there is an increased protein catabolism.
9. Protein catabolism is increased during emotional stress also.
10. Malabsorption syndrome can seriously affect the digestion and absorption, therefore, increases the protein requirement.

Protein Quality

Protein quality is not only the quantity of protein, which is important but also the quality. This depends mainly on the type of amount of particular amino acids present in the particular protein. There are 22 amino acids, which are needed by the human body out of which eight are called 'essential'. It is because the body cannot synthesize them; therefore, they must be obtained from the diet. Rest of the amino acids are termed as 'non-essential' as they can be synthesized in our body. Essential amino acids are isoleucine, leucine, lysine, methionine, phenylalanine, threonine, tryptophan and valine. In addition to these infants require histidine for growth.

Based on the quality of proteins, they can be classified into three classes:

1. Complete protein (first class).
2. Partially complete proteins (second class).
3. Incomplete proteins (third class).

Complete Proteins

Complete proteins contain all the essential amino acids in sufficient quantities, so that a normal rate of growth can be maintained by the body. Mainly proteins from animal source belong to this class, i.e. milk, meat, eggs, fish and poultry. Wheat germ and dried yeast have a biological value approaching that of animal sources.

Partially Complete Proteins

Partially complete proteins can maintain life, but they lack sufficient amount of some of the amino acids necessary for growth. Proteins from plant source like pulses, wheat and nuts belong to this class.

Incomplete Proteins

Incomplete proteins can neither promote growth nor maintain life because they lack many of the amino acids or even if they contain, it is in very small amounts, gelatin and zinc, which is found in corn are the examples, which belongs to this class.

Supplementary Value of Proteins

Supplementary value is the capacity of one protein to make good the deficiency of another protein. This is also known as the 'mutual supplementation effect'. The chief source of protein in diets for most of the world's people is from plants. Just because plant foods, when fed alone do not provide necessary quota of essential amino acids is no reason to condemn them as protein sources. However, four possibilities exist for improving the quality of protein:

1. First, is to feed some amount of animal or complete protein with second and third class protein, e.g. to include little amount of animal protein at each meal.
2. Second, to use a combination of various vegetable proteins so that they would make up the deficiency of each other, e.g. mixture of cereals and pulses.
3. Third, to add the lacking essential amino acids synthetically.
4. Fourth, by germination and fermentation, e.g. sprouting of pulses, cereals, etc.

Digestion of Proteins

1. There are no proteins-splitting enzymes in saliva and so in salivary digestion protein is not affected.

2. Hydrolysis of protein begins in the stomach. The enzymes secreted by gastric glands in the stomach, breaks down proteins into proteoses and peptones.
3. Milk proteins are first converted to casein by a special enzyme called rennin. Casein combines with calcium to form calcium caseinate, pepsin converts into peptones. All the peptide linkages are not broken by gastric digestion.
4. A stronger enzyme of pancreatic and intestinal juice contains trypsin and chymotrypsin. They hydrolyze peptones and proteoses into polypeptides.
5. The final breakdown of all protein fractions to amino acids is brought about by erepsin secreted by intestinal mucosa.
6. Amino acids are absorbed by the small intestine and they are carried to the tissues or to the liver a small amount.

Protein Metabolism

The metabolism of proteins may be conveniently discussed under the following heads:
1. Breakdown and synthesis of tissue proteins.
2. Nitrogen balance.
3. Oxidation of amino acids.

Breakdown and Synthesis

Digestion: It involves the following:
1. The digestion and absorption takes place in the stomach and intestines. As a result of digestion, the proteins are broken down to amino acids and absorbed.
2. Gastric digestion: The proteolytic enzyme present in gastric is called pepsin. It acts medium and hydrolyses them to simpler compounds known as polypeptides.
3. Intestinal digestion: The digestion of proteins is further carried on in the intestines by the action of proteolytic enzymes (trypsin, chymotrypsin and peptidases) present in the pancreatic and intestinal juices. The polypeptides

produced by gastric digestion are hydrolyzed to free amino acids by the above enzymes.

4. The amino acids are absorbed in the small intestines and enter the blood circulation through the portal vein.

Utilization of proteins in the body: The amino acids from digested proteins are absorbed rapidly into the blood and passed onto different tissues to meet their needs.

Some non-essential amino acids are synthesized in the liver and also released into the circulation. The amino acids released by hydrolysis of tissue proteins are also added to the amino acid pool in the body. The protein metabolism of mammals is in a dynamic state and the synthesis and breakdown of tissue protein takes place constantly. The unwanted amino acids are oxidized in the liver to yield energy and urea. The dynamic aspects of protein metabolism are represented as follows.

Sources

There are two main dietary sources of proteins (Table 2.4):

1. **Animal sources:** Milk and milk products excluding butter, ghee, eggs, meat, fish and poultry.
2. **Plant sources:** Pulses, e.g. soybean, Bengal gram, red gram dal, green gram, black gram dal; cereals, e.g. wheat, maize, rice, barley, jowar, bajra and nuts, e.g. peanuts, almond, cashew nuts. Fruits and vegetables are poor sources.

Protein Allowance per Day

The protein requirements vary from individual to individual. Apart from age and physiological conditions, factors like emotional disturbances, infection and stress can affect a person's protein requirement. For proper utilization of protein, energy intakes should be adequate. Maximum amount of protein per kilogram of body weight is required during infancy, i.e. till 1 year of age. The requirement per kilogram of body weight slowly decreases as one reaches the adulthood and then it is stable, i.e. 1 g/kg of desirable body weight (Table 2.5).

CHAPTER 2: Review of Macro- and Micro-nutrition

Deficiencies

Protein energy leads to kwashiorkor. In Greek word, it means the displaced child when the next baby is born. This is widely prevalent among weaned infants and preschool children due of lack of protein, calories, vitamins and minerals. It usually occurs in the age group of 1–4 years. The following symptoms are observed. They are muscles wasting, mental change, edema, moon face, gray hair, necrosis, vitamin A deficiencies, anemia, fatty liver, nervous irritability, diarrhea, low-serum level, disturbances of GIT.

Treatment

High-quality protein and adequate amount of calories are required. Protein of 3–5 g/day in the form of milk is required.

Calories: 140–150 kcal/kg body weight.

Vitamin A: 50,000 international units.

Iron: Iron salts and tablets of folic acid are prescribed.

Electrolytes: Potassium chloride 3–4 g, magnesium chloride 5 g to be given daily.

Marasmus

In Greek word, it means withering. It is usually occurring

Table 2.4: Sources of proteins

Sources	Percentage
Plant sources	
Soybean	43%
Roasted groundnut	26%
Skimmed milk	38%
Field bean	25%
Black gram dal	24%
Green gram dal	24%
Peas (dried)	24%
Cowpea	24%
Moth beans	23%
Almond	20%
Bengal gram	20%
Wheat	12%
Agathi greens	8%
Sundakkai (dried)	8%
Wood apple	7%
Animal sources	
Chicken	25%
Cheese	24%
Fish (seer/vanjaram)	22%
Prawn	19%
Mutton	18%
Pork	18%
Egg	13%
Cow milk	3.2%

Table 2.5: Protein requirement of various age group

Sl No	Age group	Requirements
1.	0–3 month	2.3 g/kg
2.	3–9 month	1.8 g/kg
3.	9–12 month	1.5 g/kg
4.	1–3 year	22 g/day
5.	4–6 year	29 g/kg
6.	7–9 year	36 g/day
7.	10–12 year	43 g/day
8.	13–15 year	47.5 g/day
9.	16–18 year	48.5 g/day
10.	Adult	1g/kg body weight
11.	Pregnancy	+ 14 g/day
12.	Lactation	+ 25 g/day

in earlier age than kwashiorkor. Marasmus is caused by both protein and calories, widely prevalent among infants in the age group of 0–12 months. Signs and symptoms are growth failure more severe than kwashiorkor, edema is absent, acid stool, dehydration, lack of subcutaneous fat and apathy (lack of interest in surrounding).

Marasmic Kwashiorkor

In this condition, both kwashiorkor and marasmus symptoms are noticed. So, calories and protein allowances are required in adequate amounts (Table 2.6).

▶ LIPIDS

Lipids are more commonly known as fats and oil, which are integral part of our food. They are insoluble in water, but soluble in organic solvents. They occur in both plants and animals. Lipids are concentrated sources of energy.

The term 'lipids' is applied to a group of naturally occurring substance and are characterized by:

CHAPTER 2: Review of Macro- and Micro-nutrition

Table 2.6: Clinical features of kwashiorkor and marasmus

Clinical features	Kwashiorkor	Marasmus
Weight (growth for age)	Below normal, may be marked by edema	Very much below normal
Muscles	Thin upper arms can be marked by edema	Very thin upper arms
Edema of feet and legs	Present	Not present
Hair color and texture	Bright than in others or reddish and brittle	Lighter, but softer than others
Skin	Stretched and taut, flaking off of skin, pale patches	Shriveled and wrinkled
Appetite and behavior	Poor appetite looks miserable or irritated weak cry	Usually accepts food offered, alter but looks anxious
Stools	Often loose, motion may also be constipated	Sometimes loose, motion may also be constipated
Diarrhea	Often	Sometimes
Anemia	Sometimes	Sometimes
Vitamin deficiencies	Usually found	Sometimes found

1. Their insolubility in water.
2. Greasy feel.
3. Solubility in some organic solvents.

Fats are solid at 20°C and they are called 'oils' if they are liquid at that temperature. They are classified as:

1. Simple lipids, e.g. triglycerides.
2. Compound lipids, e.g. phospholipids.
3. Derived lipids, e.g. cholesterol.

Composition

Fat as a complex molecule constitutes a mixture of fatty acids and an alcohol, generally glycerol. It contains carbon, hydrogen and oxygen, but differs from carbohydrates, in that it contains more carbon and hydrogen and less oxygen. When one gram of fat is oxidized it yields 9 kcal.

Classification

Lipids are classified into simple, compound and derived lipids, which are further subdivided as follows.

Simple Lipids

Fats and oils are included in this type. At room temperature, oils are liquids and fats are solids. Fats and oils contain esters of fatty acid and glycerol, a form in which lipids are present in food.

Compound Lipids

Compound lipids are esters of fatty acids containing phosphorus carbohydrate or protein. Phospholipids contain a phosphoric acid in addition to the alcohol and fatty acids. Glycolipids contain a fatty acid, carbohydrate and a nitrogenous base. Phospholipids and glycolipids form part of the cell membrane and the nervous system. Lipoproteins are macromolecular complex of lipids with proteins.

Derived Lipids

Derived lipids are substances liberated during hydrolysis of simple and compound lipids, which still retain the properties of lipids. The important members of this group are sterols, fatty acids and alcohol.

Sterols

Sterols are solid alcohols and form esters with fatty acids. In nature, they occur in the free state in the form of esters. Based on their origin, sterols are classified as cholesterol (animal origin) and phytosterol (in plants).

CHAPTER 2: Review of Macro- and Micro-nutrition

Cholesterol is a complex type of lipid that is regularly synthesized by and stored in the liver. It is present in all animal products.

Fatty Acids

Fatty acids are the main building blocks of fat. They have a methyl group (CH_3) at one end and a carboxyl group (COOH) at the other end with a chain of carbon and hydrogen atom in the middle. They have a general formula $CH_3(CH_2)n$ COOH. Where, 'n' denotes the number of carbon atoms, which may vary from 2 to 21. Fatty acids can be classified into:

1. **Saturated fatty acids (SFA):** The fatty acids that are unable to absorb more hydrogen. They are usually stiff and hard fats, e.g. ghee, butter.
2. **Unsaturated fatty acids (UFA):** They have one or more double bond in their molecule and are thus not saturated with hydrogen. They are liquid at room temperature, e.g. sunflower oil. Unsaturated fatty acids may be monounsaturated or polyunsaturated depending on the number of double bonds:
   a. *Monounsaturated fatty acids (MUFA):* They have only one double bond in their molecule, e.g. oleic acid found in olive oil, peanut oil.
   b. *Polyunsaturated fatty acids (PUFA):* They have two or more double bonds in their molecule, e.g. linoleic acid, linolenic acid. They are present in corn, safflower, soybean, sunflower oils and fish oil. Monounsaturated and polyunsaturated fats are usually soft or liquid at room temperature.

Triglycerides

Fatty acids combine with glycerol to form a glyceride, when only one fatty acid combines with glycerol, it forms a monoglyceride, diglycerides have two fatty acids and triglycerides have three fatty acids attached to glycerol. Most of the fatty acids present in the body and absorbed from foods occur in the form of triglycerides. During digestion triglycerides are hydrolyzed to form free fatty acid, monoglycerides and glycerol, which are absorbed by the intestinal wall and the majority of these are rebuilt as triglycerides:

1. **Long- and short-chain fatty acids:** The number of carbon atom in fatty acids decides the chain length. Thus, short-chain fatty acids contain 4–6 carbon atoms, medium chain 8–12 carbon atoms and long-chain fatty acid have 14–18 carbon atom.
2. **Essential fatty acids:** It is those, which cannot be synthesized by the body and need to be supplied through diet. Linolenic acid, linoleic acid and arachidonic acid are essential fatty acids.
3. **Non-essential fatty acids:** They are those, which can be synthesized by the body and which need not be supplied through the diet. Palmitic acid, oleic acid and butyric acid are examples of non-essential fatty acids.

Functions

Lipids perform several important functions:

1. They are the concentrated fuel reserve of the body.
2. Lipids are the constituents of cell membrane structure and regulate the membrane permeability.
3. They are essential for the digestion, absorption and utilization of fat-soluble vitamins like vitamin A, D, E and K.
4. Lipids are important as cellular metabolic regulators (steroid hormones and prostaglandin).
5. Lipids protect the internal organs serving as insulating materials.
6. As compounds of the mitochondria membranes, lipids (phospholipids) participate in electron transport chain.
7. Fat imparts palatability to the diet and slows stomach emptying time, thus giving a feeling of fullness. This delay of onset of hunger is called 'satiety value' of fats.
8. The calories in fat spare the proteins from being oxidized for energy.

CHAPTER 2: Review of Macro- and Micro-nutrition

9. Fat deposited in the adipose tissue serves as reserve source of energy during starvation. It acts as an insulator conserving the body heat.

Essential fatty acids, which are derived lipids, perform important functions in our body.

Functions of Essential Fatty Acids

1. Maintenance of the function and integrity of cellular and subcellular membrane.
2. Regulation of cholesterol metabolism by transporting it between the blood and body tissues.
3. Acts as precursor of hormone-like prostaglandin, which aid in regulating vascular function and help relieving pain and inflammation.
4. Delays blood clotting time.

Digestion

1. **In the mouth:** Fat digestion starts in the mouth with hard fats beginning to melt when they reach body temperature. The salivary glands at the base of the tongue release a lipase enzyme, which digests fat to a less extent in adults.
2. **In the stomach:** In the stomach fat floats as a layer above the other components of swallowed food. As a result little fat digestion takes place.
3. **In the small intestine:** When fat enters the small intestine, the hormone cholecystokinin signals the gallbladder to release bile. Bile emulsifies fat and also provides an alkaline medium for the action of pancreatic lipase and intestinal lipase. The triglycerides are acted upon by these lipases and hydrolyzed to monoglycerides and fatty acids.

The cholesterol esters are hydrolyzed to give cholesterol and fatty acids:
a. Triglycerides → Monoglyceride + Fatty acids.
b. Cholesterol esters → Cholesterol + Fatty acids.

SECTION 1: Nutrition

Absorption and Utilization

Small molecules of digested triglycerides (glycerol, short- and medium-chain fatty acids) can diffuse into intestinal cells and are absorbed directly into the bloodstream. Larger molecules (monoglycerides, long-chain fatty acids) merge into spherical complexes known as micelles. The lipid contents of the micelles diffuse into the intestinal cells. Once inside, the monoglycerides and long-chain fatty acids are reassembled to new triglycerides. Within the intestinal cells the new triglycerides and larger lipids-like cholesterol and phospholipids are placed into transport vehicle called chylomicrons.

The intestinal cells then release chylomicrons into the lymphatic system. The lymph circulation empties into the thoracic duct, which in turn enter the subclavian vein and subsequently into the bloodstream.

The blood transport lipids to the rest of the body and cells absorb them and utilize for energy. This breakdown of fat to yield energy is called lipolysis.

Majority of lipids enter via the lymph to the liver where the protein and lipid (cholesterol, triglycerides) are bound together to form lipoproteins.

There are four types of lipoproteins, they are:
1. Chylomicrons.
2. Very-low density lipoproteins (VLDL).
3. Low-density lipoproteins (LDL).
4. High-density lipoproteins (HDL).

Chylomicrons, VLDL and LDL serve to transport and deposit lipids from the intestine and liver to the tissues for absorption. Low-density lipoprotein, which has the highest cholesterol fraction favors lipid deposition in tissues including blood vessels and hence, termed 'bad' cholesterol. HDL cholesterol removes the lipids from the tissues and transports it back to liver for disposal; hence it is termed as 'good cholesterol'. High levels of LDL cholesterol indicate a high risk of cardiovascular disease. Apart from lipoproteins, triglycerides, cholesterol and phospholipids are synthesized in the liver. This is called lipogenesis.

CHAPTER 2: Review of Macro- and Micro-nutrition

Dietary fats are derived from two main sources:
1. Animal sources: It includes butter, ghee, curd, whole milk and its products meat, fish, poultry and eggs.
2. Plant sources: They include all vegetables oils, e.g. groundnut, gingelly, mustard, cottonseed, sunflower and coconut oil. Also it will include hydrogenated fats, margarine, nuts and oil seeds like cashew nut, peanuts, almonds and mustard seeds:
   a. Animal fats (fat of meat and fish, ghee, butter, milk and eggs).
   b. Vegetable fats (some of the plants store fat in the seeds, e.g. groundnut, mustard, sesame, coconut, etc.).
   c. Other sources from cereals, pulses, nuts and vegetables.

Invisible or Hidden Fats

Invisible or hidden fats are those, which form an integral part of foods and are therefore not visible. It includes the fats present in the cells, cell walls and cell membranes of both plant and animal tissues. Almost everything we eat as listed below carries some invisible fats:
1. **Plant food:** Cereals, millets, vegetables, spices, nuts and oil seeds, coconut, avocado.
2. **Animal food:** Milk and milk products (curd, cream, cheese), flesh foods, (mutton, beef, pork, chicken) organ meats (brain, liver, kidney), fish, shrimp, prawn.
3. **Sources of saturated fat:** Saturated fat is resistant to oxidation even at frying temperatures. Examples are:
   a. *Plants:* Coconut oil, hydrogenated vegetable oils and palm kernel oil.
   b. *Animals:* Butter, ghee, fats from flesh foods and organ meats.
4. **Sources of unsaturated fat:** Unsaturated fats and oils include MUFAs and PUFA in various proportions. Important sources of unsaturated fats are as follows:
   a. *Plant sources:* All common vegetable oils with the exception of coconut oils are predominantly unsaturated. The

invisible fats present in nuts, oil seeds, cereals, pulses, legumes, roots, tubers, vegetables, spices and fruits.

In most plant foods and vegetable oils linoleic acid are the predominant PUFA, but mustard and soybean oils, legumes/pulses. Fenugreek leaves and green leafy vegetables are good sources of α-linolenic acid.

b. *Animal sources:* The muscles (lean meat) of flesh foods, unlike the depot fat surrounding the tissues is mainly composed of cholesterol esters and phospholipids, both of which have a high proportion of long chain n-6 PUFAs, which are otherwise formed in the body from linolenic acid. Arachidonic acid is found in animal and human cells. Fish and fish oils provide long chain n–3 PUFA.

Hydrogenation

Hydrogenation (addition of hydrogen at double bonds) converts liquid oils into semisolid or solid fats. During hydrogenation, linoleic and α-linolenic acid present in the oils are converted to trans fatty acids and saturated fatty acids. Also, the MUFAs are converted to saturated fatty acids. Hydrogenated fats were designed to imitate ghee. It is used to prepare processed foods like biscuits and cakes. Vanaspati is produced in India by hydrogenation of vegetable oil.

Cholesterol

Cholesterol is a constituent of animal foods, but is absent in plants. Vegetable oils do not have cholesterol. In human diets, cholesterol is obtained from ghee, butter, cheese, milk, curd, egg, flesh foods, organ meats, fish and prawns. Most animal foods are good sources of both cholesterol and fatty acids.

Recommended Daily Dietary Intakes

The fat requirement mainly depends upon the energy needs of the individual. From physiological point of view there can be wide variation in fat intake and still good health can be maintained. On an average about 15%–20% of the total energy should be supplied from fats. The dietary fats should be a good source of EFAs and hence at least 50% of the dietary fat should be from vegetables oils rich in EFAs.

Effects of Deficiency

Deficiency of fat in the diet causes the deficiency of EFAs. Deficiency of EFAs leads to cessation of growth. It also results in flaky skin, development of itchy sores on the scalp. The common disorder in adults and children in India is phrynoderma or toad skin.

The condition is characterized by the presence of horny eruptions on the posterior and lateral aspects of the limbs on the back and buttocks.

Phrynoderma is cured rapidly by the administration of linseed or safflower seed oil rich in EFAs. Infants fed on an EFA deficient diet develops irritation and changes in the skin within a few weeks. The skin changes appear as dryness and desquamation with oozing in the folds. Diarrhea may also occur, supplementation of the diet with linoleic acid helps to restore the skin to normal condition.

Excess

If excessive fat is consumed it will result in obesity gastrointestinal disturbances and predisposal to many other diseases like diabetes and cardiovascular ailments. In recent years there has been a revival of interest in the nutritional aspect of excessive intake of the fat in the diet in increasing the level of cholesterol in the blood. Excessive cholesterol in blood gradually causes it to deposit under the lining of blood vessels, resulting in 'atherosclerosis' where in the blood vessels are narrowed and hardened leading to heart diseases.

SECTION 1: Nutrition

▶ VITAMINS

Introduction

The term 'vitamin' derives from the word 'vital amine', which means essential nitrogenous compounds. The term was coined by Polish scientist, Funk, who gave the name 'vitamine' to antiberiberi substance. Later on 'e' was dropped and thus the term 'vitamin' was coined. However, with the discovery of more vitamins, it was soon realized that all the vitamins are not nitrogenous compounds; but all vitamins are essential for health. Vitamins are complex chemical substances required by the body in very small amounts. They do not yield energy, but act as catalyst in various body processes. Since, vitamins cannot be manufactured in the body (at least in sufficient amounts) they have to be supplied through the diet.

Vitamins are organic substances present in small amounts in food; they are required for carrying out vital functions of the body. They are involved in the utilization of the major nutrients like proteins, fats and carbohydrates.

Though, needed in small amounts, they are essential for health and well-being of the body. When these vitamins were discovered on the basis of their function and before their chemical nature were elucidated, they were designated as B, C and D or in terms of their major functions like antineuritic, antirachitic vitamins. Vitamins are classified based on their solubility as fat-soluble vitamins and water-soluble vitamins.

Vitamins may be defined as organic compounds occurring in small quantities in different natural foods and necessary for the growth and maintenance of good health in human being and certain experimental animals. Vitamins may be classified into two groups:
1. Fat-soluble vitamins.
2. Water-soluble vitamins.

Fat-soluble vitamins, e.g. vitamin A, D, E and K. Water-soluble vitamins, viz. vitamins of the B group and vitamin C.

▶ FAT-SOLUBLE VITAMINS

Vitamin A

Vitamin A occurs only in foods of animal origin. Vitamin A activity is also possessed by carotenoids found in plants. Hence, carotenoids are called provitamin A. Vitamin A is not synthesized in the body and must by supplied by food supplements. One of the best defined roles of vitamin A is its requirements for normal vision. Vitamin A is necessary for the health of the epithelial cells. Vitamin A was the first fat-soluble vitamin to be recognized. Three forms of vitamin A are active in the body, retinol, retinal and retinoic acid. They are collectively called retinoids.

Beta carotene is the provitamin of vitamin A. Provitamins are substances that are chemically related to a vitamin, but must be changed by the body into active form of the vitamin. Vitamin A in the diet comes in two forms, retinoids (preformed vitamin A) and carotenoids. Vitamin A is present in vegetable foods, which contain yellow pigment called carotenes. It was isolated from carrots hence called carotenoids, which are provitamins of vitamin A.

Chemistry

Vitamin A occurs in several forms: As retinol, as retinal, as an aldehyde and as retinoic acid. These several forms may be referred to as vitamin A. In its pure form, vitamin A is a pale-yellow crystalline compound and occurs naturally in animals. It is soluble in fat solvents, but insoluble in water and is relatively stable to heat, acids and alkalis. It is easily oxidized and rapidly destroyed by ultraviolet radiation. The ultimate source of all vitamin A is in the carotenes, which are synthesized by plants. Animals, as well as man in turn convert a considerable portion of carotene of the foods they eat into vitamin A. Carotenes are dark-red crystalline compounds also known as 'pro vitamin A' or 'precursors of vitamin A'. The α-, β- and γ-molecules of carotene are of significance in nutrition. Each molecule of beta carotene yields two molecules of vitamin A.

SECTION 1: Nutrition

Absorption, Transport and Storage

Absorption

Vitamin A is usually complexed with proteins. Before vitamin A can be absorbed, it is hydrolyzed by proteases and pancreatic enzymes to form free retinol. In addition to this, retinyl esters must also be hydrolyzed by lipases in the small intestine to retinol and free fatty acids. Vitamin A is absorbed in two forms: As retinol, which is the preformed vitamin A from animal source and as carotene, which is a precursor from plant sources. The absorption of vitamin A and carotene is aided by bile salts, pancreatic lipase and fat. After it is absorbed into the mucosal cells, retinol is re-esterified to retinyl esters and these esters are incorporated into chylomicrons for transport through the lymph and eventually the bloodstream by way of thoracic duct. Carotenes are cleaved in the intestinal mucosa into retinaldehyde, which is then reduced to retinol. This cleavage requires an enzyme and bile salt. The conversion of dietary carotene chiefly takes place in the intestine, but some carotene is converted in liver or kidney also. The absorption of vitamin A and carotene follows the same route as that of fat.

Factors affecting vitamin A absorption

1. The absorption of vitamin A is seriously affected when the diet contains very low fat or when there is an obstruction of the bile duct.
2. The presence of vitamin E in the intestinal tract prevents the excessive oxidation of vitamin A, thus making it available for absorption.
3. The presence of mineral oil reduces the absorption because mineral oil itself is not absorbed; it carries vitamin A as well as other fat-soluble vitamins with it. Mineral oil which is used as a laxative should be taken at or around mealtime.
4. In premature infants the absorption is poor.
5. During protein-energy malnutrition the absorption may be affected due to lack of carrier protein. They have typically low circulating retinol and may not respond to vitamin A supplementation unless protein-energy malnutrition is treated.

Transport and Storage

After the absorption of preformed retinol from animal and plant sources, carotene conversion is re-esterified with long-chain fatty acids in the intestinal mucosa. Vitamin A is incorporated into the chylomicrons. It enters the bloodstream through the lymphatic system and finally carried to the liver for storage from where it is distributed to the cells as required. Liver stores vitamin A (retinol) as retinyl esters in lipid droplets. These retinyl esters are then hydrolyzed and free retinol is bound to a carrier protein, retinol-binding protein (RBP) and is delivered to cells. About 90% of vitamin A in the body is found in the liver alone and the remainder is present in the kidney, lungs, adrenal glands and adipose tissue. An average healthy adult stores enough vitamin A for several months to a year. These liver stores are reduced during periods of infectious disease. Infants and children do have such reserves; therefore they are more susceptible to develop deficiency symptoms.

Vitamin A and its products formed on hydrolysis are excreted mainly in the bile. Some amount of vitamin A is reabsorbed, but most of it is excreted in the feces. Some of these products may be excreted in the urine also.

Functions

1. **Vision:** The role of vitamin A in visual process is well-understood, it maintains the normal vision in dim light. There are two types of light receptors in the retina of the eye, i.e. the rods for vision in dim light and the cones for vision in bright light and color vision. The rods produce rhodopsin or visual purple, a photosensitive pigment and cones produce iodopsin or visual violet. When the light strikes the eye, the rhodopsin is split into its component parts, retinaldehyde (retinal) and protein opsin. Due to these changes nerve impulse is initiated, which is then transmitted to the brain by way of optic nerve. Rhodopsin is regenerated in the dark, but some retinaldehyde is lost in each cycle, therefore, it becomes necessary to maintain

SECTION 1: Nutrition

constant supply from the blood. Inadequate supply of vitamin A for the synthesis of rhodopsin causes night blindness or nyctalopia.

2. **Maintenance of epithelial tissue:** Vitamin A is associated with the maintenance of healthy tissue covering. It makes the linings of the outside of the body and inside cavities smooth. In the presence of adequate amounts of vitamin A, they form columnar, goblet-cells mucus secretion, but in the deficiency of vitamin A, they are keratinized. This secretes mucus that coats and protects the surface from invasive microorganisms and other harmful particles. The mucus lining of the stomach protects itself from digestion by the gastric juices. Vitamin A plays a role in maintaining the integrity of cell membranes. It is also essential for healthy skin.

3. **Maintenance of bone growth:** Vitamin A is essential for normal development of skeleton, teeth and soft tissues. When vitamin A is deficient, bones do not grow in length and the normal remodeling process does not occur. Vitamin A plays an important role in removing old bones and makes way for the new ones.

4. **Reproduction:** Vitamin A is also essential for normal reproduction. It is necessary for spermatogenesis in the males and normal estrous cycle in the females. In the absence of vitamin A (retinol and retinal) during fetal development various malformations occur, it also causes sterility and testicular degeneration in males and abortion in females.

5. **Antioxidant:** Beta carotene (provitamin A) acts as an antioxidant. It has the ability to protect persons from cell damage caused by free radicals. These antioxidants neutralize free radicals in the cells thus protecting the persons from oxidative stress. These free radicals are the byproducts of normal metabolism in cells or they are created by the exposure to sunlight, tobacco smoke, fumes from vehicles or X-rays. These free radicals also damage the DNA, cell membranes and cell compounds.

6. **Other roles:** Some not well-understood roles include helps in the synthesis of corticosterone hormone by the adrenal

gland; ensures normal output of thyroid hormone (thyroxin) from the thyroid gland; helps in maintaining nerve cell sheaths; assist in immune reactions; helps in synthesizing red blood cells.

Sources

Vitamin A in the human diet exists as retinol or as retinal or beta carotene, which has to be converted to vitamin A. Foods of animal origin contains retinol. Plant sources are rich in beta carotene. Only one third of the dietary beta carotene is absorbed. Beta carotene from green leafy vegetables is well-utilized than from carrots and papayas. Good sources of vitamin A are sheep liver, butter, ghee, egg, milk, curds, liver oils of shark and halibut. Good sources of beta carotene are agathi, amaranth, drumstick leaves, green leafy vegetables, mango, papaya, carrot and jackfruit.

Effects of Deficiency

Deficiency of vitamin A is manifested as nutritional blindness and increased susceptibility to infection. Nutritional blindness is an important public health problem among young children in India.

Night blindness is an early symptom of vitamin A deficiency. The individual cannot see in dim light. This can be corrected with adequate supply of vitamin A. In the absence of adequate vitamin A intake the outer lining of the eyeball loses its usual moist, white appearance and becomes dry and wrinkled called xerosis. This condition is followed by raised muddy dry triangular patches on the conjunctiva called the Bitot's spots.

Redness and inflammation of the eye and gradual loss of vision may follow. The central portion of the eye loses its transparency and becomes opaque and soft, if not treated and leads to total blindness termed xerophthalmia. Xerophthalmia encompasses all ocular manifestations of vitamin A deficiency. Increased susceptibility to infection occurs because the mucous membrane lining becomes dry and rough, which is easily invaded by the microorganism.

SECTION 1: Nutrition

Hypervitaminosis

Intake of large amount of vitamin A for prolonged periods can lead to toxic symptoms, which include irritability, headache, nausea and vomiting.

▶ VITAMIN D

Vitamin D can be synthesized in the body in adequate amounts by simple exposure to sunlight, even for 5 min/day is sufficient. It is essential for bone growth and calcium metabolism. It acts as a hormone in the body by facilitating calcium absorption and deposition in the bone.

Chemistry and Characteristic

Vitamin D is a group of sterol compounds possessing antirachitic properties, but only two are of nutritional interest:
1. Vitamin D_2 or ergocalciferol found in plants.
2. Vitamin D_3 or cholecalciferol, which occurs in animal cells and activates in the skin on exposure to ultraviolet light. Pure vitamin D is white, crystalline compounds, which are soluble in fats and fat solvents, but insoluble in water. They are stable to heat, alkalis and oxidation.

Absorption, Transport and Storage

Absorption of dietary vitamin D takes place along with other lipids into the jejunum and ileum of the small intestine by passive diffusion. The absorption of vitamin D requires the presence of bile salts because it is a fat-soluble vitamin. Vitamin D is incorporated into chylomicrons after it is absorbed and enters the lymphatic system and eventually enters the plasma from where it is transported to the liver. Any conditions, which interfere with fat absorption, will hinder the complete absorption of vitamin D. These conditions include pancreatitis, tropical sprue, colitis and malabsorption syndrome. The vitamin D made in the skin from cholesterol enters the blood and is transported by vitamin D binding protein (DBP) to the peripheral tissues. Small amount of vitamin D is stored in the liver. The major pathway of vitamin D excretion is through the bile. Daily losses of vitamin D in the urine are very small.

Functions

1. Vitamin D helps in the absorption of calcium and phosphorus by increasing the synthesis of calcium binding protein.
2. Vitamin D helps to maintain the calcium and phosphorus levels in the body by stimulating the following:
   a. Absorption in the gastrointestinal tract.
   b. Retention by the kidney.
3. Vitamin D helps in deposition of calcium in the bones. The bones grow denser and stronger.

Food Sources

The vitamin D content of food sources from animals varies with the diet, breed and exposure to sunlight of the animal. The good sources of vitamin D are cod liver oil, shrimp, liver, butter, yolk, cheese, milk, spinach and cabbage.

Requirements

The expert group of Indian Council of Medical Research (ICMR) has not recommended dietary intake of vitamin D for Indians. Only in those cases where the vitamin D requirement is not met due to inadequate exposure to sunlight, the ICMR recommends 400 µg/day of vitamin D.

Deficiency

Vitamin D deficiency occurs due to:
1. Inadequate intake.
2. Inadequate exposure to sunlight.
3. Drugs that interfere vitamin D activity.
4. Secondary causes, such as damaged liver and kidneys where its metabolism takes place.

Vitamin D deficiency causes reduced absorption of calcium and phosphorus from the small intestine, which leads to faulty or incomplete mineralization of bone and teeth. Soft bones become unable to bear the stress of weight and results in skeletal malformations. The deficiency symptoms manifest as rickets in children and as osteomalacia in adults.

Rickets

Rickets generally occurs in dark and overcrowded areas of large cities with high rise building where the sunshine does not penetrate through the fog, smoke or pollution. Rickets is a deficiency disease, which affects children. It involves incomplete or impaired mineralization of growing bones. It is not caused solely by the deficiency of vitamin D, but also due to the deficiency of calcium and phosphorus. There is a lack of calcium phosphate deposition on the bones.

Symptoms

1. Structural abnormalities of the weight-bearing bones, such as tibia, radius, ulna, humerus and ribs associated with pain and delayed walking. The child is miserable and in pain.
2. Fontanel closure is delayed. Skull becomes soft and forehead is bulging out, which gives the box-like appearance; large head.
3. Bones become soft and fragile, which leads to widening of the ends of long bones. The cartilage of the end of bones continues to grow and become enlarged without getting mineralized.
4. Bones are poorly mineralized and soft, so they bend and result in bowing of legs due to weight of the body.
5. The spine becomes curved with the projection of the sternum or 'pigeon chest'.
6. Narrowing of the pelvis.
7. Joints of wrist, knees (knock-knees) and ankle are enlarged. The gait becomes waddling due to bowed legs or knock-knees.

8. Patients show elevated plasma and serum levels of alkaline phosphatase.
9. Restlessness and nervous irritability.
10. Neuromuscular irritability. Underdeveloped muscles and lack of muscle tone. Pot belly due to weakness of abdominal muscles.

Causes

1. It affects those children who reside in dark and overcrowded areas of large cities where ultraviolet rays of sunshine do not reach due to thick fog, smoke, etc.
2. Poverty and failure to obtain required vitamin D concentrates or skin exposure.
3. Dark-skinned children are more prone to rickets as compared to white-skinned people because the skin pigmentation inhibits the penetration of ultraviolet rays.
4. Premature infants are more prone to developing rickets than full-term infants. This is because the growth rate and skeletal calcification impose additional demands for vitamin D.

Treatment

Rickets can be treated effectively by giving relatively large amounts of vitamin D concentrates orally or by giving vitamin D from natural sources, such as fish-liver oil. Fish-liver oil contains 9 µg (360 IU) of vitamin D.

Osteomalacia

Osteomalacia means bone softening. It is similar to rickets, but develops in adults so often refer to as 'adult rickets'. Due to the deficiency of vitamin D and calcium bone mineral density decreases. This deficiency occurs mostly in women who have insufficient calcium intake and little exposure to sunlight. It is also seen in women who have repeated pregnancies in quick succession and periods of lactation and also due to malabsorption of vitamin D. In osteomalacia, lack of calcium phosphate deposition decreases the bone mineral content.

Symptoms
1. Skeletal pain of the rheumatic type especially in bones of the legs and lower back.
2. Bone tenderness and spontaneous multiple fractures.
3. Muscular weakness with difficulty in walking and climbing.
4. Softening of the bones. The bones of the legs, spine, thorax and pelvis may bend and cause deformities.

Causes
1. Little exposure to sunlight. Women observing purdah, clothing, which completely shields them from sunlight and dietary calcium is not absorbed properly, ultimately leads to vitamin D deficiency.
2. Interference with fat absorption and thereby in absorption of vitamin D also.
3. Steatorrhea also reduces the absorption of calcium.
4. Chronic renal failure and disease of the parathyroid and liver. Because in the complicated process involved in the metabolism of vitamin D, any liver and kidney disease can lead to bone deterioration. Chronic kidney disease can cause osteomalacia because of the inability of kidneys to convert vitamin D to its active form. Patient on dialysis are frequently prescribed vitamin D supplementation.
5. Diet inadequate in calcium.
6. Repeated pregnancies and prolonged lactation reduces the body reserves.
7. Having dark skin.
8. Consumption of cereal grains having high-phytate content hinders calcium absorption.
9. Premature infants.
10. Elderly people who are housebound.
11. Those treated with anticonvulsants.

Treatment
Osteomalacia can be effectively treated with vitamin D_3 secondary causes can be treated accordingly.

Prevention

The occurrence of osteomalacia can be prevented with adequate intake of vitamin D, calcium and phosphorus in the diet. Moderate exposure (10–15 minutes) to sun on a clear sunny day, two to three times a week, is enough to prevent osteomalacia.

Osteoporosis

Osteoporosis is often confused with osteomalacia, but they are very different from each other. In osteoporosis bone mass is decreased, but the histologic appearance is normal. It is associated with aging. It involves impaired vitamin D metabolism and is associated with low estrogen levels. This disease is chronic and is most commonly seen in postmenopausal women, but may develop in older men also. It is a decrease in the total bone mass. The onset of the disease is quite gradual and it is asymptomatic in the early stages. The causes of osteoporosis are thought to be multifactorial, but it is also associated with aging. It involves diminished vitamin D metabolism and decreased estrogen levels. It is commonly seen in postmenopausal women and is a major cause of bone fracture. Osteoporosis can be prevented by increase intake of dietary calcium and moderate exercise daily (walking), which improves the calcium status in women. Current approaches include hormonal therapy with estrogen and vitamin D hormone. Prevention must start in youth because it is late when it is diagnosed and the treatment has little effect on reversing the disease, partly because reduced calcium absorption in elderly. Osteoporosis can be treated with hormone replacement therapy in early menopausal women.

Toxicity

Massive doses of vitamin D can be dangerous. High intake of vitamin D may cause reabsorption of calcium from the bones resulting in localized osteoporosis. Hypervitaminosis D is characterized by hypercalcemia and hyperphosphatemia. The common symptoms include headache, nausea, vomiting,

SECTION 1: Nutrition

diarrhea, excessive thirst, weight loss, polyuria, nocturia (excessive urination at night) and constipation. Laboratory tests and history of excessive intake are the basis for diagnosis. This can be treated with low-calcium diet, plenty of fluids and stopping vitamin D intake.

▶ VITAMIN E

Vitamin E is the generic name for a group of closely related and naturally occurring fat-soluble compounds, the tocopherols of these α-tocopherol is biologically the most potent. Vitamin E is widely distributed in foods. The usual plasma level of vitamin E in adult is between 0.8 and 1.4 mg/100 mL. Vitamin E is known as antisterility vitamin, because it is required for normal reproduction in animals and men.

Chemistry and Characteristic

Vitamin E consists of a group of chemical substances called 'tocopherols'. α-tocopherol is the compound possessing the greatest vitamin E activity. High temperature and acids do not affect the stability of this vitamin, but oxidation takes place in the presence of rancid fats or lead and iron salts. Decomposition occurs in ultraviolet light, alkalis and oxygen.

Absorption, Transport and Storage

Vitamin E, like any other fat-soluble vitamin and fat, is absorbed with the help of pancreatic secretions and bile salts. The absorption occurs mainly in the upper small intestine by micelle-dependent diffusion. The presence of dietary fat is essential for its absorption. The absorbed vitamin E are repackaged in the chylomicrons and transported by way of the lymphatic system into the general circulation. Vitamin E is incorporated into VLDLs and delivered to the liver and this uses a transport protein specific for vitamin E. The absorption of vitamin E is hindered by the presence of fatty diarrhea, celiac disease, intestinal resection and absence of bile. Vitamin E is stored in the liver and adipose tissue. A very small amount is excreted in the urine with the normal intake.

CHAPTER 2: Review of Macro- and Micro-nutrition

Functions

1. Vitamin E is the primary antioxidant in the body and serves to protect PUFA from oxidation in cells and maintain integrity of the cell membrane. It also prevents the oxidation of beta carotene and vitamin A. Vitamin E helps to maintain cell membrane integrity and protect red blood cells (RBCs) against hemolysis.
2. Vitamin E reduces platelet aggregation.
3. Vitamin E is essential for the iron metabolism and the maintenance of nervous tissues and immune function.
4. Vitamin E been promoted as an antiaging vitamin, because as cells age they accumulate lipid breakdown products. Vitamin E prevents this accumulation in maintaining cell health.

Food Sources

Vitamin E is widely distributed in foods. It is present in high concentration in vegetable oils and in cereal grains. Wheat gum, sunflower seeds, almonds, safflower oil, eggs, butter are good sources. Meat, fruits and vegetables contain small amounts. Sesame oil and mustard oil are good sources of vitamin E.

Requirement

The requirement of vitamin E is linked to that of EFAs (linoleic and linolenic acids). The requirement of vitamin E is 0.8 mg/g of EFA.

Deficiency

A deficiency of vitamin E in various species of animals results in reproductive failure, macrocytic anemia and shorter life span of RBC. Recently, the cytotoxic effect of vitamin E on human lymphocytes vitro at high concentrations has been reported:

1. Prolonged intake of vitamin E deficient diets produces the uncoordinated movement, weakness and sensory disturbances.

2. It causes hemolytic anemia in low-birth-weight (LBW) infants.
3. Defective functioning of the retina leading to permanent blindness in premature infants occur.
4. It leads to reproductive failure in humans.
5. Vitamin E deficiency is associated with decreased ability of the lymphocytes.

▶ VITAMIN K

Vitamin K is recognized as the antihemorrhagic factor owing to its vital role in blood clotting mechanism. Vitamin K is necessary for the synthesis of prothrombin and enzyme synthesized by the liver; prothrombin is required for normal clotting of blood. Vitamin K is found in plants. Good sources are cauliflower, spinach and soybean. In contrast fruits, cereals and animal products contain little vitamin K. It is also synthesized in the intestinal tract by the bacteria.

In the newborn babies intestinal bacteria are not sufficiently developed for the synthesis of vitamin K. Thus some infants, especially those who are immature show susceptibility to hemorrhage. Vitamin K is given to infants immediately after birth especially to those who show hemorrhagic tendency.

Chemistry and Characteristics

Vitamin K is found in nature in two forms, i.e. K_1 occurs in alfalfa and K_2 is produced by bacterial synthesis. These are soluble in fat. They are not destroyed by heat, but are unstable to alkalis, strong acids, oxidation and light.

Absorption, Transport and Storage

The absorption of phylloquinones (K_1) occurs in the small intestine, and is an energy dependent process and the absorption of menaquinones (K_2) and menadiones (K_3) takes place in the small intestine as well as colon by passive diffusion. Since, it is a fat-soluble vitamin, it requires bile salts and minimum amounts of dietary fat for its absorption. Vitamin K is incorporated in chylomicrons after it is absorbed and travels through the lymphatic system and eventually enters the portal blood from where it is transported to the liver. They are incorporated into VLDL and eventually delivered to the tissues where they are needed by LDL. Most tissues contain phylloquinones and menaquinones. Vitamin K is apparently stored in the liver in small quantities. Vitamin K is excreted in the urine after the administration of therapeutic doses.

Functions

Synthesis of blood clotting proteins and it is essential for the activation of prothrombin. This gets converted to thrombin, which in turn activates fibrinogen to form fibrin.

The process of blood clotting occurs as follows:

1. Injured tissue releases thromboplastin, which catalyses prothrombin formation.
2. Vitamin K catalyses conversion of prothrombin to thrombin.
3. This in turn causes conversion of fibrinogen to fibrin, which forms the clot.

Food Sources

Dark-green leafy vegetables are good sources of vitamin K. Fruits, tubers, seeds, dairy and meat products contain vitamin K.

Requirements

The ICMR committee considered that no recommendation is needed for this vitamin, as the synthesis of vitamin K occurs in the lower intestine by the colonic bacteria and present widely in foods.

Deficiency

Deficiency of vitamin K predominantly causes hemorrhage. Newborn infants have sterile intestinal tract, so no intestinal vitamin K is supplied during the first few days of life until intestinal microflora develops. Hemorrhagic disease may occur immediately after birth and it can be prophylactically treated by administering menadione intramuscularly at birth.

Malabsorption syndrome is the secondary cause of vitamin K deficiency. Any obstruction in fat absorption, biliary obstruction will also affect vitamin K absorption because it is a fat-soluble vitamin. Therefore, vitamin K deficiency results in prolonged blood clotting time. Patients suffering from this problem are given vitamin K before surgery. Normal bile flow is hindered after surgical removal of gallbladder with the result vitamin K is not absorbed properly.

Vitamin K is involved in several drug-nutrient interactions. An anticlotting drug (dicumerol) inhibits the action of vitamin K. Prolonged use of antibiotics kill bacteria and reduces intestinal microflora, thus reducing the main source of vitamin K.

Toxicity

Both vitamin K_1 (phylloquinones) and vitamin K_2 (menaquinones) have not shown any toxic effects. However, menadione in large amounts can be toxic. Some of the symptoms reported include liver damage, hypoprothrombinemia, renal tubule degeneration and hemolytic anemia in premature infants.

Water-soluble Vitamins

In 1911, Funk coined the term 'vitamin' for the substance, which he found effective in preventing beriberi. McCollum and Davis applied the term water-soluble B vitamins to the concentrates, which cured beriberi. It was soon discovered that vitamin B was not a single substance, but a group of compounds to which we now designate as the vitamin B complex. Some of these are discussed below:

▶ THIAMINE

Thiamine (vitamin B_1) is a water-soluble vitamin. It is essential for the utilization of carbohydrates. In thiamine deficiency there is accumulation of pyruvic and lactic acids in the tissues and body fluids. Thiamine occurs in all natural foods, although, small amounts. Important sources are whole-grain cereals, wheat gram, yeast, pulses, oil seeds and nuts especially groundnut, meat, fish, eggs, vegetables and fruits contain smaller amounts. Thiamine is known as vitamin B_1. Deficiency of thiamine leads to beriberi. This condition is widely prevalent among population whose diet contains more of polished cereals.

Chemistry and Characteristics

Thiamine hydrochloride is a white-crystalline substance. It has a faint yeast-like order and a salty, nut-like taste. It is readily soluble in water, but not in fat solvents or fats. It is readily destroyed by heat in neutral or alkaline solution; in acidic medium it is resistant to heat up to 1,200°C.

Absorption, Transport and Storage

Thiamine taken in food is available either in the free form or in bound form as thiamine pyrophosphate (TPP) or it is also present as protein phosphate complex. Before absorption it is split in the digestive tract, and then it is absorbed from the proximal duodenum by active transport and passive diffusion. Alcohol consumption interferes with transport of the vitamin and folic acid deficiency interferes with the replication of enterocytes. About 90% of thiamine is circulating as TPP and carried by erythrocytes and remaining small amounts exist as free thiamine and thiamine monophosphate (TMP) bound mainly to albumin. The bodily stores of thiamine are not so great. About 50% is stored in the skeletal muscles and some amounts are also found in the heart, kidneys, liver and brain. Thiamine is excreted in the urine and small amounts are present in the feces. If it is taken in excess, it is excreted in the urine and if small amounts are ingested the amount excreted, falls.

Functions

Thiamine functions in the release of energy from the metabolism of carbohydrate. As a result thiamine is related to the maintenance of normal appetite, normal muscle tone in the gastrointestinal tract and healthy nervous system. More advanced deficiencies result in the disease beriberi. There are two types of beriberi, i.e. dry beriberi, wet beriberi and infantile beriberi.

Role of Thiamine

1. Thiamine is converted to TPP, which is an important co enzyme in the carbohydrate metabolism.
2. It is involved in transmission of nerve impulses across the cells.
3. Thiamine as TPP is an essential cofactor for the conversion of amino acid tryptophan to niacin.

Sources

Yeast, whole wheat, millets, hand-pounded rice, parboiled rice are good sources of thiamine. The bran contains most of the thiamine in the cereals. Gingelly seeds, groundnut, soybean, cashew nuts, organ meats, pork, liver and eggs supply thiamine.

Requirements

Thiamine is involved in the carbohydrate metabolism. Its requirement is related to energy derived from carbohydrate. The ICMR expert group recommends an allowance of 0.5 mg/1,000 kcal for adults and for infants 0.3 mg/1,000 kcal is suggested.

Deficiency

Thiamine deficiency is usually associated with a low-calorie intake. But frank thiamine deficiency is usually not seen. Thiamine deficiency ultimately causes beriberi in humans.

CHAPTER 2: Review of Macro- and Micro-nutrition

Gastrointestinal disturbances and severe diarrhea vomiting may cause thiamine deficiency. The efficiency symptoms may also be seen in febrile conditions or surgery when the intake is inadequate. The symptoms of thiamine deficiency include anorexia, indigestion and severe constipation, lack of gastric muscle tone and lack of hydrochloric acid secretion.

Alcoholics are especially susceptible to thiamine deficiency. The deficiency of thiamine also affects cardiac muscles and the central nervous system (CNS) also. With continued deficiency cardiac muscles weaken and results in cardiac failure. The functioning of CNS depends on glucose for energy. Thiamine helps fulfill this need. Inadequate thiamine affects nerve activity, reflex responses are reduced and general weakness and fatigue results. Prolonged thiamine deficiency hinders lipogenesis and degeneration of myelin sheaths occurs. The symptoms include progressive nerve irritation, pain and prickly sensations. If the severe deficiency state is left untreated, paralysis will results.

Adequate amount of TPP in muscle tissue results in chronic and painful musculoskeletal condition known as fibromyalgia.

Symptoms

Deficiency affects the gastrointestinal, cardiovascular and peripheral nervous systems. Early symptoms include fatigue, lack of interest, emotional instability, irritability depression, anger and fear and loss of appetite, loss of weight and loss of strength.

Dry Beriberi

As the deficiency progresses, the symptoms become more marked, which include indigestion, constipation, headache, insomnia (inadequate sleep), tachycardia (rapid heartbeat), feeling of heaviness and weakness of the legs, cramps of the calf muscles and burning and numbness of the feet (peripheral neuritis). Eventually muscle degeneration and lack of coordination occurs. This is often referred to as 'dry beriberi'.

SECTION 1: Nutrition

Wet Beriberi

Vitamin B_1 deficiency also leads to cardiomegaly, tachycardia, mental confusion and muscle wasting. This condition of the disease is known as 'wet beriberi' because it is associated with edema.

Infantile Beriberi

Infants in the far East are especially prone to this deficiency because their mothers had decreased thiamine intake and the milk produced by them for the infants contains very small amounts of thiamine. Onset is sudden and is characterized by pallor, facial edema, irritability, vomiting, abdominal pain, loss of voice and convulsions. The progression of the disease is so fast that the infant may die within a few hours, but with thiamine treatment, recovery is remarkable.

Treatment

Thiamine deficiency can be treated with B complex vitamins rather than thiamine alone. Along with B complex vitamins, a high-calorie and high-protein diet is prescribed.

Toxicity

Little is known about thiamine toxicity. However, mega doses of 1,000 times more than the RDA of commercial preparation have caused the suppression of respiratory center and ultimately cause death. Studies have further reported that the parenteral doses of thiamine of 100 times more than the recommended levels have produced weakness, headache, convulsions, muscular weakness, cardiac arrhythmia and allergic reactions.

▶ RIBOFLAVIN

Riboflavin or vitamin B_2 is the yellow enzyme, which is heat stable unlike other B vitamins. Riboflavin in the combined form with proteins forms flavoproteins or yellow enzymes. This enzyme is of two types flavin adenine dinucleotide (FAD)

Riboflavin (vitamin B_2) is a member of B group vitamins. It has fundamental role in cellular oxidation. It is a cofactor in a number of enzymes involves with energy metabolism. Its richest natural sources are milk, eggs, liver, kidneys and green leafy vegetables. Meat and fish contain small amounts. There are no real body stores of riboflavin.

Low-dietary intake of riboflavin may result in fissures at the angle of the mouth, accompanied by the yellow cast. The tongue may exhibit glossitis, turning to purplish red in color, accompanied by a painful burning sensation.

Chemistry and Characteristics

In its pure form this vitamin is bitter tasting, orange yellow, odorless compound in which crystals are needle shaped. It dissolves sparingly in water to give a typical greenish-yellow fluorescence. It is stable to boiling in acids, but in alkaline solutions it is readily decomposed by heat. It is also destroyed by exposure to light.

Absorption, Transport and Storage

Riboflavin is either present in foods in free state, or in combination with phosphate or with protein and phosphate together. These compounds are broken down during digestion and free riboflavin is absorbed in the proximal small intestine by a carrier mediated process. This process requires adenosine triphosphate (ATP). Riboflavin is present as the coenzyme or as flavoproteins in body tissues. The absorption of free riboflavin depends on its phosphorylation in flavin mononucleotide (FMN).

Riboflavin is transported as free riboflavin and FMN in the plasma and cells by a carrier-mediated process. Small amounts are present in the liver, kidney and heart, but it is not stored in appreciable amount, thus it becomes necessary to supply riboflavin in the diet regularly. If intake increases, then the urinary excretion also increases markedly and it is excreted as such.

Functions

Riboflavin is part of two coenzymes, FMN and FAD. FMN and FAD are contained in flavoproteins. They are both oxidizing agents and take part in vital reaction points. These two act as hydrogen acceptor and form $FMNH_2$ or $FADH_2$. The enzymes are essential for the completion of many reactions in the energy cycle through which ATP is produced in which hydrogen is transferred from one compound to another and eventually it combines with oxygen to form water. These enzymes and niacin containing enzymes are closely associated.

The FMN and FAD also act as coenzymes of dehydrogenases, which catalyze the initial oxidations of fatty acid and many intermediates in carbohydrate metabolism. Pyridoxine (vitamin B_6) is converted to active form, pyridoxal phosphate (PLP) in the presence of FMN. Similarly, tryptophans can biosynthesize vitamin niacin in the presence of FAD. Riboflavin is necessary for normal growth and maintenance of tissues. It also plays an important role in the health of the eye.

Recommended Daily Allowances

The requirement of riboflavin is directly proportional to energy intake. It is 0.6 mg/1,000 kcals. The daily safe intake ranges from 0.7 to 2.2 mg/day, which depends on age, physiological status and level of activity.

Food Sources

Riboflavin is widely distributed in foods. Dairy products and meats are the best sources. Eggs, liver and green leafy vegetables are also good sources. Cereals like millets and pulses are fair sources of riboflavin, but rice is specially a poor source as more than half of the vitamin is lost when it is milled. However, the cereals can be enriched with riboflavin to increase its content.

CHAPTER 2: Review of Macro- and Micro-nutrition

Effects of Deficiency

Riboflavin deficiency is prevalent mainly among the low income groups particularly the vulnerable group and the elderly adults. Riboflavin deficiency is characterized by:

1. Soreness and burning of the mouth and tongue.
2. Lesions at the angles of the mouth called angular stomatitis.
3. The inflammation of the tongue called glossitis.
4. Dry chapped appearance of the lip with ulcers termed cheilosis.
5. The skin becomes dry and results in seborrheic dermatitis.
6. Photophobia, lacrimation, burning sensation of the eyes and visual fatigue.
7. Decreased motor coordination.
8. Normocytic anemia.

▶ NIACIN

Niacin or nicotinamide (amide form) is required by all the cells of our body. Like thiamine and riboflavin it plays a vital role in the release of energy from carbohydrates, protein, fat and alcohol.

Nicotinic Acid

Nicotinic acid contains a pyridine nucleus. It is essential for the metabolism of carbohydrate, fat and protein. Nicotinic acid is essential for the normal functioning of the skin, intestinal tract and the nervous system. Foods rich in niacin or tryptophan are liver, kidney, meat, poultry, fish, legumes and groundnut. Milk is a poor source of niacin.

Chemistry and Characteristics

Niacin occurs in white needle-like bitter tasting crystals. It is moderately soluble in hot water, but only slightly soluble in cold water. It is stable to heat, alkalis, acids light and oxidation, and unstable to reduction. In fact, it is one of the most stable of the vitamins. Niacin occurs in two forms: Such as niacin and proniacin form, i.e. tryptophan. Human body can make 1 mg of vitamin from 50 to 60 mg of tryptophan. Thus, if a diet contains large amount of tryptophan, it will provide enough niacin, even though the diet might be low in its niacin content.

Absorption, Transport and Storage

Nicotinamide and nicotinic acid are readily absorbed from the small intestine by carrier-mediated facilitated diffusion. Body reserves seem to be just enough to meet day-to-day needs. NADH and NADPH, both are transported in the plasma and they are taken up by tissues through passive diffusion. Niacin, if taken in excess is excreted in the urine in different forms, N-methylnicotinamide and N-methylpyridine. During deficiency state, such as pellagra, the urine content of the metabolites either diminish or are absent altogether.

Functions

1. Nicotinamide is essential for tissue metabolism. The active forms of nicotinamide are nicotinamide adenine dinucleotide (NAD) and nicotinamide adenine dinucleotide phosphate (NADP).
2. NAD and NADP are involved as coenzymes in large number of reversible oxidation-reduction reactions.
3. Nicotinic acid enhances stomach secretion.
4. NAD is involved in catabolic reactions and NADP is involved in anabolic reaction in our body.

Food Sources

Dried yeast, liver, rice polishing, peanut, whole cereals, legumes, meat, fish are good sources. Tryptophan present in dietary protein is converted to niacin in humans. 60 mg of tryptophan yields 1 mg of niacin.

Recommended Daily Allowances

Niacin is expressed in milligrams or niacin equivalent (NE). Its requirement is affected by:
- Metabolic rate and physical excretion
- Daily tryptophan intake in the diet
- Age and growth periods
- Pregnancy and lactation
- Illness and tissue trauma
- Body size and physical activity.

The estimated requirement of niacin is 6.6 mg niacin equivalent per 1,000 kcal.

Effects of Deficiency

Nicotinic acid deficiency causes the disease 'pellagra' in human being. This disease is characterized by three D's such as dermatitis, diarrhea and dementia.

The dermatitis and diarrhea are two distributions and occurs in the hands, feet and neck.

Dermatitis

Pellagra comes from Italian 'pelle means skin' and 'agra means rough'. Marked changes occur in the skin especially in the skin exposed to sun and friction areas like elbows, surfaces of arms, knees. Lesions are symmetrically distributed in the affected parts. At first there is reddening, thickening and pigmentation of the skin. Later on there is exfoliation leading to ultimately parchment of skin—butterfly-like appearance.

Diarrhea

Diarrhea enhances the deficiency state. There are structural and absorptive defects in the small intestine. Tongue appears raw and mucous membrane of the tongue is inflamed.

Dementia

Dementia is irritability, depression, poor concentration and loss of memory. Delirium is a common mental disturbance.

▶ PYRIDOXINE

Pyridoxine (vitamin B_6) exists in three forms, i.e. pyridoxine, pyridoxal and pyridoxamine. It plays an important role in the metabolism of amino acids, fats and carbohydrates. Rice dietary sources are dried yeast rice polishing, wheat gram and liver. Pyridoxine is essential for maintaining the nerves in normal condition. Pyridoxal phosphate (PLP) acts as coenzyme in the metabolism of amino acids. Pyridoxine is unique among B complex vitamins in that it functions primarily in protein metabolism. Pyridoxine denotes related substances, such as pyridoxine, pyridoxal and pyridoxamine are three forms in which it is present in our body.

Chemistry and Characteristics

Vitamin B_6 consists of a group of related pyridines they are pyridoxine, pyridoxal and pyridoxamine. Vitamin B_6 is soluble in water and relatively stable to heat and to acids. It is destroyed in alkaline solutions and is also sensitive to light.

Absorption, Transport and Storage

Vitamin B_6 is absorbed from the small intestine, especially from the jejunum and ileum by passive diffusion of the dephosphorylated forms (pyridoxine, pyridoxal and pyridoxamine). Muscle is the major depot and contains 80%–90% of the total body vitamin and stores in the form of PLP bound to glycogen phosphorylase.

All three vitamins are easily interconverted metabolically by phosphorylation-dephosphorylation, oxidation-reduction and amination-deamination reactions. They are excreted in the urine, but 4-pyridoxic is the principal metabolite excreted. Body stores of B_6 are small, because it is a water-soluble vitamin.

Functions

In Protein Metabolism

Pyridoxal phosphate is the coenzyme involved in several reactions in amino acid metabolism, for example:

1. **Decarboxylation:** The removal of carboxyl group from amino acid is accomplished in the presence of the coenzyme, PLP. Every amino acid is decarboxylated by a specific enzyme.
2. **Transamination:** The amino group is removed from one amino acid and is transferred to a new carbon skeleton to form a new amino acid. The non-essential amino acid is formed by this reaction only.
3. **Deamination:** In this reaction amino group is removed from amino acid, such as serine and threonine.
4. **Transsulfuration:** In this reaction sulfur groups are removed from sulfur containing amino acids, such as cysteine in the presence of transulfurases.
5. **Conversion of tryptophan to niacin:** There are several steps that take place in this reaction and one of these reactions requires PLP.
6. **Synthesis of hemoglobin:** This vitamin is essential for the formation of delta-aminolevulinic acid in the synthesis of heme, the chief non-protein core of hemoglobin.
7. **Amino acid transport:** It effectively transports amino acids from the intestine into the circulation. From here it enters the cells.

In Carbohydrate and Fat Metabolism

Through decarboxylation and transamination reactions, PLP supplies metabolites for generating energy in the citric acid cycle. It is also required to convert EFA, linoleic acid to fatty acid and arachidonic acid.

Recommended Daily Allowances

The need for pyridoxine depends on the amount of protein in the diet. High-protein diet increases the requirement, since it is essential for amino acid metabolism. The requirement of vitamin B_6 has not been established for Indian population. However, a range has been suggested as daily intake, i.e. 0.6–2.5 mg for various age groups, which would meet the requirement.

Food Sources

Meat, pulses and wheat are rich sources. Other cereals are fair sources of this vitamin. Fruits and vegetables are poor sources. Cooking and processing of food causes loss of this vitamin.

Deficiency

The clinical symptoms of vitamin B_6 deficiency include:

1. **Anemia:** Certain types of anemia's, such as hypochromic (deficient content of RBCs) and microcytic (smaller than normal erythrocytes and less circulating hemoglobin) occur even when the serum iron levels are high or adequate.
2. **Central nervous system disorder (CNS):** Pyridoxine controls neurological conditions related to the brain activity. Due to the deficiency of the vitamin CNS disorders show abnormal electroencephalogram (EEG) readings. In infants, the deficiency of vitamin B_6 causes hyperirritability, which progresses to convulsive seizures. This condition arises in infants who are fed commercial milk formula, because most of the pyridoxine is destroyed by high-temperature autoclaving.
3. **Drugs:** Isoniazid used for tuberculosis is an antagonist to pyridoxine.
4. **Pregnancy:** Along with maternal metabolic demands, fetal growth increases the pyridoxine requirement.
5. **Oral contraceptives:** Women who are on estrogen-progestin oral contraceptives require more vitamin B_6. It causes

abnormal tryptophan metabolism, which contributes to the increased requirement.

▶ PANTOTHENIC ACID

Pantothenic acid (B_5) is one of the vitamins of the vitamins B_2 complex, which can prevent or cure a specific type of dermatitis (chick pellagra) in chicks fed on vitamin B_2 deficient. Pantothenic acid in the form of coenzyme A takes part in the metabolism of carbohydrates and fats. It is essential for the oxidation of pyruvic acid.

Burning feet syndrome was observed in prisoners of war during World War II in Japan and Burma. This syndrome was associated with neurological and mental disturbances. Gopalan (1946) found that burning feet syndrome observed in Indian subjects responded to treatment with calcium pantothenate (20–40 mg).

▶ FOLIC ACID

Folic acid was known under different names from 1933 by its curative effects in deficiency states in man and in different experimental animals. It is essential for the maturation of RBCs. It acts as a coenzyme in the synthesis of methionine, and of purine and pyrimidine rings. Foods such as liver, meat, dairy products, eggs, milk, fruits and cereals are as good dietary sources as leafy vegetables. Folic acid was first extracted from dark green leafy vegetables. It forms yellow crystals, and is a conjugated substance made up of three acids namely pteroic, para-aminobenzoic acid (PABA) and glutamic acid:

1. Simple folate deficiency results in the bone marrow producing immature cells (megaloblasts cells) and few matured RBCs. These results in reduced oxygen carrying capacity causing anemia termed megaloblastic anemia.
2. Folate deficiency during pregnancy causes neural tube disorders of the fetus.
3. Folate deficiency impairs the ability of the immune system to fight infection.

SECTION 1: Nutrition

Characteristics

Folain is a generic term for folic acid, pteroylglutamic acid and other compounds having the activity of folic acid. It consists of three-linked components such as a pteridine grouping, PABA and glutamic acid, an amino acid. Pure folic acid occurs as a bright-yellow crystalline compound, only slightly soluble in water. It is easily oxidized in an acid medium and is sensitive to light.

Absorption, Transport and Storage

Free folate is generally absorbed throughout the small intestine, but most of it is absorbed mainly in the jejunum by active transport. About 75% of dietary folate is in polyglutamyl forms. Before it can be absorbed, these are normally hydrolyzed to free folate by conjugase present in small intestine. Alkaline pH of the intestine and intake of sodium bicarbonate collectively decrease the absorption of folic acid. The liver is the principal depot for folate.

Ascorbic acid maintains an adequate level of the folate for metabolic purposes by preventing the oxidation of tetrahydrofolic acid (active form). Small amounts are lost in the feces and urine.

Functions

1. Folic acid coenzyme is essential in bringing about transferring single carbon units for many interconversions. A number of key compounds are formed by these reactions like:
    a. Purines, which are essential constituents of living cells.
    b. Thymine, which is essential compound, forms a key part of DNA.
    c. The formation of heme group of hemoglobin.
2. The conversion of phenylalanine into tyrosine.

Food Sources

Green leafy vegetables, liver, kidneys, gingelly seeds, cluster beans are rich sources of folic acid.

Deficiency

Overcooking destroys much of folic acid and thus contributes of folate deficiency in man. Nutritional megaloblastic anemia in adults, the classical studies of Wills (1931) in India showed that the megaloblastic anemia prevalent in pregnant women of the low-income groups substituting on poor vegetarian diets. Megaloblastic anemia has been reported to occur among malnourished children in the developing countries.

▶ CYANOCOBALAMIN

Cyanocobalamin (vitamin B_{12}) is a form of cobalamin which was found effective in curing pernicious anemia when administered intramuscularly in small quantities (5–10 mg) for the absorption of vitamin B_{12} from the intestines, a factor called 'intrinsic factor' (IF) secreted by the stomach is essential vitamin B_{12} is stored in fair amount in the liver. Until 1926, pernicious anemia was a fatal disease of unknown origin with an unknown cure. In 1926, Minot and Murphy found that pernicious anemia could be cured by feeding a patient at least 0.3 kg of raw liver per day. Also in 1926 Castle noted that patients with pernicious anemia had a low level of gastric secretion. He suggested that the antipernicious anemia factor had two components. An 'extrinsic factor' found in food and an 'intrinsic factor' within normal gastric secretions. The extrinsic factor is now known as vitamin B_{12} or cobalamin.

Characteristics

Vitamin B_{12} is the only cobalt containing substance essential for health. It occurs as dark red needle-like crystals, which are slightly soluble in water. This vitamin is absorbed from the ileum only. Its absorption depends on the presence of a mucoprotein enzyme produced by the gastric mucosa. The enzyme is called intrinsic factor.

Absorption, Transport and Storage

Vitamin B_{12} is absorbed in the ileum in pH of 6.8. However, it must be released from its protein complex by pepsin and by gastric HCl in the stomach before it can be absorbed and then it must be bound to a specific glycoprotein IF secreted by gastric mucosal cells. IF is then released and the vitamin is attached to another cobalamin-binding protein carrier and transported to the cells. In well-nourished individuals, vitamin B_{12} is stored in great amounts in the liver, kidneys, heart, muscles, pancreas, testes, brain, blood, spleen and bone marrow, but mainly in the liver. The liver accumulates a substantial amount enough for 5–7 years. On an average a normal individual excretes about 30 pg of vitamin B_{12} each day in the urine.

Functions

Vitamin B_{12} functions as coenzyme in two different forms adenosylcobalamin and methylcobalamin. Adenosylcobalamin is essential for the conversion of homocysteine into methionine and for the conversion of L-methylmalonyl-CoA to succinyl-CoA. Thus, the deficiency of cobalamin causes two genetic disorders in children, i.e. homocystinuria and methylmalonic aciduria. These forms of vitamin play very important roles in metabolism of all cells. Cobalamin and folic acid are metabolically inter-related and the deficiency of either causes megaloblastic anemia. Cobalamin provides an activated form of folate for hematopoiesis.

Recommended Dietary Allowances

Vitamin B_{12} is measured in micrograms. Though the requirement is considerably small, but the suggested intake is sufficient for normal hematopoiesis and good health.

Food Source

Vitamin B_{12} is synthesized by the intestinal bacteria in the colon, but it is not absorbed. The richest sources of dietary cobalamin include liver, kidney, lean meat, milk, egg and cheese. Plant foods contain vitamin through contamination or bacterial synthesis. Pure vegetarians who do not include even milk in their diet are at a greater risk of developing vitamin B_{12} deficiency.

Deficiency

Vitamin B_{12} promotes the maturation of RBCs. It acts on the narrow elements, and is involved in the formation of WBCs and blood platelets. It cures the neurological symptoms of pernicious anemia. It acts as a coenzyme in the synthesis of methionine. Vitamin B_{12} deficiency causes the disease 'pernicious anemia':

1. Pernicious anemia is the major problem arising from an inadequate amount of vitamin B_{12}.
2. Pernicious anemia is a condition characterized by very large, immature RBCs with normal amounts of hemoglobin.

▶ VITAMIN C

The chemical name for vitamin C is ascorbic acid. It was discovered in 1747 by the British physician Lind and demonstrated that citrus fruit juices prevented and cured scurvy.

Chemistry and Characteristics

Vitamin C is a white crystalline compound of relatively simple structure and closely related to monosaccharide sugars. It can be prepared synthetically at low cost from glucose. Of all the vitamins, vitamin C is the most easily destroyed. It is highly soluble in water, heat, light, alkalis, oxidative, enzymes and trace.

Absorption, Transport and Storage

Some species, which do not biosynthesize this vitamin, need it from dietary sources. Ascorbic acid is easily absorbed from the small intestine by active transport and passive diffusion. Vitamin C is concentrated in the adrenal gland and the retina, but appreciable amounts are present in the spleen, intestine, bone marrow, pancreas, thymus, liver, pituitary and kidney also. Vitamin C is better absorbed in the oxidized form (dehydroascorbic acid) than in the reduced form (ascorbate or ascorbic acid). It is transported in the plasma in the reduced state. Vitamin C is distributed throughout body tissues and if there is any excess, it is slowly excreted in the urine. The plasma concentration of vitamin C is usually lower in cigarette smokers and in women on oral contraceptive pills. The absorption of vitamin C is hampered by the lack of hypochloric acid or by bleeding from the gastrointestinal tract.

Normally, kidneys control the excretion of vitamin C. If the tissues have reached the saturation (greater than 0.6 mg/dL), vitamin C taken in excess will be excreted and if tissue stores are depleted, very small amount of vitamin C is excreted. The urinary excretion of ascorbic acid increases during periods of emotional, psychological or physiological stress.

Functions

1. Ascorbic acid is essential for formation of cement substances and collagen, which is found in blood vessels, teeth and bones.
2. It helps in the biosynthesis of non-essential amino acids, e.g. hydroxyproline, tyrosine.
3. It is required for absorption of iron as it reduces ferric to ferrous form, which is easily absorbed.
4. Vitamin C is essential for the formation of collagen a major structural protein of connective tissues.
5. It is required for normal wound healing, because it helps in the formation of connective tissue.
6. Vitamin C is required for carnitine synthesis, which aids in the transport of fatty acids in the cell.
7. Vitamin C is essential for the synthesis of norepinephrine a neurotransmitter.

8. It activates hormones, e.g. growth hormone, gastrin releasing peptide, calcitonin, gastrin oxytocin.
9. Drug detoxifying metabolic systems in the body requires vitamin C for its optimal activity.
10. Vitamin C is an excellent antioxidant. It combines with free radicals oxidizing them to harmless substances that can be excreted.

Food Sources

Vitamin C is widely distributed in plant foods, especially in fresh fruits and vegetables. But of all the vitamins, it is most easily destroyed by the oxidation. Since, it is a powerful reducing agent, it is rapid, oxidized in the air. Due to this reason, dry and stale vegetables lose considerable amount of vitamin C. Similarly, if vegetables are cut and left exposed to air, most of the vitamin is destroyed. Therefore, it is advisable that fruits and vegetables should be eaten fresh, whenever possible. Meat, fish, poultry, milk and milk products, and eggs contain very little amounts. Dry grains are devoid of vitamin C. Germination of dry pulses considerably increases the vitamin C content. Sprouted green gram contains three times more vitamin C as compared to sprouted Bengal gram.

Excellent Sources

Amla, guava, citrus fruits, such as oranges, lemon, mausami, kinnu, fresh strawberries, cantaloupe and pineapple. It is advisable to eat orange sections with thin white peel because it has comparatively more vitamin C than the same amount of strained orange juice.

Excellent-to-good Sources

Broccoli, Brussels sprouts, capsicum, cabbage and turnips.

Small Amounts

Peaches, pears, apple, bananas.

Deficiency

Prolonged deficiency of vitamin C results in scurvy. Symptoms become evident only after 45–80 days of vitamin deprivation. It is seen in individuals who are either unable to synthesize the vitamin or have deficient intake for a prolonged period of time.

Symptoms

Since the vascular tissue is weakened in the absence of vitamin C, the capillary walls lose their firmness and rupture easily. This result in diffused bleeding, easy bruising, pinpoint bleeding, bone and joint hemorrhages, easy bone fracture. Other characteristic symptoms of adult scurvy include swollen, bleeding gums and eventually loss of teeth, lethargy, fatigue, anemia, muscular atrophy, skin lesions and some psychological changes. The symptoms of infantile scurvy include pain, tenderness and swelling of the thighs and legs. The baby is not interested to move and stay in one position with legs flexed. Symptoms frequently seen are pallor, irritability, loss of weight, fever, diarrhea, vomiting and the baby cries when handled. Swollen, tender and hemorrhagic gums are observed when the teeth have started erupting. Bone matrix does not develop properly due to faulty bone calcification. The chances of bone displacement are greater.

There is enlargement of ends of long bones and ribs as in rickets. Adult scurvy responds to vitamin C supplementation of 100–200 mg for a few days.

Toxicity

High doses of vitamin C in humans results in gastrointestinal disturbances and diarrhea. The breakdown of vitamin C yields oxalates, which may increase the risk of causing oxalate stones in the kidney.

▶ VITAMIN DEFICIENCIES

Retinol (Vitamin A) Deficiency

The deficiency of vitamin A is usually manifest clinically as:
1. Night blindness.
2. Xerophthalmia.
3. Bitot's spots and keratomalacia.

The commonest cause of blindness among children is vitamin A deficiency. The age group most affected is 1–4 years. This condition is closely associated with protein calorie malnutrition.

Xerophthalmia

Xerophthalmia is a disease of the eye in which the cornea and conjunctive become dry. The conjunctive becomes rough and wrinkled. Swelling and redness of the lids, pain and aversion to light are also noticed. Grayish, silvery or chalky, white patches (Bitot's spots) appear on the conjunctive on either side of the cornea. The child favors to keep his/her eyes away from light or closed. If not treated in time the cornea becomes soft and ulcerated (keratomalacia) resulting in total blindness.

Beriberi (Thiamine Deficiency)

Beriberi usually occurs among communities that consume overmilled rice. Two types of beriberi are described, based on age such as infantile and adult beriberi. Infantile beriberi usually occurs during the 1st year of life. Convulsive disorders, respiratory difficulties and gastrointestinal troubles like constipation and vomiting are seen among children. Adult beriberi occurs among youngsters who experience physiological stress like pregnancy, lactation, etc. It may be in dry or wet form according to the absence or presence of edema.

Riboflavin Deficiency

Important clinical manifestations of riboflavin deficiency are:
1. Angular stomatitis.
2. Cheilosis.
3. Scrotal dermatitis.
4. Corneal vascularization.

In angular stomatitis, the angles of the mouth are fissured and ulcerated. In cheilosis, the lips get fissured vertically.

Pellagra (Niacin Deficiency)

Pellagra is caused due to deficiency of niacin (B complex vitamin). The natural characteristics of pellagra are:
1. Gastrointestinal disturbances.
2. Stomatitis.
3. Dermatitis.
4. Neurological changes.

Gastrointestinal disturbances include indigestion, weight loss and diarrhea. Stomatitis is swelling and reddening of the tongue. Neurological changes include mental apathy, depression, etc.

Scurvy (Vitamin C Deficiency)

Scurvy is associated with vitamin C (ascorbic acid) deficiency. The condition is not generally seen among breastfed children because they get enough supply of vitamin C from mother's milk. Cow's or buffalo's milk does not contain vitamin C after boiling. Important symptoms are irritability, tenderness of bones and spongy and bleeding gums. The skin becomes dry and rough and scaly raised areas develop around the hair follicles in the skin. Hemorrhages into the cavities of joints causing heat, painful swelling and immobility may also occur.

CHAPTER 2: Review of Macro- and Micro-nutrition

Rickets (Vitamin D Deficiency)

The disease is caused due to deficiency of vitamin D, and is directly related to impaired metabolism of calcium and phosphorus. The main defect is failure of calcification of the growing portions of the bones. There is enlargement of the long bones at the ends particularly in the wrist and ankles. The bone being soft bends under pressure on standing or walking. The knees touch each other. The forest legs and assumes a bow shape. Adult form of rickets is known as osteomalacia.

Vitamin K Deficiency

Vitamin K is easily available in nature particularly from various green leaves. It is also synthesized by intestinal bacteria. Deficiency of vitamin K causes hemorrhagic disease. Vitamin K is necessary for the synthesis of prothrombin by the liver. This being an important blood clotting mechanism, is not produced hemorrhaging may occur.

▶ MINERAL ELEMENTS

There are a number of minerals or inorganic elements that play an important role in nutrition. Mineral elements are present in organic compounds, such as hemoglobin, phospholipids, thyroxin as inorganic compounds in sodium chloride and calcium phosphate and as free ions. They enter the structure of every cell of the body. Hard skeletal structures contain the greater proportions of some elements, such as calcium, phosphorus and magnesium, while soft tissues contain relatively higher proportions of potassium.

Mineral elements enter into numerous regulatory activities of the body. The contraction of muscles, the normal response of nerves to stimulation, the control of water balance, the maintenance of acid-base equilibrium and the water balance of the foodstuffs are few functions. Sodium, potassium, calcium, phosphorus and chloride are the essential constituents of body fluids. Calcium, magnesium, phosphorus and others are bone constituents. Iron, copper and cobalt function in an intendated manner together with protein, vitamin B_{12} and other nutrients for the synthesis of hemoglobin and RBCs.

Minerals may be defined as those elements, which remain largely as ash when plant and animal tissues are burnt. The human body contains more than 19 minerals, all of which must be derived from foods. A total of 4% of the body weight is made up of minerals. Some of the important minerals found in our body include calcium, phosphorus, iron, iodine, sodium, potassium, zinc and chloride. All these minerals are derived from the food we eat. Of these calcium, phosphorus, sodium, potassium, chloride and magnesium are the minerals required in larger amounts by the body. Calcium and phosphorus account for 3–4 of the minerals present in the body and five other elements account for most of the rest. Many of these elements are present in such minute amounts that they are referred to as a trace elements or micronutrients.

Minerals are important for the body in various ways. They are required to form such organic compounds like phosphoproteins, hemoglobin and thyroxin. Hard skeletal structures are formed with the help of elements like calcium, phosphorus and magnesium, whereas soft tissues contain a relatively high proportion of potassium. Mineral elements are also required in the constitution of enzymes; for maintaining osmotic pressure, and water balance between intracellular and extracellular compartments; for proper functioning of the nervous system; for muscular contraction and so on.

▶ CALCIUM

Calcium (Ca) is an essential element required for several life processes. The requirements of Ca and phosphorus (P) are considered together as their function and requirement are closely linked. Over 99% of the Ca and P present in the bones and the remaining 1% in the body fluids.

The Ca and P are present in the ratio of 2:1 in our body. In the skeletal system Ca and P is present in the form of hydroxyapatite crystals.

Hydroxyapatite is a compound made up of Ca and P that is deposited into the bone matrix to give it strength and rigidity.

Absorption and Excretion

Absorption

The absorption of minerals is not as efficient as of vitamins and the macronutrients. It is not necessary that all the minerals taken as a part of our food are available to the body. The extent to which the body utilizes a particular nutrient is called bioavailability of a nutrient. This depends on many factors. Ca absorption takes place in all parts of the small intestine, but mainly in the duodenum because of its acidic pH (< 7) as compared to the other parts of the intestine—normally, only 10%–30% of dietary Ca is absorbed by the adults.

Calcium is absorbed by two mechanisms:

1. Active transport, which mainly works when the luminal concentration of calcium ion is low.
2. Passive transfer or paracellular movement, which mainly works when the luminal concentration of calcium ion is high.

The active transport mainly takes place in the duodenum, but jejunum has a limited capacity. Also it is controlled by the action of 1, 25-dihydroxyvitamin D or vitamin D. This hormone enhances the uptake of Ca at the brush borders of the intestinal mucosal cell. This mechanism is not well-understood. The passive transfer mechanism occurs throughout the small intestine. When a single meal supplies large amount of Ca much of it is absorbed through passive transfer. The active transport mechanism plays an important role when Ca intakes are low due to which the body requirements are not being met. Ca is absorbed in ionic form only. The unabsorbed Ca is excreted in the feces as Ca oxalates and Ca soaps.

Excretion

If the intake of dietary Ca exceeds the requirements, it remains unabsorbed in the intestine and is secreted in the feces. Normally, approximately 50% of the ingested Ca is excreted in the urine daily. Urinary Ca excretion continues to change throughout the life cycle, but during the growth periods it is very low. Ca excretion increases markedly during menopause, but in postmenopausal stage, if the woman is on estrogen therapy, less Ca is excreted. After the age of 65 years, Ca excretion decreases, may be because of diminished intestinal absorption of Ca. A diet high in sodium decreases renal resorption of Ca and increased urinary Ca losses. Under normal conditions the losses of Ca from the skin are very small. Approximately 15 mg of Ca is lost in sweat each day. During increased physical activity, when sweating increases, Ca losses also increase even if the ingested Ca is low.

Factors Increasing Calcium Absorption

1. **Body needs:** During the growth periods, such as infancy, childhood, during pregnancy and lactation more Ca is absorbed. In elderly persons especially in postmenopausal women the calcium absorption is reduced.
2. **Concentration:** The higher concentration of Ca in the intestine the greater the absorption.
3. **Dietary protein:** When the diet is high in protein, higher percentage of Ca is adsorbed, but this higher amount of Ca absorbed results in higher renal excretion after which a negative Ca balance follows. This means that high-protein diets increase calcium requirements to maintain Ca balance.
4. **Lactose:** It is enhances Ca absorption through the action of lactobacilli, which produces lactic acid and this in turn reduces the pH.
5. **Acidity:** The acid medium (lower pH) enhances the absorption of Ca. The HCl secreted in the stomach during a meal, increases Ca absorption, therefore it is advised to take Ca supplements with a meal especially in older adults.

CHAPTER 2: Review of Macro- and Micro-nutrition

6. **Body mechanisms:** The two most important mechanisms that control the Ca absorption involve vitamin D and the parathyroid hormone (PTH). The low-blood calcium concentration triggers the secretion of PTH. PTH then stimulates the kidneys to synthesize calcitriol, which is the active form of vitamin D. Due to this, metabolite increases the absorption from the intestine and along with PTH it also mobilizes calcium from the bones.

Functions of Calcium

Formation and Maintenance of Bone and Teeth

An adult human body has approximately 1,200 g of Ca, out of which 99% is maintained in the skeletal tissue and used for developing bones out of cartilage. They form salts, which provide structural rigidity to bones and teeth as hydroxyapatite. Small amounts of magnesium, sodium, carbonate, citrate, chloride and fluoride are also present in bone salts. The bones not only provide the rigid structure and framework to the body but are also a storehouse for Ca, which is mobilized to maintain serum levels constant at all times. The remaining 1% of Ca is distributed throughout the extracellular and intracellular fluids of the body.

Growth

Calcium is essential for the growth of children.

Enzyme Activation

Calcium activates many enzymes, such as pancreatic lipase, adenosine triphosphatase (ATPase) and some protein splitting enzymes.

Nerve Impulse Transmission

Nerve impulse transmission is needed for the synthesis of acetylcholine, which is necessary for transmission of nerve impulse.

Muscle Contraction and Relaxation

Each muscle fiber contains hundreds of myofibrils, which are small contractile units. These myofibrils are composed of muscle protein filaments myosin and actin. Each myofibril has T-tubules and sarcoplasmic reticulum along its sides. Ca is firmly bound to these reticulums. Whenever the body receives a signal, Ca is suddenly released, ionized and mobilized. This free Ca ion acts as an activator for the chemical reaction between actin and myosin filament, and a large amount of energy in the form of ATP is released and brings about muscle contraction. The Ca ions again attach themselves back to sarcoplasmic reticulum and cause relaxation. Minerals like magnesium and potassium also play a role in this process. Ca also regulates the heartbeat and is necessary for the functioning of heart muscle.

Cell Membrane Permeability

Calcium increases the cell membrane permeability, therefore helps in the process of absorption. Ca ions control the passage of fluids through cell membranes.

Absorption

Calcium aids in the absorption of vitamin B_{12} from the ileum.

Blood Clotting

Calcium ions catalyze several steps in the process of blood clotting. The inactive form of blood coagulation protein (prothrombin) is catalyzed by Ca^+ and converted to an active form (thrombin). Thrombin then catalyzes the next protein (fibrinogen) to form fibrin (the clot).

Recommended Dietary Allowances

The dietary requirement of Ca has been studied extensively universally, but there is no general agreement among the experts. Some studies on Western population have indicated much higher requirements of Ca (1 g) whose diet consists of high levels of milk and milk products. On the other hand, people residing in developing countries take about 500 mg without any symptoms of deficiency. The FAQ/WHO committee has recommended 400–500 mg Ca as 'practical allowance' adults.

Deficiency

Calcium related health problems occur due to inadequate intake, improper absorption or utilization of Ca.

Osteoporosis

Osteoporosis is a condition found primarily among middle aged and elderly woman, where the bone mass of the skeleton is diminished.

It is a condition of multiple origins. It results due to the following reasons:
- Prolonged dietary inadequacy
- Poor absorption and utilization of Ca
- Immobility
- Decreased levels of estrogen in postmenopausal women
- Hyperparathyroidism
- Vitamin D deficiency.

Osteomalacia

Osteomalacia is a condition in which the quality, but not the quantity of bone is reduced. This condition is discussed in detail under deficiency of vitamin D.

Tetany

Tetany occurs when Ca in the blood drops below the critical level. There is a change in the stimulation of nerve cells resulting in increased excitability of the nerve and uncontrolled contraction of the muscle tissue. Hence, Ca and P ratio in the diet should be maintained at 1:1 for proper utilization of Ca in the body.

Importance of Calcium

1. Body contains Ca in greater amount than other minerals.
2. About 2% of the body weight of an adult is due to Ca, out of which about 99% is contained in bones and teeth.
3. Calcium is the most important factor in building skeleton and teeth is more important during growing years.
4. Normal behavior of heart, nervous system and blood clotting process, etc. depend on the presence of calcium.
5. Human body at different levels of intake has suggested the desirability of a daily intake of about 0.4–0.6 g of Ca by an adult, the case of growing children and pregnant and lactating mothers and the requirement is 1.0 g/day.
6. Milk and milk products are the richest sources of calcium. Green leafy vegetables such as spinach, amaranth are rich in Ca, but at the same time they are oxalate-rich foods.

▶ PHOSPHORUS

1. Phosphorus (P) takes a second place with regard to the total amount of minerals present in the body and constitutes about one fourth of all body minerals.
2. About 80% of the P is found in bones combined with Ca and the rest is found in bones combined with Ca, and the rest is found in soft tissues and body fluids.
3. Phosphorus plays an important role in the formation of teeth and bones, maintenance of acid-base balance of the blood and supplying energy to the muscles for contraction.
4. Phosphorus is found in good amount in the foods, which are rich in protein and Ca. Thus milk, cheese, egg yolk, meat and fish are good source of P.
5. Deficiency of Ca and P causes rickets in children is generally contributed to lack of vitamin D. Osteomalacia, the

adult rickets may also be due to a Ca deficiency, but usually, the situation is complicated by deficiency P and vitamin D as well as other factors.

Functions

Phosphorus is one mineral, which performs widely differing functions. These are:
1. It combines with calcium to form insoluble compound, Ca and P, which gives strength and rigidity to bones.
2. The P containing lipoproteins facilitate the transport of fats in the circulation.
3. Phosphorus is a constituent of nucleoproteins, the basic genetic material.
4. Phospholipids are constituents of cell membranes, thus regulating the transport of solutes into and out of the cell.
5. Phosphorylation is the key reaction in many metabolic processes.
6. Phosphorus captures and store vital energy in the cells of many tissues by forming a high-energy compound. Muscle tissue is a prominent example where P helps in energy store and thus fuel muscle contraction.
7. Inorganic P in the body fluids constitutes an important buffer system in the regulation of body neutrality.

Food Sources

Phosphorus is widely distributed in foods; the milk and meat groups being important contributors. Whole grain cereals and flours contain much more P that refined cereals and flours. Vegetables and fruits contain only small amount of P.

Deficiency

A deficiency of P is generally not seen in human beings, because diets having cereals as major food are seldom inadequate in phosphorus.

▶ MICROMINERALS

Microminerals are also known as trace elements. The microminerals are iron (Fe), iodine (I), zinc (Zn), copper (Cu), fluoride (F), selenium (Se), chromium (Cr), manganese (Mn), cobalt (Co) and molybdenum (Mo). However, only the deficiency of few of these elements is observed in humans. Iron and iodine deficiencies are widespread, while deficiency of Cu, Zn, Cr and Se has been reported in recent years.

Iron

The total body iron is 4 g in adults. Fe exists in a complex form in our body. It is present as:

1. Iron porphyrin compounds: Hemoglobin in RBC, myoglobin in muscle.
2. Enzymes: Peroxidases, succinase dehydrogenase and cytochrome oxidase.
3. Transport and storage forms: Transferrin and ferritin:
   a. Amount of Fe in the adult body is about 3–5 g of which 70% is in circulating hemoglobin, 4% in the myoglobin of the muscles and 25% in the stores held in liver, bone marrow, spleen and kidneys.
   b. Iron is essential for oxidation of the body. Hemoglobin combines with oxygen in the lungs to form oxyhemoglobin and is carried to the tissues by blood circulation.
   c. Iron-containing oxygen in the muscles makes the oxidation of carbohydrate, fat and protein possible within the intact cell.
   d. Iron is stored chiefly in the liver, spleen and bone marrow. The amount is variable, ranging from 1 to 2 g.
   e. Recommended allowances based on the availability and utilization of Fe, it is recommended that 20–30 mg of Fe per day is sufficient for an adult. The requirements increase in special conditions-like pregnancy.
   f. Nutritional anemias are due to the deficiency of Fe and folic acid.

CHAPTER 2: Review of Macro- and Micro-nutrition

g. Liver is an excellent source of Fe. Other meat products and egg yolk also have generous amount of this mineral.

Functions

The chief functions of Fe in the body are:

1. Iron forms a part of the protein: Hemoglobin, which carries oxygen to different parts of the body.
2. It forms a part of the myoglobin in muscles, which makes oxygen available for muscle contraction.
3. Iron is necessary for the utilization of energy as part of the cells metabolic machinery.
4. As part of enzymes Fe catalyzes many important reactions in the body. For example:
    a. Conversion of beta carotene to active form of vitamin A.
    b. Synthesis of carnitine, purines, collagen and neurotransmitters.
    c. Detoxification of drugs in the liver.
5. Iron is a major constituent of a red-colored compound called hemoglobin (Hb) present in the blood. Fe is present in the hemoglobin. Hemoglobin is necessary for transport of oxygen to various parts of the body. Hb carries oxygen from the lungs to the tissues, and in turn helps in carrying carbon dioxide from the tissue to the lungs. From the lungs carbon dioxide is then exhaled out.

Food Sources

The Fe present in food can be as heme and non-heme iron depending upon the source from which it is obtained. Heme iron is obtained from animal tissues; non-heme iron is obtained from plant foods.

Sources of non-heme iron are ragi, green leafy vegetables, dried fruits and jaggery. Liver, fish, poultry, meat, eggs, dates are good sources of heme iron.

Heme iron is absorbed and utilized better than the non-heme iron. Fe absorption from Indian diets is only 3% as it is mainly cereal-based diet.

Lean meats, deep green leafy vegetables and whole-grain cereals are good sources. Egg yolk and organ meats are also among good sources. Liver is an excellent source of Fe. Other vegetable and fruits are fair source. Milk, cheese and ice cream are poor sources. Jaggery contains a good amount of Fe.

Deficiency

Dietary Fe deficiency leads to nutritional anemia. Nutritional anemia is defined as the condition that results from the inability of the erythropoietic tissue to maintain a normal hemoglobin concentration.

Anemia occurs when the hemoglobin level falls below 12 g /dL in adult man and woman. During pregnancy hemoglobin level below 11 g/dL is termed as anemia.

Nutritional anemia is the common form of anemia affecting women in reproductive years, infants and children, which are mainly due to poor intake and absorption.

Iron deficiency (anemia) is widespread in our country; the prevalence varying from 45% in men and 70% in women and children. The major cause of anemia in India is because of Fe and folic acid deficiency.

Nutritional anemia is manifested as:
1. Reduced hemoglobin level (less than 12 g/dL).
2. Defects in the structure and function of the epithelial tissues.
3. Paleness of skin and the inside of the lower eyelid is pale pink.
4. Finger nails becoming thin and flat, and eventually (spoon-shaped nails) koilonychia develops.
5. Progressive untreated anemia results in cardiovascular and respiratory changes leading to cardiac failure. The general symptoms include lassitude, fatigue, breathlessness on exertion, palpitations, dizziness, sleeplessness, dimness of vision and increased susceptibility to infection.
6. Iron is also present in the muscle in the form of myoglobin. Myoglobin has the capacity to store oxygen. This oxygen is used for muscle contraction and for other immediate needs of the muscle cells.

7. Iron facilitates the complete oxidation of carbohydrates, fats and proteins within the cell.
8. Iron plays an important role in maintenance of specific brain.
9. Iron forms a vital component of certain enzymes and substances that aid in metabolism.
10. Iron has protective function. It helps in preventing the infections.

Zinc

Zinc (Zn) is primarily intracellular substance. Its total quantity in the body is 2.3 g. Largest stores of Zn are present in the bones. Zn forms a constituent of the blood. Zn is an important element performing a range of function in the body as it is a cofactor for a number of enzymes.

Functions

1. Zinc is a constituent of enzymes, such as carbonic anhydrase, alkaline phosphatase and lactic dehydrogenase.
2. It is a constituent of the hormone insulin.
3. It plays a major role in the synthesis of DNA and proteins.

Sources

Meat, unmilled cereals and legumes are good sources. Fruits and vegetables are poor sources.

Requirements

The daily requirement of Zn in adults is 15.5 mg/day as recommended by the ICMR expert group. Apart from iron, iodine, zinc, copper, selenium and fluoride are essential trace elements. Copper is an essential element in iron absorption.

Selenium is an essential element along with vitamin E for maintaining integrity of the liver cells. Fluoride is required in minimum amounts to prevent dental caries. Excessive consumption leads to mottling of teeth.

SECTION 1: Nutrition

Iodine

About one third of iodine present in an adult body variously estimated from 25 to 50 mg is found in the thyroid gland. The concentration in thyroid tissue is 2,500 times as great as is any other tissue, all of which contain traces:

1. Iodine is considered to be an important dietary nutrient because normal functioning of thyroid gland depends upon adequate supply of it in the body. It is an essential component of thyroxine and other iodine containing compounds of thyroid glands.
2. Primary function of thyroxine is to influence the rate of oxidation in the cells of the body. Thyroxine also helps in normal growth and development in the Young's all the species.
3. Sources of iodine vary widely under different soil and fertilizer conditions. Marine or deep-sea fish and shellfish are high in iodine content. The leaves and flowers of plants have higher concentration of iodine than roots.
4. The recommended daily allowances of iodine have been reported to be about 100–150 mg.
5. Prolonged deficiency of iodine not only develops goiter but also causes sterility in many cases. Development of goiter enlargement of thyroid gland, during pregnancy indicates special requirement of iodine.

Functions

The only known function of iodine is as a constituent of thyroglobulin, a protein complex of several iodine-containing compounds. The thyroid hormone regulates the rate of oxidation within the cells and in doing so, regulates the physical and mental growth; the functioning of nervous and muscle tissues, circulating activity and the metabolism of all nutrients.

CHAPTER 2: Review of Macro- and Micro-nutrition

Food Sources

Iodine is supplied by food and water; the variations are wide depending upon the iodine content of the soils from which they come. People living in coastal areas and eating locally grown foods ingests enough iodine for their use. In hilly areas where there is a deficiency of iodine in food and drinking water, iodization of the salt is the only technique available to make good this deficiency in order to prevent goiter.

Recommended Daily Allowances

The daily requirement of iodine is 0.14 mg for an adult man and 0.10 mg for an adult woman. Growing children, pregnant and lactating women may need more.

The ICMR recommended dietary allowance for iodine is 150 µg/day.

Iodine is an essential constituent of the thyroid hormone produced by the thyroid glands. It occurs as free iodide ions or as protein bound iodine in our body. About 15–23 mg of iodine is present in the adult human body. The body store of iodine is predominantly present in thyroid gland and also in salivary gland, mammary glands, gastric glands and in kidneys to a certain extent.

Deficiency

Iodine deficiency in the diet causes enlargement of the thyroid gland called 'goiter'. Goiter occurs in people staying in hilly regions where the iodine content of water and soil is comparatively less.

In India, goiter is common in hilly districts of Himalaya. Goiter can be treated by administration of iodine. If treatment is given in early stages goiter can be corrected.

Severe iodine deficiency in children leads to hypothyroidism resulting in retarded physical and mental growth. This condition is known as cretinism.

SECTION 1: Nutrition

Goitrogens are substances present in foods, which cause goiter. These substances react with iodine present in the food making it unavailable for absorption. Foods like cabbage, cauliflower, radish contain goitrogens.

Fluoride

Fluoride (F) occurs normally in the body primarily as a Ca salt in the bones and teeth. It is not essential for life, but small amounts of fluoride bring about striking reductions in tooth decay:

1. Fluoride is found primarily in the bones and teeth. Small amount F brings about striking reduction in teeth decay, because this mineral makes tooth enamel more resistant to the action of acid.
2. Dental caries is reduced more resistant to the action of acid, water at the rate of 1 part per million (ppm).
3. Source of F: Food as well as water by fluoridation of the water at the rate of 1 ppm.
4. The recommended level of F in drinking water in this country is accepted as 0.5–0.8 mg/L.
5. Fluoride is often called double-edged sword. Prolonged ingestion of F through drinking water in excess of the daily requirement is associated with dental and skeletal fluorosis and inadequate intake with dental caries.

Functions

A proper intake of F is essential to prevent dental caries. It is required for normal mineralization of bones.

Food Sources

The main source is drinking water. It occurs in traces in many foods and in good amounts in shellfish, cheese, etc.

CHAPTER 2: Review of Macro- and Micro-nutrition

Deficiency and Excess of Fluoride

On one hand F is required for deposition of F on teeth, and discourages the solubility of minerals and growth of acid forming bacteria. If there is a deficiency of F during the growing period, it will result in dental caries and tooth decay. On the other hand, when taken in excess it could damage teeth and bones. The enamel on the teeth loses its luster, becomes patchy, chalky white and pits appear on its surface. This condition is known as dental fluorosis.

Sodium

An adult body contains approximately 120 g of sodium (Na) of which about 50% of the body's Na is present in the extracellular fluid, 40% in bones and 10% or less in intracellular fluid (intracellular fluid refers to fluid inside the cell).

Functions

1. Sodium is required for maintenance of normal osmotic pressure and water balance.
2. It is also required for maintaining the permeability of cell membrane.
3. Sodium 'pump' helps to maintain the electrolyte difference between intracellular and extracellular fluid compartments.

Food Sources

Common salt or sodium chloride is the chief source of sodium in the diet. One teaspoon of salt provides almost 2,000 mg sodium. It is universally used to flavor the food we eat and is also used for preserving food for long periods. Numerous sodium compounds are used in food processing and preparation; baking soda, baking powder, sodium alginate, sodium propionate, sodium citrate.

Sodium is a naturally occurring constituent of animals food including milk, egg, meat poultry and fish and in certain vegetables as spinach, celery, beet greens and fenugreek. Most vegetables, fruit, cereals, legumes are naturally low in sodium.

Recommended Daily Allowances

A 5–10 g of salt (sodium chloride) is sufficient for an average adult. An individual doing hard labor may need more.

Sodium Imbalance

Osmotic pressure and the pH are seriously affected when there is a disturbance in the concentrations of sodium in the extracellular fluid of the body tissues. When there is retention of sodium in the tissue, edema occurs. In cardiac and renal failure sodium excretion gets reduced. Excess sodium losses occur during the hot weather causing muscular weakness, cramps, fatigue, vomiting and loss of appetite. In this case, a small amount of salt may be added to liquid intake.

Potassium

An adult body contains about 250 g of potassium (K) of which about 97% of the potassium in the body is in intracellular fluid (intracellular fluid refers to fluid inside the cells), while the remainder being in the extracellular fluid compartments (extracellular fluid refers to fluid outside the cells):

1. The adult human body contains about 250 g of potassium, which is present almost in the cells of different tissues, muscle, etc.
2. The functions of potassium is regulation of pH of cell contents, regulation of the osmotic pressure of cell contents and potassium ion increases the relaxation of heart muscle, which is antagonized by calcium ion.
3. Potassium deficiency causes weakness and muscular paralysis. In animals, hypertrophy of the heart has been observed.
4. In consumption of excessive amounts of potassium causes muscular weakness and apathy; symptoms similar to those of potassium deficiency.

Functions

1. Within the cell it maintains the osmotic pressure and fluids balance.
2. It is required for the synthesis of proteins.
3. It is required for enzymatic reactions taking place within the cell. Some potassium is bound to phosphate and is required for the conversion of glucose to glycogen.
4. It is required for the transmission of nerve impulse and for contraction of muscle fibers.

Food Sources

Potassium is widely distributed in foods. Meat, poultry and fish are good sources. Fruits, vegetables and whole grain cereals are especially high in potassium. Banana, potatoes, tomatoes, carrots, orange juice, grapefruit juice are rich sources.

Recommended Daily Allowance

The exact amount of potassium required is not known. A normal diet provides this mineral in sufficient amount.

Deficiency

Primarily the deficiency of potassium is not seen. Impaired appetite, severe malnutrition, chronic alcoholism and burn injuries can disturb the acid-base balance and lower osmotic pressure.

Magnesium

The amount of magnesium in the body is much smaller than that of calcium and phosphorus, i.e. about 20–35 g in the adult body. Of this about 60% are carbonates and phosphates at the surfaces of the bones. Most of the remaining magnesium is within the cells:

1. Magnesium is a constituent of bones and is present in all body cells.

2. Human adult body contains about 25 g of magnesium of which about half is found in the skeleton.
3. It appears that magnesium is essential for the normal metabolism of calcium and potassium.
4. Magnesium deficiency may occur in chronic alcoholic, cirrhosis of liver, toxemias of pregnancy, protein-energy malnutrition and malabsorption syndrome.
5. The principal clinical features attributed to magnesium deficiency are irritability, tetany, hyperreflexia and occasionally hyporeflexia.
6. The requirements are estimated to be about 200–300 mg/day for adults.

Functions

1. Magnesium is required for numerous biological reactions involving the release of energy.
2. It is a constituent of bone. It is involved in bone mineralization.
3. It is also essential for normal metabolism of calcium and phosphorus.
4. Its presence in the extracellular fluids regulates the transmission of nerve impulses.
5. It activates the enzyme responsible for breakdown of glycogen.

Food Sources

Dairy products excluding butter provide enough magnesium. Flour and cereal products, dry beans, soybeans, peas and nuts are good sources of magnesium. Green leafy vegetables are excellent sources, because magnesium is a part of chlorophyll.

Effect of Imbalances

Under normal conditions of health and food intake magnesium deficiency is not likely to occur. A deficiency of it may result from malabsorption syndrome, chronic alcoholism and toxemia of pregnancy or after intake of diuretics. Deficiency of magnesium results in neuromuscular irritability, tetanic convulsions, twitching, tremors and convulsions. In excess, it results in extreme thirst, excessive heat in the body, decrease in neuromuscular.

Chlorine

Chlorine exists in the body almost entirely as chloride ion. Most of the 100 g or so of chloride ion is present in the extracellular fluid, but it also occurs to some extent in the RBCs and to a lesser degree in other cells.

Functions

1. Chlorine is important in regulation of osmotic pressure, water balance and acid-base balance.
2. It activates the gastric enzymes and the digestion in the stomach.
3. It is one of the several activators of salivary amylase.

Recommended Daily Allowances

The requirements for chlorine have not been ascertained, but if sodium chloride is taken liberally, it ensures the adequate intake of chloride as well.

Chloride Imbalance

Severe vomiting, drainage or diarrhea leads to large loses of chloride and an alkalosis, because of the replacement of chloride with bicarbonate.

▶ TRACE ELEMENTS

Copper

1. The healthy human adult body contains about 100–150 mg of copper (Cu). Cu is present in the blood in the form of copper protein complex; hemocuprin in RBCs and ceruloplasmin in plasma.
2. Anemia produced in infants fed exclusively on milk can be cured only by giving copper salts along with Fe. The estimated average daily intakes in adult diets range from 2 to 3 mg.
3. The high intake in Indian diets may be due to contamination of Cu from brass vessels used in cooking.

Zinc

1. Zinc is active in the metabolism of glucides and proteins, and is required for the synthesis of insulin by the pancreas and for the immunity function.
2. Zinc is present in small amount in all tissues. Zn plasma level is about 96 mg/100 mL for healthy adults and 89 mg/100 mL for healthy children.
3. The average adult body contains 1.4–2.3 g of Zn. Zn deficiency in the diet has been reported to the cause of anemia, growth retardation and delayed genital maturation (dwarfism) in children.
4. Zinc is a constituent of insulin; the hormone present in the islets of Langerhans of pancreas.

Cobalt

1. Cobalt (Co) occurs in small amounts in all tissues, highest concentration occurring in liver and kidneys. Most of the Co is present in vitamin B_{12}.
2. It is suggested that Co may be necessary for the first stage of hormone production. Co may interact with iodine and affect its utilization.

CHAPTER 2: Review of Macro- and Micro-nutrition

Chromium

1. The chromium (Cr) content of an adult human body is estimated to be 6 mg. Most adult tissues contain 0.02–0.4 ppm of Cr on dry basis. The blood contains about 0.009–0.055 ppm.
2. Chromium plays an important role in carbohydrate, lipid and protein metabolism.
3. Chromium deficiency is characterized by impaired growth and disturbances in glucose, lipid and protein metabolism.

Selenium

1. Selenium (Se) administration to children with kwashiorkor resulted in significant weight increase.
2. Studies indicate that human Se deficiency may occur in protein-energy malnutrition.
3. Selenium deficiency especially when combined with vitamin E deficiency reduces production.

▶ CONCLUSION

Micronutrients are in our diets, but in very small amounts. These can be found in vitamins, minerals and trace elements. Micronutrients, just like water do not provide energy, however they are still needed in adequate amounts to ensure that all our body cells function properly. Even though their presence is in minute amounts it should be no way diminish their importance to nutrition. Most of micronutrients are known to be essential nutrients, meaning they are those which are dispensable to life processes and what the body cannot make itself. In other words meaning these essential nutrients can only be obtained from the food in which we eat.

Chapter 3

Balanced Diet

▶ INTRODUCTION

There is no one single food or type of food that provides all the nutrients that the human body needs to function efficiently. A balanced diet will depend on the types of food eaten over a period of time and the nutritional needs of the particular individual. The wider variety of foods eaten, the more nutrients will be provided by them. It is now known that some health problems are caused by dietary intake, such as too much fat causing heart disease and too much salt contributing to strokes. Balanced diet is one that contains different types of foods such as cereals, pulses and vegetables in such quantities, and proportions so that the need for calories, proteins, minerals, vitamins and other nutrients is adequately met and a small provision is made for extra nutrients to withstand short duration of leanness. A balanced diet should provide around 60%–70% of total calories from carbohydrate, 10%–12% from protein and 20%–25% from fat.

▶ IMPORTANCE

A balanced diet is important to maintain health and a sensible body weight. No single food will provide all the essential nutrients that the body needs to be healthy and function efficiently. A balanced diet should contain proteins, fats, carbohydrates and fiber in the form of fresh vegetables and fresh fruit, all in the right amounts providing with a good supply of essential amino acids, essential fatty acids, vitamins, minerals and of course fresh drinking water.

In addition, the nutritional value of a person's diet depends on the overall mixture or balance of food that is eaten over a

CHAPTER 3: Balanced Diet

period of time, as well as on the needs of the individual. A diet that includes a variety of different foods is most likely to provide all the essential nutrients.

▶ DEFINITION

A balanced diet is one that provides the body with all the essential nutrients, vitamins and minerals required to maintain cells, tissues and organs as well as to function correctly. A diet that is lacking in nutrients can lead to many different health problems ranging from tiredness and lack of energy to serious problems with the function of vital organs and lack of growth and development.

▶ MEANING

A balanced diet needs to contain foods from all the main food groups in the correct proportions to provide the body with optimum nutrition. It should also be made up of the correct number of calories to maintain a healthy weight and be low in processed foods. Every person is different and hence the correct diet for health may vary from person to person. However, by following a diet that is varied, covers all foods groups and is low in undesirable nutrients such as sodium, saturated fats and sugar are well on the way to a healthy body.

▶ ELEMENTS

The food pyramid divides the foods we eat into the categories of grains, vegetables, fruits, milk, meat and beans, oils and discretionary calories (Fig. 3.1).

Grains

Grains, including wheat, rice and oats, can be either whole grains, which contain the entire grain kernel or refined grains in which the bran and germ have been removed. Refined grains lack the rich fiber, iron and vitamin content of whole grain. The United States Department of Agriculture (USDA) recommends

SECTION 1: Nutrition

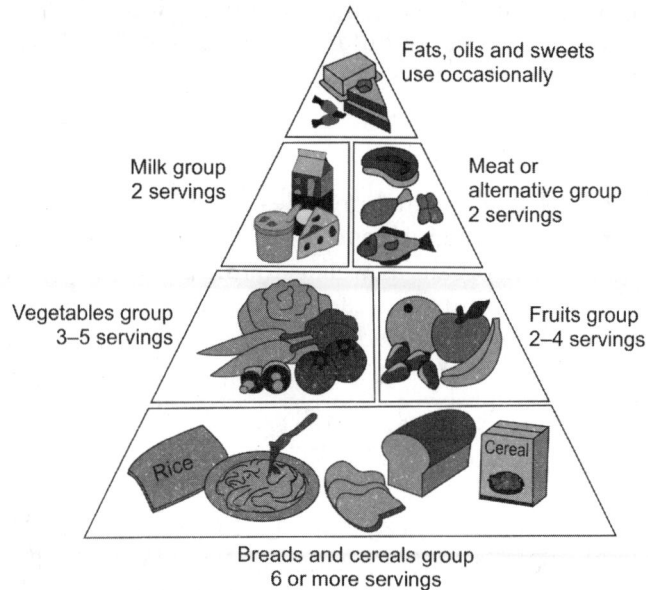

Fig. 3.1: Diagrammatic representation of elements of balanced diet

making whole grains at least half of the daily grain intake. Recommended daily amounts vary depending on age, sex and level of physical activity; recommended servings range from three daily for toddlers to eight servings daily for young men.

Vegetables

Vegetables are a crucial component of a well-balanced diet. The USDA divides vegetables into the categories of dark green vegetables, orange vegetables, starchy vegetables, other vegetables and dry beans and peas. Incorporating more fruits and vegetables into the diet may reduce the risk of some chronic diseases. Vegetables are a rich source of many important nutrients, including potassium, dietary fiber, folate and vitamins A, E and C. Vegetables are low in calories and can help in weight management. Young women should strive to eat at least 2½ cups of vegetables daily and women 51 or older should aim for 2 cups. Men should eat 3 cups, then aim for 2½ cups once they turn 51. Over the course of a week, people should eat vegetables from all categories.

CHAPTER 3: Balanced Diet

Fruits

Fruits are cholesterol free and low in fat, sodium and calories. Like vegetables, fruits are important sources of a number of key nutrients, including potassium, dietary fiber, vitamin C and folate. Fruit juice is a good way of incorporating fruit into the diet, but it lacks the dietary fiber found in whole fruit. Fruits that is particularly rich in potassium, which can help control blood pressure, include bananas, prunes, cantaloupe and honeydew. Young men and women should eat at least 2 cups of fruit daily. When women turn 31, this can be cut back to 1½ cups daily.

Milk, Yogurt and Cheese

As with all the food groups, daily dairy needs vary by age. Dairy products provide calcium, vitamin D and potassium. Calcium is important in building and maintaining bone mass and consuming dairy products is important to help prevent osteoporosis later in life. For men, women and children age 9 and up, recommended daily dairy intake is 3 cups. Children younger than age 9 should consume 2 cups.

Meat and Beans

Nutrients found in meat, poultry, fish, dry beans and peas, eggs, nuts and seeds include proteins, vitamin B, vitamin E, iron, zinc and magnesium. Fatty meats and eggs should be eaten in limited amounts, as they can raise the cholesterol levels. This recommendation is echoed by the American Heart Association's guidelines for a heart healthy diet. Fish, nuts and seeds are good sources of monounsaturated and polyunsaturated fatty acids. The USDA recommends 6½ daily servings from this group for young men and 5½ daily servings for young women. After age 31, women should consume 5 servings and men should eat 6 serving. Men 51 and older should cut back even further to 5½ servings daily.

Oils

The USDA recommends getting most of the dietary fat from fish, nuts and vegetable oils. Most oils have high levels of monounsaturated or polyunsaturated fats and low levels of saturated fat. Oils from plant sources, such as vegetable and nut oils are cholesterol free. Daily intake recommendations range from 3 teaspoon for toddlers to 7 teaspoon for young men.

Discretionary Calories

In the USDA pyramid plan, discretionary calories are allotted based on the food choices. These discretionary calories can be used to eat more foods from any food group than the food guide recommends, eat higher-calorie forms of foods, add fats or sweeteners to foods, or consume items such as such as candy, soda, wine and beer. For a physically active young man, discretionary calories should make 410–510 calories of a 2,600–3,000 calorie diet.

▶ COMPONENTS OF HEALTHY BALANCED DIET

Dairy

Dairy includes cheese, milk and yogurt. Dairy foods are usually high in saturated fat so to reduce fat and calories it is best to choose low fat or fat-free varieties. Dairy is essential in the diet to provide calcium for strong bones as well as protein and vitamin D. For those who do not consume dairy products it is essential to use a replacement such as soy or nut-based milks or supplement calcium in the diet.

Proteins

Protein is main containing in food groups and includes lean meat and poultry with visible fat and skin removed, as well as fish, beans, lentils, peas, nuts and seeds, eggs and soy proteins such as tofu and tempeh.

Meat and poultry are high in iron, whilst legumes are a rich source of fiber and eggs provide a multitude of vitamins and minerals. Fish should be included regularly, particularly oily fish high in omega-3, fatty acids such as salmon, mackerel and sardines. Cooking methods should be low fat such as grilling, poaching, dry frying or steaming to minimize extra fat added during the cooking process. It is also important to avoid processed meats such as sausages and sandwich meats where possible as these are high in fat and sodium.

Fruits

Fruit is virtually fat free, low in calories, high in fiber and very nutritious. Aim to include a variety of fruits to get a wide range of vitamins and minerals. This could also include dried fruits 100% and fruit juices, however, it is important to choose unsweetened varieties. Both dried fruit and juices are concentrated sources of calories, so make sure that portion sizes are controlled.

Vegetables

Vegetables generally contain the least calories, and the most vitamins and minerals, hence they are an excellent option for filling up on. Make sure to include a wide variety in the meals as different vegetables are rich in different vitamins. Try to use low fat cooking methods such as steaming or grilling. 100% vegetable juices can also be included and are the great ways to get a few serves of vegetables into the diet. If struggling to include enough vegetables in day-to-day meals, try adding grated of finely chopped vegetables to mixed dishes such as pasta sauces, burger mince or lasagnes, chances are you will not even notice the difference.

Grains

Grains group is the major carbohydrate source in a balanced diet and includes bread, cereals, pasta and rice. Try to choose wholegrain varieties as these are higher in fiber and contain more B vitamins than white versions. Enriched cereals and breads, for example with iron, calcium or omega-3 can also be a good way to add some extra nutrition to diet. Avoid sugary or toasted breakfast, cereals and sweetened breads made with refined flour as these contain little fiber, and are higher in calories and fat.

Fats and Oils

Whilst some fat is necessary in our diets for the body to function correctly, it is important that these are the right types of fats. Saturated and trans fats should be minimized as these are unhealthy for the heart. These should be replaces with vegetable fats such as canola, olive or sunflower oil or spreads. All fats do contain a high amount of calories however, so it is important to keep added fats to a minimum in order to maintain a healthy body weight. Opt for light or low-fat salad dressings and mayonnaise, and use vegetable oils for cooking and baking. Other good sources of unsaturated fats include nuts, avocado and fish.

Treats and 'Sometimes' Food

Food that does not fit into the above groups are generally considered to provide no or little nutritional benefit and are therefore not required in a balanced diet. Foods such as candy, chocolate, cakes, chips and other 'junk' foods should be avoided. If do indulge in a treat, try to choose one that is less than 145 calories.

▶ FACTORS INFLUENCING

Dietary needs will vary for each individual. As we have seen from the information above, dietary needs will differ according to age, but other factors will come into play. Such factors include:

- Level of exercise taken
- Type of job a person does
- Religious or cultural decisions
- Likes and dislikes
- A person's health
- Availability of food.

Religion/Culture

Religion and culture will play a large part in the food that people eat. Various foods are forbidden in certain religions. In general, Jews and Muslims do not eat pork, Hindus do not eat beef and Buddhists are vegetarian [refer Chapter 1 for Religious factors (Table 1.2), which shows the general food rules for different religions]. Asian groups, particularly teenage girls, may be deficient in vitamin D, which is known as the sunshine vitamin. Because their religion requires them to cover most of their body, they do not get the opportunity to expose their skin to the sunlight. This can result in conditions known as rickets and osteomalacia. The most common sign of this is bowed legs.

They should ensure that they eat a diet that is high in vitamin D. They may also be more at risk of becoming anemic as a traditional Asian diet may not provide enough iron.

Social Class

There is some evidence to suggest that differences in social class will play a part in influencing dietary choices. In general, people from social classes I and II tend to eat more healthy food and poorer people eat fewer fruit and vegetables and more high-fat, high-sugar foods (Scottish Health Survey—Eating Habits, 1998). Women (not men) in the lower social classes are more likely to be obese than women in the upper social classes. People in lower social classes generally earn less money than those in the higher social classes and because of this are more likely to substitute cheap, processed food for fresh food.

Personal Preference

Personal preference plays a part in the choices an individual makes about food. This may not just be linked to likes and dislikes, but other factors, for example people who choose not to eat meat because of the implications of killing animals for food. Personal preference is also influenced by taste, texture, cultural and social habits.

Peer Pressure

Peer pressure can have an effect on the food choices that are made especially by children and teenagers. Many young people develop a stereotyped view of people who eat healthy and unhealthy foods, and may choose less healthy options such as fast food to fit in with what their friends eat because they do not want to seem different.

Media

Information publicized in the media can be another factor that influences food choice. Food scares can often be caused by reporting of facts in the press and in news bulletins. Two examples of this were the egg scare in 1988 and 'mad cow disease' in 1995. In 1988, a junior health minister, Edwina Currie said that the majority of eggs in the UK were contaminated with salmonella. This had a huge impact on the sale of eggs 400 million eggs and 4 million chickens were destroyed. In 1996, beef exports to Europe were banned when a link between eating beef and a brain disease, Creutzfeldt-Jakob disease, was established. Again, this had a huge impact on beef sales and consumption of beef and beef was banned from school menus.

Position in the Family

There is little evidence available to suggest that there is a difference in food choice depending on the position hold in the family, but it is known that mothers will often give more protein or fruit and vegetables or larger quantities to their husband/partner or children. They will then fill upon lower quality food and their nutritional status may suffer as a result. Choice may also be related to, who in the family does the shopping and cooking. For example, if you do most of the family shopping and do not like a particular food, even if others in the family do like it you are less likely to buy it.

Geographic Location

Where we live will have an effect on the diet we have. Although there is enough food in the world, it is not evenly distributed. More wealthy countries can afford to buy food and so have a greater variety than countries that are poor. Food that is grown

CHAPTER 3: Balanced Diet

in poor soil will contain fewer minerals and so the quality of the diet will be poorer.

Availability of Food

Many developing countries suffer from poor soil conditions, flooding and drought, which result in repeated years of lost harvests. People have access to restricted diets that are high in carbohydrates and not so rich in protein and fats. This can lead to undernutrition. In developed countries, people have access to a good variety of food. Much of it is home grown and the increase in air travel means that most foods are available all year round. As a result, the population of developed countries is more likely to suffer from overnutrition.

Other factors influenced by geographical location will be where people live and how easily they can get food. Greater variety is available in large supermarkets generally situated on the outskirts of large towns. Small corner shops in rural areas tend to have less variety and less fresh fruit and vegetables.

Financial Resources

The ability to afford food is linked to social class (see above). People who are in the higher social classes have more money to spend on food and tend to buy better quality food and eat out more. People who have low incomes are more likely to buy food that is high in salt, fat and sugar, and provide concentrated sources of energy.

▶ CALCULATION

Steps in Planning

1. **Identify the individual and his/her specific characteristics:**
    a. Age.
    b. Sex.
    c. Activity level (for adults).

SECTION 1: Nutrition

    d. Income, socioeconomic status.
    e. Religion.
    f. Region where residing.

    The above mentioned information will help decide the kind of diet to be planned. The background of income, socioeconomic status, religion and region will decide the kind of foods to be included in the plan. The age and sex play very important role in deciding the number of calories and proteins to be given. The diet must suit the pocket of the person.

    Religion is a sensitive issue and should not be ignored while planning diet. Different regions of the country have different staple foods, which the planner must be aware of keeping in mind not to include foods that are not available in local markets.

2. **Consult for recommended dietary intake (RDI) for energy and protein:** Generally, if the diet contains required amount of energy and protein as per the RDIs, it provides sufficient amounts of other nutrients as well. Careful selection of foods with inclusion of rich sources of vitamins and minerals will help meet the needs.

3. **Decide the total amount of specific food groups:** The selection of specific foods will depend on the income and personal preferences. The foods should be selected from each food group as mentioned earlier. The amount and selection of foods should be done carefully so as to meet the requirement of energy and protein.

4. **Decide on number of meals to be consumed:** Meal frequency is influenced by various factors such as income, occupation, school timings and convenience. People of more affluent society have more meals. The number of meals consumed may be a three meal, a four meal, a five meal or a seven to eight meal pattern. Traditionally most regions in India follow 3–5 meal pattern, which include three major meals (breakfast, lunch and dinner) and two small meals (midmorning and late afternoon). The frequency of meals may vary according to the age.

5. **Distribute total amount between decided meals:** The total amounts of foods from each food group should be distributed over the day's meal.
6. **Decide the items and their amounts within each group for each meal:** In other words plan the menu. The dishes to be included from each food group must be decided. This means selecting specific foods for a particular dish or a meal.
7. **Check day's diet for inclusion of each food group and the amounts decided:** In step 6 the menu was planned. In this step we must check whether all the food items decided in step 3 are included or not.

▶ EFFECTS OF UNBALANCED DIETS

Malnutrition

A balanced diet is based on the consumption of appropriate amounts of nutrients and energy. Malnutrition can result from people eating too much or too little of some nutrients over a period of time. Insufficient intake can result in undernutrition or starvation and excessive intake can result in overnutrition and obesity.

Overnutrition

There are some conditions that are related to eating too much of a certain nutrient. Coronary heart disease occurs as a result of eating too many foods such as animal proteins that are high in saturated fats. Fatty deposits build-up in the coronary arteries in the heart and this can lead to the formation of a clot that will stop the supply of blood to part of the heart muscle, which then dies. This is known as a heart attack. Symptoms of a heart attack can include shortness of breath and pain in the chest, jaw and left arm.

Obesity results from eating too much food. Any food that is eaten in excess will ultimately be converted to fat and stored in the body, which leads to overweight and obesity.

Type 2 diabetes, also known as late or adult onset diabetes, is today seen in children as young as 9 years old. It is caused by eating too much fat and sugar in the diet. The pancreas is either unable to produce enough insulin to allow the cells to absorb glucose from the blood or the body becomes resistant to the insulin that is produced. Symptoms of type 2 diabetes include thirst, excessive urination and extreme tiredness.

Undernutrition

Undernutrition can result from the general lack of nutrients, particularly protein and energy or from the lack of a particular nutrient. Two conditions that are seen in underdeveloped countries and that particularly affect children are kwashiorkor and marasmus. The differences between them are detailed in Chapter 2 (Table 2.6).

▶ SPECIFIC NUTRITIONAL DEFICIENCIES

Anemia

Anemia is caused by iron deficiency. Iron is used for making red blood cells and in the body's use of oxygen. Symptoms include:
- Fatigue/lack of energy
- Weakness
- Brittle fingernails
- Tooth decay.

Tooth decay or dental caries cannot be strictly described as undernutrition, as it is caused by an excess of sugar in the diet. Sticky deposits called plaque are deposited on the teeth. Plaque is acid and overtime it will dissolve the enamel on teeth, causing cavities. If they remain untreated, they can kill the tooth's nerve and blood supply, and eventually the whole tooth will die. It is important that sugary foods and drinks are kept to a minimum and good dental hygiene is observed.

Rickets

Rickets is caused by vitamin D deficiency, which controls calcium metabolism. In elderly, adolescents and women who have repeated pregnancies, may suffer from osteomalacia (the adult form of rickets) because they absorb too little calcium from a low-calcium diet. There is also some ethnic evidence of a difference in vitamin D metabolism.

In children, long bones are not calcified enough, and their legs bend and they tend to have very tiny chests. The four main plates of the skull are not ossified—this is known as the hot cross bun sign in newborn babies.

Night Blindness

Night blindness is caused by a lack of vitamin A. It is also known as xerophthalmia or dry eye. In its early stages, it can be cured by providing sufferers with vitamin A supplements such as palm oil or other foods high in vitamin A. However, in its later stages it is incurable and leads to complete blindness and in some cases death.

Beriberi

Beriberi is vitamin B_1 or thiamine deficiency—this vitamin is needed to metabolize carbohydrates.

Scurvy

Scurvy is known as vitamin C deficiency and only occurs when fresh food, especially citrus fruits is not available. Symptoms include swelling of gums and teeth falling out, bleeding and slow wound healing.

▶ CONDITIONS WITH SPECIFIC DIETARY REQUIREMENT

Coronary Heart Disease

People who suffer from coronary heart disease should modify their diet in order to prevent further damage to the heart. Sufferers should be advised to make the following changes to their diet:

SECTION 1: Nutrition

1. Eat at least in five portions of fruit and vegetables a day.
2. Reduce the total amount of fat in the diet and substitute saturated fats for poly and monounsaturated fats such as vegetable and olive oil.
3. Eat oily fish such as mackerel, sardines, herring, tuna and salmon, 2–3 times a week.
4. Introduce nuts and seeds into the diet.
5. Maintain a healthy weight.
6. Reduce the amount of salt in the diet to a maximum of 6 g/day.
7. Drink alcohol in moderation 1–2 units per day.
8. Take exercise—a minimum of 30 minutes three times a week.

Obesity

The best way to combat obesity is to maintain a diet low in fat and sugar, and high in complex carbohydrates and fruit and vegetables. Regular exercise will also help to burn up any excess energy intake.

Type 2 Diabetes

People who suffer from type 2 diabetes can do a lot to help the levels of blood glucose by maintaining a diet low in fat and sugar. Complex carbohydrates should form a part of the diet, as low carbohydrate diets can be high in fat. There is a, relatively high incidence of coronary heart disease in diabetics' sufferers in the UK.

Lactose Intolerance

Lactose intolerance is an inability to digest lactose, the sugar found in milk and milk products. It is particularly common in people of African and Asian origin, and can lead to digestive disturbance such as cramps, diarrhea and wind. Milk should be avoided in the diet, but often sufferers can tolerate yoghurt and cheese because the lactose is converted to lactic acid during manufacture.

CHAPTER 3: Balanced Diet

Food Allergies

Allergic reactions to food vary in intensity and similar symptoms and illnesses can be triggered by different allergens as well as the same allergens causing very different reactions in different people. Symptoms can include eczema, asthma, urticaria (hives) and other health problems.

Anaphylaxis is an extreme reaction, which must be treated by adrenaline injections. Failure to treat this promptly can result in death. Avoidance of food that causes allergies is the only way to prevent the onset of symptoms.

Genetic Disorders

Certain genetic disorders can cause problems that can be relieved by diet. Cystic fibrosis is a disorder that causes thick, sticky mucous to coat the pancreatic duct. Pancreatic enzymes needed to digest food cannot pass into the small intestine and sufferers are given these enzymes in powdered form sprinkled onto their food. Phenylketonuria is a rare inherited condition in which there is a buildup of phenylalanine in the body. Phenylalanine is an amino acid—a building block of protein. A low-protein diet is essential for sufferers and has to be supplemented with artificial protein that does not contain phenylalanine. If this diet is not followed, learning difficulties can result.

Religion/Culture

The Table 3.1 shows the main dietary rules for some world religions, some people choose not to eat meat and become vegetarian or vegan. Vegetarians do not usually eat meat, poultry, game or fish. However, most will eat eggs and dairy products. Vegetarians will be healthy as long as they eat a varied diet and combine plant proteins.

Vegans eat no animal foods at all and have to be careful about the plant proteins they eat to ensure that they have a balanced diet. There is a possibility that they may suffer from vitamin B_{12} deficiency as this is mainly found in animal products, although yeast extract is a good source.

SECTION 1: Nutrition

Table 3.1: Elements of balanced diet

Group	Examples and serving size	Daily servings
Grains	Breakfast cereals, rice, pasta, bread and noodles Emphasize on whole grains 1 ounce equivalent equals: 1 slice of bread or small muffin 1 cup of dry cereal ½ cup cooked cereal, rice, pasta	6–8 ounce equivalents (the lower number is the servings for a 2,000 calorie diet and the higher number is for 2,400 calorie diet)
Vegetables	Tomatoes, potatoes, carrots, green peas, squash, broccoli, spinach, green beans, sweet potatoes 1 cup raw leafy vegetables = ½ cup	2.5–3.5 cups
Fruits	Apricots, bananas, dates, grapes, grapefruit, oranges, orange juice, mangoes, melons, peaches, pineapples, plums, berries	1.5–2 cups
Dairy	Milk, yogurt and cheese The following count as 1 cup: 1½ ounces of natural cheese 2 ounces of processed cheese	3 cups
Meat, eggs, nuts and beans	Meat, poultry, fish, eggs, dry beans and nuts 1 ounce equivalent equals: 1 ounces of cooked lean meat, poultry or fish 1 egg ½ oz of nuts or seeds 1 tablespoon peanut butter ¼ cup cooked dried beans or tofu	5.5–6.5 ounce equivalents
Oils	Soft margarine, low-fat mayonnaise, light salad dressing, vegetable oil (olive, canola, safflower, corn)	27–31 g
Discretionary calorie allowance	After selecting nutrient dense foods from the list above there is room for a few more calories Fat and added sugars are always counted as discretionary calories	267–362 calories

CHAPTER 3: Balanced Diet

▶ NURSES HEALTH PROMOTION ROLE

The general population needs to have a balanced, healthy diet as it provides the energy and nutrients required to survive and stay healthy. Combining a healthy diet with an active lifestyle has huge benefits, and helps reduce the risk of heart disease, cancer and obesity. Registered dietitians and nurses can work together to advice people on healthy eating. All nurses play a vital role in the promotion of healthy eating. Primary care nurses, in particular practice and school nurses are well-placed to promote healthy eating.

▶ CONCLUSION

We eat a variety of foods to satisfy our needs everyday because it is important for our body. It is important that we eat the right amount of each type of food. There are different types of food. Each type of food performs specific functions in our body. To stay healthy, we are advised to eat food, which contains a combination of many types. Some food can give us energy while others can make us grow. A combination of essential foods is called balanced diet. It is generally believed that you are what you eat. Balanced diet means eating the right amount of foods from all available food groups. It refers to the intake of edibles, which can provide all the essential constituents necessary for growth, development and maintenance of the body. While prescribing balanced diet following points must be considered. A balanced diet leads to proper growth and development in organism hence everyone should take balanced diet.

Chapter 4

Meal Planning

▶ INTRODUCTION

Meal planning means planning diets, which will provide all nutrients in required amounts and proportions, i.e. adequate nutrition. As the family's well-being and health are depended on how well they are fed. It is a challenge to every meal planner to meet it and when well-done, it proves to be a satisfying and rewarding experience.

Besides others factors such as digestibility, palatability, economy, family customs, related to religion, food fads, etc. it also determines whether the food can be actually supplied and utilized by the individual.

What are the characteristics of a well-planned meal? First of all it should be remembered that food has to be palatable before it can become nutritious, as majority of people will not eat something they do not like, even if it has excellent nutritive value. We should remember that appetite is the pleasurable anticipation of foods and depends not only on hunger but also on taste, texture, appearance and attractiveness of the foods, pleasantness of the surrounding, and a cheerful frame of mind.

Meal planning thus is both an art and a science; an art in the skillful blending of colors, texture and flavor, and a science in the wise choice of food for optimum nutrition and digestion.

▶ IMPORTANCE

The meal planning helps to make the best use of the material, time and financial resources. To obtain meals that meets the physical, social and psychological needs of the individual and families. It is very important to plan family meals in order to fulfill the nutritional requirement of the family members. This is essential to keep them strong, healthy and free from any disease and deficiency of any kind. Meal planning is of utmost importance because it economizes on time, labor and fuel.

While planning meals, the methods of working can be carefully throughout, so that there is maximum retention of nutrients and minimum losses.

Meals can be planned according to the budget of the family. Then there can be maximum utilization of money, if it is spent in the best possible way. Once can have a rich diet without buying expensive foods. Meal planning therefore encourages one to plan within the family means. Meal planning allows one to select different foods from the same food group and avoid monotony. Besides, use of variety of foodstuffs is important from nutritional points also.

Meal planning determines the adequacy of the diet, the kinds of foods purchased, its quality and cost, the way it is stored, prepared and served.

▶ OBJECTIVES

1. To satisfy the nutritional needs of the family members.
2. To keep expenditure within family food budget.
3. To take into account the food preference of individual members.
4. Using methods of cooking to retain maximum nutrients.
5. To economize on time, fuel and energy.
6. To serve attractive and appetizing meals.

▶ GOALS

1. **Achieving nutritional adequacy:** The first goal is good nutrition. It is essential to satisfy the nutritional needs of the family members according to their age, activity level and occupation.

SECTION 1: Nutrition

2. **Matching meals to the budget for foods:** It is necessary to ensure that the meals do not cost too much. Spending money on foods must be planned and should stay within the family's food budget. Purchase foods from each food group.

3. **Achieving meals the family wants and likes:** Meals must be so planned that it should be accepted, eaten and enjoyed by the family members. The kind of meals we eat is influenced by ethnic background, family customs, region of residence, socioeconomic status, education, religion and the previous experiences. Family size must also be considered.

4. **Matching meals to available time:** Meals must be planned according to the time and energy available. Time is required for planning and organizing the manual work of meal. Time and energy are required for shopping, meal preparation and clean up after meals.

▶ FACTORS AFFECTING

Meal planning whether for the simplest family meal or for an elaborate company dinner, involve consideration of a number of factors.

Nutritional Adequacy

Meal pattern must fulfill the family needs, so that the nutrition requirement of each individual in the family are met. These requirements differ from person to person according to age, sex, activity and physiological condition; therefore, due consideration should be given to each member of the family. The best way to ensure nutritional adequacy of a diet is to select the food from all the five food groups. The different requirements for different family members do not mean that separate cooking is to be done for all of them. But the diet can be planned in such a way that while cooking the same food, the nutritional requirements of all the members can be catered, e.g. by increasing or decreasing the amount of certain foodstuff by including some extra protein food for growth periods. For instance, the same salad can be used for both the overweight and the underweight members of the family if the dressing is omitted for the former.

Economy

The amount of money available, depending upon the socioeconomic status also effects the meal planning. The major part of the income is spent on food. Therefore, one should spend economically to get maximum utilization. Although the budget of a family of moderate income group may not provide for foods of the luxury class, it can still offer variety and opportunity for choice. Food budgets in lower income families permit even more limited choice and it may become increasingly necessary to depend on cereal foods for the main or substantial part of the meal. Then the problem faced is the supplementation of this cereal with foods necessary for a balanced diet. Although it may become difficult to plan, it is nevertheless possible. Thereby, it is very important to know the less expensive alternative for the more expensive recommended foods, having high nutritive value. Such recipes and foods should be included in meal preparation like using cereal pulse combination, e.g. khichdi, paushtik roti, seasonal vegetables, butter milk, jaggery, pickle and chutney.

Facilities and Help Available

The time spent in cooking depends on other facilities and other help availability of servant, using readymade foods, using labor saving devices. However, time like money needs to be budgeted for its best use. Time management in the preparation of foods is essential for the homemaker who is also employed outside the home.

Satiety Value

Any individual meal should provide enough satiety value, so that one does not feel hungry till it is time for the next meal.

Proteins and fats have greater satiety value as compared to carbohydrates, e.g. a breakfast of just tea and toast will not provide enough satiety value till lunch, whereas, a breakfast of milk, cereal, eggs and fruit will provide enough satiety value till lunch.

Personal Likes and Dislikes

Although the recommended dietary allowances for each of the classes of food should be followed, there is room for individual preference amongst the foods in each class. Some people make personal likes and dislike the only basis for the inclusion or exclusion of certain foods in their meals the failure to include milk is a common practice. It is always better to change the form of the food rather than to completely omit it. For example, milk can be given in the form of curd, cheese, custard or other sweet dish, soybeans in the form of soya flour chapatis mixed with wheat flour.

Religions, Traditions and Customs

Religions, traditions and customs are important in determining the food included in the diet, type of meal and the dishes served to the individual of family. For instance, Muslims do not eat pork, whereas Hindus do not eat beef. Rice is considered an auspicious dish at festivals and marriages. Widows are generally not served fish in Bengal. Therefore, religion, traditions and customs should be kept in view, while planning meals for a family.

Food Fads and Fallacies

Food fads and fallacies often receive more publicity than sound nutrition information. Therefore, while planning the meals, one must try and remove these foods fads, so that notorious meals are provided.

Availability of Foodstuffs and Climate

In earlier times, the dietary habits depended mainly upon the foods produced in a particular area or community, but today with improved methods of foods preservation and distribution, even the most perishable foods are available over large areas. The wide variation in dietary patterns throughout the world depends largely upon the available food supply and, which depends on the climate. Thereby, only seasonal foods should be included in the diet. Also, the season of the year requires some consideration for the type of dishes selected, e.g. inclusion of hot soups, chilled salads, etc. in cold winter days and juices in summers.

Variety

Variety is very important, because nobody likes to eat even stuff favorite food over and over again. Therefore, to introduce variety, do not repeat same food items during day meal. Also variety in meal planning is the sum total of many kinds and classes of food served in pleasing color combinations with judicious mixture of soft and crisp foods, blunt and sharp flavors, hot and cold dishes. It ensures better nutrition and also results in more interesting meals with an attractive variety of texture, color, taste and appearance, which in turn stimulates appetite and pleases the palate. Various methods of working can also introduce a variety, a meal consisting of tandoori roti, dal and seasonal green vegetable also with a crisp salad.

Schedules of Family Members

When planning meals, one need to think of the schedules (time table) of the family members—mealtimes and the number of meals eaten at home and those that are eaten away from home. If packed lunches are made the menus need to be modified to ensure that the items can be packed and the menu is appetizing even when cold.

Family Size and Composition

The family size affects the foods that can be served. It is known that the money spent for food per person decreases as the family size increases, when the family income remains constant.

Staples such as wheat and rice are bought in larger amounts, but quantity of milk, vegetables and fruits is lowered. Thus, the quality of the diet is affected. Family composition affects the kind and amounts of mood needed and pattern of meals served, e.g. when children are below 5 years of age, more milk is required, the numbers of meals are more, as the child cannot take large amount at a time.

As the child grows the meal pattern changes to accommodate the school hours and the need to pack lunch or snack may arise. Older members of the family may require change in consistency of food due to faulty teeth.

Mealtimes

Mealtime is also an important factor in meal planning. The meals should be planned according to the time for meal, i.e. whether it is breakfast, lunch or dinner. Normally, while planning the meal for whole day, it is seen that one third of day's requirement are met by lunch one third by dinner and one third by breakfast and evening tea, but this is not a rigid schedule and can be changed according to individual requirement, but as long as the total nutritional requirements are being met.

Occasion

For daily meals, the first importance is given to nutritive value. However, for special occasion, special importance has to be given to color, appearance, number of dishes to be included, but at the same time nutritive value cannot be ignored. Similarly each festival has its specific food item, which should always be given importance e.g. preparing sweets for Deepavali, cake for Christmas, seviyan for Eid, gujiya for Holi, etc.

▶ STEPS IN MEAL PLANNING

1. **Preparing a list:** One should make shopping list of foods available in the market from each food group. This would save time and energy.

2. **Compare the prices:** Compare the prices in the market and decide which food suits the budget.
3. **Estimating daily needs:** Develop skills in estimating the daily needs of the family members and then calculate for the month.
4. Divide the shopping list into four:
   a. Foods to be purchased monthly.
   b. Fortnightly.
   c. Weekly.
   d. Daily.
5. Planning menus according to the requirements of the family.
6. Choose an appropriate cooking method to prepare meals.

▶ MEAL PLANNING FOR DIFFERENT MEALS IN A DAY

Breakfast

Breakfast is very important meal as taken after 10–12 hours long gap between dinner and breakfast the next day. It should be well planned, nutritious attractive and should provide 1/3rd–1/4th of the day's requirements, but do not make it very heavy, which would lead to lethargy. The school children usually miss breakfast and as a result, they cannot concentrate on studies after some time. Breakfast should include the following:

- Fruit or fruit juice
- Cereal preparation: Paratha, puri, toast, porridge
- Protein food: Eggs, sausages, milk.

Low Cost Menu

- Banana (any seasonal fruit)
- Cereal and protein food—'missi' roti
- Tea/butter milk/milk.

Middle Cost Menu

- Apple or orange
- Paratha (stuffed) with curds or toast and butter, milk/tea and pickle or puri, vegetable preparation and a glass of milk lassi.

Western Menu/High Cost Menu

- Fruit juice (orange, pineapple)
- Porridge (cornflakes, rice, flakes, oatmeal, etc.) with milk
- Fried eggs with sausages/poached egg/paneer sabzi
- Buttered toast
- Coffee/tea.

Lunch

Lunch is the main meal, hence an important meal. About one third of the total day's requirements should be provided. The members, who are not at home for the lunch, should be given packed lunch, which should be nutritious, easy to carry, attractive and with some variety.

Packed Lunch Menu (for School Children)

- Dal/paneer stuffed paratha
- Fruit, e.g. orange
- Piece of cake.

Or

- Sandwiches (paneer/egg/beans)
- Sweet (peanut chikki/besan ladoo/halwa/burfi).

For children foodstuff should have variety, but it has to be handy too.

Packed Lunch Menu (for Adults)

- Parathas/chapatis
- Dry vegetable

CHAPTER 4: Meal Planning

- Dry dal
- Salad/fruit.

However, on holidays when everyone is at home, menu with difference is prepared.

Normal Lunch Menu (on Holidays)

- Soup
- Cereal preparation: Rice/pulav/chapati/puri/paratha
- Meat curry/egg curry/kabuli chana, pulse preparation, etc.
- Vegetable preparation: Carrot, pea, sabzi/koftas
- Curd preparation
- Salad
- Dessert/fruit: Custard/kheer/carrot halwa/soufflé/pudding/fruit salad.

The selection of food items and number of dishes can vary according to the socioeconomic status. On the other hand, where normally lunch is eaten at home, the menu should be simpler. Also dishes such as curries, rice, curd, etc. can be included, which are otherwise difficult to carry, some of the examples are:

- Moong whole, brinjal bharta, rice/chapati, curd fruit
- Stuffed tandoori paratha, curd, potato and pea curry, fruit
- Chapati, pea paneer curry, pumpkin sabzi, curd fruit
- Rice, sambar, sweet curd mixed with fruits.

Evening Tea

Evening tea is generally light and usually includes snacks, sweets, pakoras, cutlets, mathri and tea/coffee/juice. For children something heavy should be given such as sandwiches, ladoos, burfi, cakes, etc. It tea time is special occasion, 3–4 snacks and beverage can be served.

Evening Tea Menu (Normal)

- Pakoras, tea
- Tomato sandwich, tea

- Mathri, ladoo, tea
- Biscuit, vadas, tea
- Jalebi, wafers, tea.

Evening Tea Menu (for Special Occasion)

- Rainbow sandwich, coconut rolls, cashew nuts fried, tea
- Cutlets, rasgullas, chirwa, biscuit, tea
- Chocolate burfi, samosa, pastry, wafers, tea
- Coconut burfi, khandvi, gulab jamun, moong dal, tea
- Cashew nut burfi, peanut cutlets, chocolate cake, chirwa, tea.

Dinner

Dinner is also the main meal and should provide one third of day's requirements and should make up for all deficiencies in person's meal, e.g. if curd has not been taken in the morning, include it in the dinner.

Menu has to be elaborate when someone is invited. Otherwise, menu is like lunch. For festivals, prepare particular food according to sanity of festivals, e.g. various sweets on Deepavali, cake on Christmas, seviyan on Eid, gujiya on Holi, etc.

Suggestions for Menu Planning

1. Consider whole day as a unit rather than individual meals.
2. Try to distribute carbohydrates, fats and proteins throughout the day, so that no meal has predominance of any kind of foodstuff.
3. Use seasonal foods because they are best in flavor and cheap, however, avoid giving the same foodstuff and especially in the same meal, e.g. do not give tomato soup, tomato macaroni and tomato salad for the same meal. But during the day, things such as cereals, butter, milk has to be repeated.
4. Take care of color, flavor and texture by giving contrast in each meal, e.g. keep the color combination of dishes

in mind, while planning the meal. The dishes can be garnished to bring about more colors in diet. Flavor of food should be blended with each other. There should also be some contrast in texture, e.g. some dishes can be soft and some dishes can be crisp, like with the soup toasted bread can be given, etc.
5. There should be a balance between the dishes like some dishes should be light and some should be heavy, e.g. filling soup can be served with light main meal and vice versa.
6. Include the favorite foods of the family at different meals, but at the same time do not be limited to only these foods and try to introduce new dishes, so that food habits can be expanded.

Money can be saved on food: By following methods:
- Buying bigger packs
- Compare the prices before buying
- Wholesale markets are cheaper than retail ones
- Cook just the required amounts, if food is left over then make use of it by converting to another dish, etc.
- Use seasonal fruits and vegetables
- Keep accounts.

Time can also be saved: By following methods:
- Plan meal for several days at a time
- Buy dry ingredients together at least for a month
- Avoid going market during crowded hours
- Arrange things properly in kitchen so as to save the time, while working
- Use pressure cooker
- Plan your time, while working
- Use labor saving devices, e.g. mixer, but possible only in case the money is available to purchase them.

▶ **BUDGET FOR FOOD**

Budgeting the food means to provide budget for the nutritional requirements of an individual, a family or a community.

The practice of family budget in India is almost non-existent because of lack of education and traditions. So much that, even during times of requirement, a cut in meals time and a cut in expenditure on diet is the tendency of people. Under these circumstances, food budgeting is difficult to imagine yet it cannot be underestimated. Budgeting of food is becoming important in view of the greater literacy percentage of women. Food budgeting is becoming an important factor in family budgeting in the service class or in fixed-income group families.

Importance of Food Budget

1. To decide the expenditure on food in relation to income.
2. To receive subsidy in food planning, fulfillment of special nutrition for vulnerable classes, e.g. in children, in pregnancy and lactation, and in old age.
3. Prebudgeting for contingencies like, guests and parties.
4. Possibility of changes in diet, keeping in mind the nutritional requirements as per budget.
5. To raise the health status of the individual or the family by food budgeting, so as to minimize the spending on disease and treatment.

Factors Affecting Food Budget

1. Lack of nutrition education/less literacy.
2. Poverty/unemployment.
3. Less individual income or low per capita income.
4. Fluctuation in market prices of food, especially in dearness and inflation.
5. Lack of tradition of family and food budgeting.
6. Disturbances of family budget due to tradition of entertaining guests and arranging parties.

Food Expenditure

The nutritionists are not unanimous on the percentage of expenditure on food budget, out of the family budget. There is no any definite principle, formula or ratio about this. However, 50% of total income should be spent on food. Higher classes spend more on.

Plans for Food Budget

In practice, one must make daily menus for a week and base the food purchase on them. This step is essential whether the plan is for a single person, a family or an institution. Food purchase is guided by nutrient needs and the food budget. The planning helps to make the best use of available money to meet the needs of the family. The food choices within a group can be guided by ones food budget. The step, which help to get the best returns for food money include:

1. Buying the staple food, dals and pulses in bulk, when the prices are competitive just after the harvest.
2. Buying milk and milk products from government daily outlets.
3. Buying fruits and vegetables from main markets at competitive rates.
4. Buying seasonal vegetables and fruits.
5. Buy sugar, jaggery in bulk from wholesale dealers.
6. Buy oils from whole sale depots in bulk.
7. Make butter and ghee at home.
8. Buy spices in bulk and prepare the spices mix at home.

There are several government programs, which subsidize foods for the various socioeconomic strata. These include rationed food grains, food given to children in grade schools to ensure attendance, school level programs and supplementary feeding of expectant and nursing mothers. These programs help to meet the nutritional needs. To some extent, these reduce the food budget of the family.

Planning of a Balanced Diet

A balanced diet is the one, which contains various groups of foodstuffs such as energy yielding, body building and protective foods in the correct proportion and also make provision for extra nutrients to withstand short duration of leanness. The components of balanced diet will differ according to age, sex, physical activity, economic status and physiologic state namely pregnancy, lactation, etc.

Balanced diet at high cost: It can include liberal amounts of costly foods such as mile, fish, fruits, meat, egg and moderate amounts of cereals and pulses.

Balanced diet with moderate cost: It includes moderate amounts of cereals, pulses, nuts and green leafy vegetables.

Balanced diet with low cost: It includes large amounts of cereals, pulses and vegetables, but small amounts of milk, eggs, fish and meat.

A balanced diet has become an accepted means to safeguard the population from nutritional deficiencies. Its goals are:
1. The requirements of protein should be met, which amounts to 15%–20% of daily energy needs.
2. Fat should be limited to 20%–30% daily energy needs.
3. Carbohydrates rich in natural fiber stored constitute the remaining food energy.

Ways to Save on Food Budget

1. Eat meals at home or carry packed meals to workplace whenever possible. Eating out in a restaurant is always more expensive than home, cooked foods.
2. Buy foods when they are in plenty. Take advantage of special offers, such as special of the week, buy one get one free, etc.
3. Plan meals in advance and make use of food guides to ensure good nutrition.
4. Plan meals according to the preference of the family. Introduce new varieties of dishes and serve attractively.
5. Limit the use of ready-to-eat foods and prefer home-prepared foods from scratch.

6. Limit the amount of money to be spent on snacks and aerated drinks. This will only increase the expenditure without providing any nutrients.
7. Substitute foods with other foods of equal value if they are cheaper. Avoid impulsive buying.
8. Read labels for dates and nutrition facts. Compare the prices.
9. Try to purchase family packs as anything in bulk is always economical.
10. Avoid food wastage at home by properly storing to maintain their freshness; avoid loss of nutrients by using appropriate cooking methods and use leftovers within 24 hours.

▶ CONCLUSION

Enjoying meals together as a family is highly valued among Indians. Eating together as a family has many nutritional, social and psychological benefits. Studies show that children who eat with their families have higher intakes of vegetables, fruit, and dairy products, which are foods we often do not eat enough of. The advantages of meal planning are numerous. Planning meals helps to manage the time better and makes meal preparation easier. It can turn a hectic week into one that is nearly stress free. It also helps to improve own personal health and the health of the family. Meal planning is so important, fitness experts and those preparing for fitness competitions consider it a must.

Chapter 5

Food Hygiene/Sanitation

▶ INTRODUCTION

Food sanitation implies cleanliness in the producing, preparing, storing and servicing of food and water. Food sanitation is essential aspect of food preparation. It needs to emphasize at every stage of food handling and preparation. Some of the items, which need particular attention to ensure that food is safe for consumption, are a safe and portable water supply.

Selecting wholesome ingredients and hygienically handling to prevent the entry of pathogenic organisms, and spoilage both during preparation and serving. In addition, all equipment during come in contact with food supply is scrupulously clean the surrounding should be clean, and there should be a proper and safe method for the disposal of waste. Inculcation of hygienic habits would help in preventing foods from being contaminated during handling.

▶ DEFINITION

The World Health Organization (WHO) has defined food safety/food hygiene as all conditions and measures that are necessary during the production, processing, storage, distribution and preparation of food to ensure that it is safe, sound wholesome and fit for human consumption (Table 5.1).

▶ HYGIENE

Food Hygiene

Food is a potential source of infection and is liable to contamination by microorganisms and any point during its journey

CHAPTER 5: Food Hygiene/Sanitation

Table 5.1: Terminology used in food hygiene

Sl No	Term	Description
1.	Clean	Free from dirt, dust, grease, waste, food residues and all other foreign visible materials as well as objectionable odor
2.	Contamination	Foods exposed to conditions, which permit: a. Introduction of foreign matters including dust, dirt, chemicals and pests b. Introduction or multiplication of disease-causing microorganisms or parasites c. Introduction or production of toxins
3.	Cross-contamination	Transfer of microorganisms or contaminants from one food (usually raw) to another food either directly when one food touches another, or indirectly through hands or equipment
4.	Equipments	Apparatus, vessels, containers, utensils, machines, instruments or appliances used for storing, handling, cooking and cleaning of food
5.	Food-contact surfaces	Surfaces that will come into contact with food in a food premises
6.	Food handler	Any person who engages in the handling of food, equipments or utensils that will come into contact with food in a food business
7.	Food premises	Any place where food is supplied, prepared, processed, handled, stored, packaged, displayed, served or offered for sale for human consumption
8.	Open food	Uncooked perishable food and food not contained in containers as to exclude risks of contamination
9.	Pathogen	A disease-causing microorganism
10.	Pest	Any animal or insect that may contaminate food or a food contact surface; this includes rats, mice, cockroaches and flies
11.	Potable	Suitable for human to drink or ingest

Contd...

Contd...

Sl No	Term	Description
12.	Potentially hazardous food	Food that requires temperature control to minimize the growth of any pathogenic micro-organisms that may be present or to prevent the formation of toxin
13.	Poultry	Any domesticated bird whether live or dead (chickens, ducks, geese, quails, etc.) commonly used for human consumption
14.	Ready-to-eat food	Food that is ready for immediate consumption at the point of sale; it could be raw or cooked, hot or chilled and can be consumed without further heat treatment
15.	Utensils	Articles, vessels, containers or equipment used in the handling, preparation, processing, packaging, displaying, serving, dispensing, storing, containing or consumption of food

from the production to the consumer. Food hygiene in its widest sense implies hygiene in the production, handling, distribution and serving of all types of food. The primary aim of food hygiene is to prevent food poisoning and other foodborne illnesses, which can be grouped under the following headings.

Milk Hygiene

Milk is an efficient vehicle for a great variety of disease agents, the source of infection or contamination of milk may be the dairy animal, human handler or the environment. For example, a contaminated vessel, polluted water, flies, dusts, etc.

▶ PRINCIPLES OF FOOD SANITATION

1. The food handlers are free from any communicable diseases.
2. Human air, nasal discharge, skin can also be source of microorganisms therefore persons handling food, must wash hands with soap before starting preparation and refrain from touching hair or wiping nose during food preparation.

CHAPTER 5: Food Hygiene/Sanitation

3. Personal hygiene—a high standard of personal hygiene among individuals engaged in the handling, preparation and cooking of food is needed.
4. Food handling techniques—the handling of ready-to-eat food with bare hands should be reduced to a minimum.
5. Sanitary conditions—sanitation of all work surfaces, utensils and equipment must be ensured. Food premises should be kept free from rats, mice, flies and dust.

▶ SOURCES OF FOOD CONTAMINATION

1. Water used for washing or cleaning is not potable.
2. Soil adhering to foods grown close to ground in not completely removed.

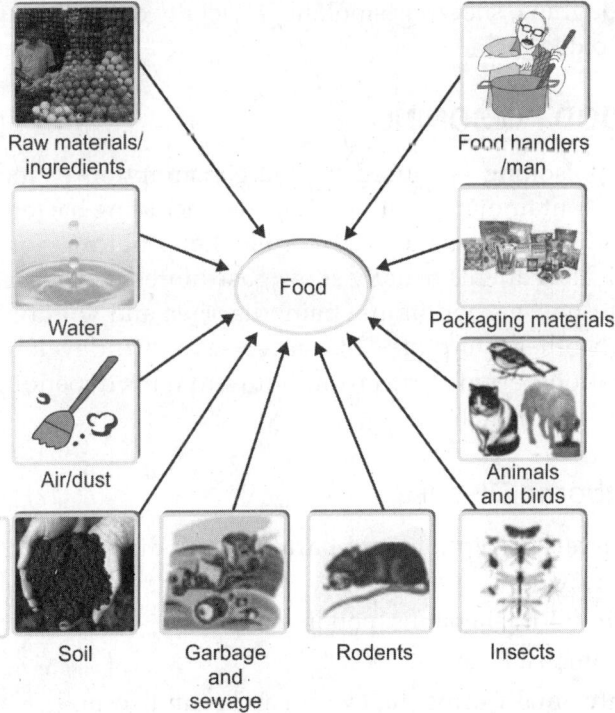

Fig. 5.1: Sources of food contamination

3. Container or utensils used for storage and preparation are not clean.
4. Personnel handling food have unhygienic habits.
5. Personnel handling food suffer from communicable diseases (Fig. 5.1).

Hygienic Practices of Food Handlers

1. Hand should be washed properly and should be clean always.
2. Fingernails should be kept short and free from dirt.
3. Head covering should be used to prevent loose hair falling into the food.
4. Aprons should be worn.
5. Coughing, sneezing, smoking in vicinity of food should be avoided.

▶ FOOD POISONING

Food poisoning is caused by the consumption of food or drinks contaminated with pathogens (including bacteria, viruses and parasites), bacterial or biochemical toxins or toxic chemicals. Patients usually show gastrointestinal symptoms such as nausea, abdominal pain, diarrhea and vomiting, although other symptoms like fever may also develop. The incubation period varies from hours to days depending on the causative agent.

Foodborne Disease

1. **Bacterial:** Typhoid and paratyphoid, diarrhea and dysentery.
2. **Viral:** Viral hepatitis, poliomyelitis.
3. **Protozoa:** Amebas.
4. **Intestinal worms:** Tapeworm and roundworm.
5. **Others:** Food poisoning.

CHAPTER 5: Food Hygiene/Sanitation

Bacterial Food Poisoning

Common Types of Bacterial Food Poisoning

In Hong Kong, bacterial food poisoning caused by pathogenic bacteria is the commonest type of food poisoning. There are various kinds of bacterial food poisoning (Table 5.2), but the following are the most prevalent.

Table 5.2: Various kinds of bacterial food poisoning

Sl No	Name of bacteria	Common foods involved
1.	Salmonella species	Raw or undercooked egg and egg products (e.g. tiramisu), undercooked meat, poultry and their products (e.g. barbecued and preserved meat, goose intestines, etc.)
2.	Staphylococcus aureus	Foods, which have been subject to a large amount of handling with no subsequent cooking or reheating (e.g. lunch boxes, cakes, pastries, sandwiches, etc.)
3.	Vibrio parahaemolyticus	Raw or undercooked seafood, shellfish, marine products and salted food (e.g. jellyfish, cuttlefish, salted vegetables, smoked knuckles, etc.)
4.	Bacillus cereus	Leftover cooked rice, fried rice, meat products and vegetables
5.	Clostridium perfringens	Cross-contaminated and inadequately cooked meat and meat products (e.g. stew, meat pies, etc.)

Common Contributing Factors to Bacterial Food Poisoning

1. **Contamination of cooked food:** Cooked food has been contaminated by food handlers, raw food, food contact surfaces or pests.
2. **Improper storage of cooked food:** Cooked food has been stored between 4°C and 60°C for a prolonged period.
3. **Inadequate cooking of food:** Raw food has not been cooked thoroughly to reduce any pathogen present.

4. **Inadequate reheating of cooked food:** Cooked food has not been reheated to 75°C.
5. **Inadequate thawing of food before cooking:** Insufficiently thawed food, which still has a high bacteria count or pathogen content and which needs a longer time to reach the temperature that kills the bacteria and pathogens in cooking, has not been cooked for sufficiently long time.
6. **Preparation of food too early in advance:** Food has been prepared too early in advance, but has not been stored under proper temperature control.
7. **Infected food handlers:** Food handlers infected with communicable diseases have engaged in handling food.
8. **Consumption of raw food:** Food (e.g. shrimps) that usually has a high bacteria count or pathogen content has been eaten in a raw state without cooking.
9. **Use of unsafe food source:** Food has been purchased from an unapproved or unreliable source such as hawkers.
10. **Use of leftovers:** Use of food leftovers (e.g. cooked rice) that have been stored between 4°C and 6°C for a prolonged period.

Prevention of Bacterial Food Poisoning

In principle, the best way to avoid bacterial food poisoning is to ensure safe food production. Essential measures include the following.

Purchase of food
1. Do not buy foods that are not properly protected (e.g. siu mei and lo mein that has been exposed to the open air during transportation or cooked food that has not been covered properly).
2. Do not purchase food from unlicensed sources, especially for cooked or cold food (because the place and ways in which they cook their foods are usually not hygienic).
3. Do not buy any food, which looks abnormal (e.g. swollen or dented canned foods).

4. Food to be eaten raw, such as sashimi and rock oysters, should be obtained from a reliable and reputable source to ensure their quality.

Handling of food
1. Food should be thoroughly cooked before being served to customers (both meat and marine products should be well-cooked).
2. Cooked food should be prepared and stored separately from raw food (to avoid cross-contamination).
3. Food handlers should thoroughly wash their hands after going to the toilet and before handling food (to prevent the soiled hands from contaminating the food). In any case, do not touch cooked food with bare hands.
4. Anybody suffering from diarrhea, vomiting, sore throat or inflamed wounds (unless properly bandaged with waterproof plastic tapes) should not handle or touch any food, so as to prevent the food from being contaminated by food poisoning bacteria.

Storage of food
1. Food should be served once it is prepared (that means food should be served either hot or cold. Food that is neither hot nor cold is conducive to the growth of bacteria).
2. Leftovers should best be discarded. Otherwise, it should be properly stored in refrigerators (4°C or below) and thoroughly reheated to 75°C or above before being served to customers.
3. Any food that is not to be served immediately should be stored at a temperature below 4°C or above 60°C. Do not store food at room temperature, which is favorable to bacterial growth or production of toxins.

▶ **PRACTICAL RULES FOR FOOD SANITATION**

1. Tie hair neatly before starting food preparation, use hair net or cap if necessary. Wash hands thoroughly with soap and water before starting preparation.

SECTION 1: Nutrition

2. Wash fruits, vegetables, cereals and beans thoroughly before preparation with portable water. Boil milk in a clean container as soon as possible after receipt and keep covered.
3. Use portable water in food preparation.
4. Boil water used for drinking or for preparation of cold beverages, if the purity of water is not guaranteed.
5. Utensils and equipments used for preparation should be scrupulously cleaned.
6. Cooked food should be stored covered, preferably in the container in which it is cooked.
7. Leftover foods such as rice, vegetables should be stored either in a refrigerator or kept in a pan of cold water. Reheating before use is advisable.

▶ **HYGIENE CONTROL**

Hygiene control is essential when working with food. This is because food must be kept safe. This is done by:

1. Protecting food from contamination by harmful bacteria.
2. Preventing bacteria from multiplying to dangerous levels.
3. Destroying harmful bacteria in or on food by thorough cooking.
4. Disposing of harmful food safely.

Basic Rules of Food Hygiene

Always wash hands before touching food, particularly after visiting the toilet, after touching animals and our own skin and hair and after touching raw food:

1. Always cover any break in the skin of hands or sores or spots with a waterproof adhesive dressing (preferably a highly colored one so notice it if it comes off).
2. No smoking during the preparation of food.
3. Avoid preparing food if you have any illness (particularly skin, nose or throat infections and sickness and diarrhea).
4. Do not allow animals into the food preparation area.
5. Cover food to protect it from flies and other insects.

CHAPTER 5: Food Hygiene/Sanitation

6. Wrap all food waste and dispose of it in a covered waste bin.
7. Clean as go. Wash surfaces with hot water and detergent.
8. Wipe spills up immediately with kitchen tissue and place this in a covered bin.
9. Serve food as soon as possible after preparing it.
10. Never allow raw food to come in contact with cooked food; common ways in which cooked food is contaminated from raw food are through the hands, knives and working surfaces.
11. Wear clean clothing and be clean ourselves.
12. Do not cough or sneeze over food.

Temperature Control

Control of temperature is very important in the cooking and storage of food. The Food Safety (temperature control) Regulations, 1995, sets out the safe temperatures for the storage, heating and chilling of food, as given below:

1. Freezer: 18°C–22°C.
2. Refrigerator legal requirement: 8°C; good practice: 5°C–6°C.
3. Hot holding food: Hot food must be maintained at a temperature of 63°C.
4. Reheating of commercially manufactured food that has been cooked once during manufacture and the temperature of reheated food must reach a minimum of 82°C.

Pest Control

A food pest is any animal that can live on or in food, causing damage or contamination. The main types of pests are:

1. Insects such as flies, cockroaches and weevils.
2. Birds.
3. Rodents such as rats and mice.

Flies land on food and carry bacteria on their bodies. In addition, they defecate on food and regurgitate half-digested

SECTION 1: Nutrition

food from a previous meal onto the food. They can also lay eggs and their dead bodies can be found in food.

Cockroaches can deposit feces on food and spread bacteria and small insects such as weevils live in stored foods and food products such as flour and cereals.

Rodents such as mice and rats carry bacteria, and pass these on by either walking on the food or on work surfaces. Mice particularly have a tendency to urinate on food.

Some birds can also carry bacteria. Food can be contaminated by droppings and feathers, and by insects that they carry on their bodies. Some birds will contaminate milk by pecking through the foil tops of bottles left on the doorstep.

Protecting premises where food is stored or manufactured is the most important way of preventing possible infection of or damage to food. The owner of the premises must ensure that the building is kept in good repair with no obvious points of entry for pests. Food pests tend to like warm, dark, damp undisturbed places, so it is important for food storage and preparation areas to be cool, clean and dry.

▶ EFFECTS OF UNSAFE PRACTICES

Food can be contaminated in a variety of ways—both physical and chemical. Physical contaminants include bones, shells or pips and stalks food, food packaging, nut or bolt from equipment, jewelry, hair, fingernails, plasters, dust and dirt, insects and their droppings and eggs.

Chemical contamination can be caused by cleaning chemicals, if they are not kept separate from food and food preparation areas and agricultural chemicals, for example on fruit and vegetables if they have been sprayed. They must be cleaned thoroughly or peeled before eating.

Leftover food or drink from metal containers should always be transferred to a non-metallic container and stored covered in a refrigerator. Acidic and salty food can attack the metal once a can is opened, which then affects the food.

CHAPTER 5: Food Hygiene/Sanitation

Biological contamination is contamination by bacteria or viruses where they multiply on the food to dangerous levels or by molds, which cause toxins on food. When they are eaten, they cause illness.

▶ LEGISLATION, REGULATIONS AND CODES OF PRACTICE

Food safety legislation requires that establishments preparing and serving food ensure that food is safe to eat. Three of the main laws and regulations are detailed below.

Food Safety Act 1990

The Food Safety Act is the main piece of legislation that governs the safety of food. The act says that it is illegal to sell or keep for sale food that is unfit for people to eat or causes food to be dangerous to health or is not of acceptable content or quality or is labeled or advertised in any way that misleads the consumer. If prosecuted, people who work with food must show that they have taken all reasonable steps to avoid causing any of the above.

Food Safety (General Food Hygiene) Regulations 1995

Food Safety Regulations cover the basic hygiene principles that businesses must follow and relate to staff, premises and food handling. They affect anyone who owns manages or works in a food business, whether it is a caravan in a lay-by selling tea, coffee and snacks or a five-star hotel. The regulations cover the following:

1. The supply and selling of food in a hygienic way.
2. Identification of possible food hazards.
3. Control of identified hazards to prevent harm to customers.

4. The establishment of effective control and monitoring procedures to ensure that harm does not come to customers.

Food Safety (Temperature Control) Regulations 1995

Food Safety Regulations cover the following aspects of food hygiene:
1. The stages of the food chain that is subject to temperature controls.
2. The temperatures at which certain foods must be kept.
3. Which foods are exempt from specific temperature controls?
4. When the temperature controls allow flexibility.

The safe temperatures are given under the heading temperature control (page 174).

▶ HAZARD ANALYSIS AND CRITICAL CONTROL POINT

Hazard analysis and critical control point (HACCP) is a universal food safety system. It aims to protect food from contamination by:
1. Identifying critical points in the food handling process that might cause contamination.
2. Putting controls in place to prevent microbiological, chemical and physical contamination of food.
3. Monitoring the critical points to ensure that contamination does not occur.

This means that all potential hazards at each stage of food handling, from delivery of raw products to the serving of fully prepared food, must be identified. The whole process is designed to ensure that any problems can be dealt with before they cause any problems or illness.

► CONCLUSION

The term 'food hygiene' is used to describe the preservation and preparation of foods in a manner that ensures the food is safe for human consumption. This term typically refers to these practices at an individual or family level, whereas the term 'food sanitation' usually refers to these types of procedures at the commercial level within the food industry, such as during production and packaging, or at stores or restaurants. Food hygiene in the home kitchen includes things such as the proper storage of food before use, washing one's hands before handling food, maintaining a clean environment when preparing food and making sure that all serving dishes are clean and free of contaminants. Food hygiene also includes keeping preparation areas clean and germ free. Mixing bowls, spoons, paring knives and any other tools used in the kitchen should be washed thoroughly before they are used, as well as after. Kitchen countertops and cutting boards also should be cleaned and sterilized from time to time. Keeping the workspace is sanitary decreases the chance that food will be contaminated and make people sick. Preventing cross-contamination also is an important aspect of food hygiene.

Chapter 6

Food Adulteration

▶ INTRODUCTION

Adulteration of food consists of a large number of practice, e.g. mixing, substitutions, concealing the quality, putting up decomposed foods for sale, misbranding or giving false labels and addition of toxicants. A good example is addition of water to milk.

Adulteration may be intentional or incidental. The former is willful act on the part of the adulterator intended to increase the margin of profit. Incidental contamination is usually due to ignorance, negligence or lack of proper facilities. Adulteration food may endanger health if the physiological functions of the consumer are affected due to either addition of a deleterious substance or the removal of a vital component.

▶ DEFINITION

Definition of Food

Any article used as food or drink for human consumption other than drugs and water and includes:

1. Any article, which ordinarily enters into or is used in the composition or preparation of human food.
2. Any flavoring matter or condiments.
3. Any other article, which the Central Government may having regard to its use, nature, substance or quality, declare, by notification in the official gazette as food for the purpose of this act.

CHAPTER 6: Food Adulteration

Definition of Adulteration

Adulteration is defined as the process by which the quality or the nature of a given substance is reduced through the addition of a foreign or an inferior substance and the removal of a vital element:

1. If the product sold by a vendor is not of the nature, substance or quality demanded by the purchaser or which it purports to be.
2. If the product offered contains any substance or if it is so processed as to injuriously affect its nature, substance or quality.
3. If any inferior or cheaper substance has been substituted wholly or partly in the product or any natural constituent has been wholly or partly abstracted from it, to affect its quality.
4. If the product had been prepared, packed or kept under unsanitary conditions, has become contaminated, injurious to health or is unfit for human consumption.
5. If the container of the product is composed of any poisonous or deleterious substance, which renders its contents injurious to health.
6. If the product contains any prohibited coloring matter, preservatives or contains any permitted coloring matter or preservatives in excess of the prescribed limits.
7. If the quality or purity of the product falls below the prescribed standard or its constituents are present in proportions other than those prescribed, whether or not rendering it injurious to health.

▶ CONCEPT OF ADULTERATION

An article of food shall be deemed to be adulterated:

1. If the article sold by vendor is not of the nature, substance or quality demanded by the purchaser.
2. If the article contains any other substance, which affects the substance or quality thereof.

SECTION 1: Nutrition

3. If any inferior or cheaper substance has been substituted wholly or in part for the article so as to affect the nature, substance or quality of the product.
4. If any constituent of the article has been wholly or in part extracted to affect the quality thereof.
5. If the article has been prepared, packed or kept under unsanitary conditions whereby it has become contaminated or injurious to health.
6. If the article consists wholly or in part of any filthy, putrefied, rotten, decomposed or diseased animal or vegetable substance or is insect-infested or is otherwise unfit for human consumption.
7. If the article is obtained from a diseased animal.
8. If the article contains any poisonous or other ingredient, which renders it injurious to health.
9. If the container of the article is composed, whether, wholly or in part of any poisonous or deleterious substance, which renders its contents injurious to health.
10. If any coloring matter other than that prescribed in respect thereof is present in the article or if the amounts of the prescribed coloring matter, which is present in the article are not within the prescribed limits.
11. If the article contains any prohibited preservative or permitted preservative in excess of the prescribed limits.
12. If the quality or purity of the article falls below the prescribed limits of variability which renders it injurious to health.
13. If the quality or purity of the article falls below the prescribed standard or its constituents are present in quantities not within the prescribed limits of variability, which renders it injurious to health.

▶ MEANING OF FOOD ADULTERATION

Food adulteration is a growing menace; unscrupulous traders, and manufacture all over the world indulge into exploit gullible consumers to make quick and easy money. In all free market societies where legal control is poor or non-existent with respect to monitoring of food quality by authorities, usage of adulterants is common and rampant. Every nation on earth has suffered cases of adulteration at one time or other. Government authorities with great efforts have succeeded in reducing the recurrent occurrences, but have not been able to eliminate it. Only an aware and an informed consumer will be able to eliminate it conclusively by continuous routine monitoring. The dictionary defines food adulteration as an act of intentionally debasing the quality of food, offered for sale by either the admixture or substitution of inferior substances, or by the removal of some valuable ingredient.

▶ FOOD ADULTERATION AND HEALTH

Food adulteration has become a very common practice in our country and we are consuming these foods almost every day, which have numerous harmful effects to our health. Food adulteration means anything adding or subtracting with food making it injurious to health. This adulteration may be done intentionally or unintentionally. Intentional adulteration is a criminal act and punishable offense. Food adulteration with poisonous chemical like formalin is widespread and regularly applied on fish, fruit, meat and milk product that causes different types of cancers, asthma and skin diseases.

Coloring dyes, calcium carbide, urea, brunt engine oil and even some permitted preservatives are used in excessive amount that affect multiple organs of human body. Mostly it causes cancer-like colon, peptic ulcer diseases and chronic liver diseases including cirrhosis and liver failure, electrolyte imbalance and eventually kidney failure. Heart diseases, blood disorders and bone marrow abnormality are also detected. Chance of malignancy increases and neurological impairment or brain functions are also often compromised. Skin problems are frequently seen including allergic manifestation. We know it is a punishable offense and it creates health hazards and can kill human beings, even then we forget everything just for business interest.

SECTION 1: Nutrition

▶ ADULTERANTS

Any material, which is/could be employed for the purposes of adulteration.

Types

Common types of food adulterants (Table 6.1) are given below:

1. **Intentional:** These adulterants are those substances that are added as a deliberate act on the part of the adulterer with the intention to increase the margin of profit. For example, sand, marble chips, stones, mud, chalk powder, water, dyes, etc. These adulterants cause harmful effects on the body.
2. **Incidental:** These adulterants are found in food substances due to ignorance, negligence or lack of proper facilities. It is not a willful act on the part of the adulterer. Examples include pesticides, droppings of rodents and larvae in food.
3. **Metallic contamination:** Arsenic from pesticides, lead from water, mercury form effluents of chemical industries, tin from cans.

Food Materials and Common Adulterants

- Cereals (wheat and rice): Mud, grits and soapstone bits
- Dal: Coal tar dyes, khesari dal
- Black pepper: Dried seeds of papaya
- Chili powder: Sawdust, brick powder
- Milk: Extraction of fat, addition of starch and water
- Ghee: Vanaspati
- Sweet meats: Non-permitted colors
- Fresh green peas in packing: Green dye
- Coffee powder: Date husk, tamarind husk, chicory
- Tea dust/leaves: Black gram husk, tamarind seeds powder saw dust, used tea dust
- Butter: Starch, animal fat.

CHAPTER 6: Food Adulteration

Table 6.1: Simple tests for the detection of adulterants present in foods

Sl No	Substance	Adulterant	Test
1.	Asafetida (hing)	Resin or gum scented and colored	Pure asafetida dissolves in water to form a milky white solution. Pure asafetida burns with a bright flame on being ignited (burning)
2.	Sugar	Chalk powder	Dissolve in a glass of water; chalk will settle down in the bottom
3.	Cardamom	Oil is removed and pods are coated with talcum powder	On rubbing, talcum will stick to the fingers; on testing, if there is hardly any aromatic flavor, it indicates removal of essential oil
4.	Turmeric (haldi)	Metanil yellow coloring	When concentrated hydrochloric acid is added to a solution of turmeric powder, it turns magenta, if metanil yellow is present
5.	Chili powder	Sawdust and color	Sprinkle on the surface of water, sawdust floats; added color will make the water color
6.	Coffee	Chicory	Shake a small portion in cold water; coffee will float, while chicory will sink, making the water brown
7.	Coriander powder	Horse dung powder	Soak in water; horse dung will float, which can be easily detected
8.	Cloves (lavang)	Oil may be removed	If so, cloves may be shrunken in appearance
9.	Cumin seeds (jeera)	May contain grass seeds colored with charcoal dust	If rubbed in hand, fingers will turn black

Contd...

SECTION 1: Nutrition

Contd...

Sl No	Substance	Adulterant	Test
10.	Ghee	Vanaspati	Dissolve 1 teaspoon of sugar in 10 cc of hydrochloric acid and 10 cc of the melted ghee and shake thoroughly for 1 minute; allow it to stand for 10 minutes; if vanaspati has been added, the aqueous layer will be red in color
11.	Jaggery	Metanil yellow	Hydrochloric acid added to a solution of jaggery will turn its color to magenta
12.	Suji (rava)	Iron filing to add weight	Pass magnet through the suji; iron filings will cling to it
13.	Betel nut powder (supari)	Sawdust and artificial color	Sprinkle in water; sawdust will float and the added color will dissolve in water
14.	Milk	Mashed potato, other starched water	Add a drop of tincture of iodine, which is brown in color, if starch is present, turns blue Put a drop of milk on a polished vertical surface and allow to flow; pure milk flows slowly leaving a white trail, but adulterated milk will flow immediately without leaving a mark
15.	Tea dust	Used tea leaves dried, powdered and artificially colored	Sprinkle the dust on a wet white filter paper; spots of yellow, pink and red appearing on the paper indicates that tea is artificially colored
16.	Edible oil	Argemone	A reddish-brown precipitate is formed when oil and hydrochloric acid are gently mixed with ferric chloride solution, if argemone is present

Contd...

CHAPTER 6: Food Adulteration

Contd...

Sl No	Substance	Adulterant	Test
17.	Saffron	Maize fibers dried, colored and scented	Genuine saffron is tough; spurious saffron is brittle and breaks easily; dissolves easily in water, giving aroma of saffron
18.	Sago	Sand and talcum	Gritty feel in mouth; pure sago swells on burning and leaves hardly any ash
19.	Black pepper	Dried seeds of papaya fruit	Papaya seeds are shrunken oval in shape and greenish-brown in color and have a repulsive flavor distinct from the bite of black pepper
20.	Coconut oil	Any other oil	Place a small bottle of oil in refrigerator; coconut oil solidifies leaving the adulterant as a separate layer
21.	Bajra	Fungus (ergot infested)	Immerse in salt water; fungi will float to the top
22.	Cinnamon (dalchini)	Cassia bark	Added color comes off in water when adulterated cinnamon is added to water
23.	Common salt	White powdered stone, chalk	Stir a spoonful of simple salt in a glass of water; the presence of chalk will make the solution white
24.	Honey	Molasses (sugar and water)	A cotton wick dipped in pure honey when lighted with a match stick burns, if adulterated it will not burn and will produce a cracking sound
25.	Peanut oil	Cottonseed oil	Mix 2.5 mL of oil or fat with 2.5 mL Halphen's reagent; lightly screw cap and heat in boiling water for 30 minutes; the test is positive if a rose color is obtained

SECTION 1: Nutrition

Tests for Detecting Adulterants

Simple tests for the detection of adulterants present in foods are given in Table 6.1 and Figure 6.1.

▶ PACKAGING MATERIALS AND HAZARDS

Materials Used for Packing

The conventional methods of packing, which are prevalent even now to a large extent, are tin or aluminum containers, glass bottles and jars, paper and waxed paper wrappings, paper cartons, cardboard and certain plastic containers. Tin and aluminum containers have become costly and glass bottles though very good in many respects, have problems associated with breakage and heavy transportation charges on account of weight. Continued use of paper in increased volume, dwindles the natural resources.

Against the conventional materials there has emerged increased usage of newer materials derived synthetically. Some polymeric plastic materials are polystyrene, polyvinyl, polyvinylidene and derivatives, vinyl acetate, polyethylene, polypropylene and polyesters.

Folding cartons and paperboard boxes are used extensively in the food industry. Tin plate containers, the cylindrical open top variety are mostly used for processed foods. Aluminum is used principally as foil, e.g. chocolates. It is also used as bottle caps and closures and easy open tops for cans.

Polystyrene is principally made into tubs for ice creams, packs for eggs, sausages and small packages for butter, jam and cheese. Bags made from the simplest of all plastic polymers namely polyethylene or 'polythene', as commonly known have relatively low preserving

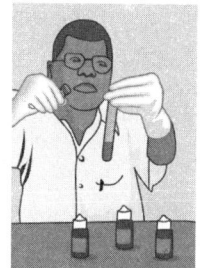

Fig. 6.1: Tests for the detection of adulterants

qualities. Material such as polyesters vinyl acetate derivatives and multilayer films made out of a combination of different materials has good preserving characteristics for food products.

Timber crates are used extensively for packing weights above 100 kg. Plastic crates are well-established in the dairy industry and for the transportation of bottled beer, mineral water and soft drinks. High-density polythene is used for milk crates.

Shrink wrap packaging is a system where heat-shrinkable thermoplastic film is wrapped around an article or a group of articles. The film is made to shrink around it by the application of heat to achieve a skin light package. Canned food products, bottles and jars of all types can be shrinking wrapped.

Nowadays it is expected that packaging material be environment friendly or eco-friendly that is it should not pose many problems for mankind and hazards to the environment. For example, corrugated boxes are eco-friendly and are preferred for exporting. They can be effectively replaced for conventional wooden boxes, which need to destroy the trees. Recyclability of packaging is desirable, so as to preserve the resources of the packaging material for future generations.

Packaging Hazards

Plastics such as cellulose acetate, polyamide, polyethylene, polypropylene and polyvinyl chloride are often used as packing materials because they are light in weight, and are resistant to diffusion due to solvents and high temperatures.

However, care should be taken; only food grade plastic packing materials should be used for packaging foods to prevent the following packaging hazards:

1. Production of noxious thermal breakdown products, which are injurious to health.
2. Formation of toxic residues that result when subjected to heat treatment for sterilization of the contents.
3. Unfavorable reactions between acid and oil content of the food and the packaging material.

SECTION 1: Nutrition

▶ FOOD LAWS AND STANDARDS

Prevention of Food Adulteration Act

Purposes

The Prevention of Food Adulteration (PFA) act, 1954 operated by the Directorate General of Health Services, Ministry of Health was designed for the following purposes:

1. It formulates and monitors the standard of quality and purity of foods, which emphasis 411 on prevention of adulteration of foods.
2. It is the basic structure intended to protect the common consumer against the supply of adulterated foods.
3. It makes provision for prevention of adulteration of food and lays down the rule that no person shall manufacture for sale, store, sell or distribute any adulterated or misbranded food or food, which contravenes the provision of act or rules.
4. It has set the yardstick to ascertain adulteration. According to this act, a food is deemed to be adulterated, if:
    a. It is not of the nature, substance and quality, which the food ought to be.
    b. It contains any other substance, which affects or if the article is so processed so as to affect injuriously the nature, substance and quality of the food.
    c. It contains added inferior or cheaper substance that affects the nature and quality of the food.
    d. Any constituent of the food is removed so as to affect injuriously the nature, quality and substance of the food.
    e. It is prepared, packed and stored under unsanitary conditions.
    f. It contains any filthy, disgusting, rotten, decomposed substance of a diseased animal or vegetable substance or is insect infested or otherwise unfit for human consumption.

g. The article is obtained from a diseased animal.
h. The article contains a poisonous ingredient or any other ingredient injurious to health.
i. The container renders the food injurious to health.
j. It contains excessive or prohibited colors.
k. It contains excessive or prohibited preservatives.
l. It does not satisfy the standards prescribed by the authorities.

Rules

Under the provision of the PFA act, the Government of India has promulgated PFA rules, which specify the following details:

1. Qualification, duties and functions of food analysts, food inspectors and central food laboratory.
2. Procedure for drawing test samples and sending them to the analyst and laboratory.
3. Specification for the identity and purity of food.
4. Tolerance for contaminants, preservatives, emulsifiers and other additives.

Objectives

1. To protect the public from poisonous and harmful foods.
2. To prevent the sale of substandard foods.
3. To protect the interests of the consumers by eliminating fraudulent practices.

Amended Prevention of Food Adulteration Act

The PFA act was amended in 1964, 1976 and lately in 1986 to make the act more stringent. A minimum imprisonment of 6 months with minimum fine of ₹ 1,000 is envisaged under the act for cases to proven adulteration, whereas for the cases of adulteration, which may render the food injurious to cause death or such harm, which may amount to grievous hurt (within the meaning of section 320 of IPC) the punishment may go up to life imprisonment and fine, which shall not less than ₹ 5,000.

Agmark Standard

The word 'Agmark' is derived from the words 'agricultural marketing'. It is a standard of quality based on the physical and chemical characteristics of food, both the natural and those acquired during processing. Products graded under Agmark include vegetable oils, ghee, butter, rice, groundnut, pulses and spices. These standards ensure accurate weight and correct selling price.

Bureau of Indian Standards

The Bureau of Indian Standards (BIS) lays down criteria for standardization of vegetables and fruit products, spices and condiments, animal products and processed food. Manufacturers are allowed to use the BIS label on each unit of their product, if their products conform to the standards laid down by BIS. The products are checked for quality by laboratories certified by BIS. BIS is also known as Indian Standard Institution (ISI).

Some of the items, which require compulsory BIS certification under PFA act include artificial food colors, natural food colors, food additives, infant formula; milk- and cereal-based weaning foods, milk powder and condensed milk.

▶ CONSUMER PROTECTION

A number of laboratories are authorized by the central government to collect samples of food suspected to the adulteration and analyze them. They can prosecute the manufacturers of these foods if they find the food to be adulterated. The various laboratories engaged in the collection of samples and analyses of such food are given below:

1. Municipal laboratories in big cities.
2. Food and Drug Administration laboratories of states.
3. Central Food Testing Laboratory of the Government of India.
4. Laboratories of the Export Inspection Council.
5. Central Grain Analysis Laboratory.

CHAPTER 6: Food Adulteration

Food adulteration is a social evil. The general public has lack of awareness of the dangers of adulteration and disinterest it occurs continuously. Unless the public rises up against the trades and unscrupulous food inspectors, the evil cannot be curbed.

▶ SALE OF CERTAIN ADMIXTURES IS PROHIBITED

Sale by themselves or by their servant or agent is prohibited in case of:
1. Cream, which has not been prepared exclusively from milk or, which contains less than 25% of milk fat.
2. Milk, which contains added water.
3. Ghee, which contains any added matter not exclusively derived from milk fat.
4. Selling skimmed milk as whole milk.
5. Mixture of two or more edible oils as edible oil.
6. Vanaspati to which ghee or any other substance has been added.
7. Any article of food, which contains any artificial sweetener beyond the prescribed limit.
8. Turmeric containing any foreign substance.
9. Mixture of coffee and other substance except chicory.
10. Dahi or curd not made out of milk.
11. Milk or milk products containing constituents other than of milk.

▶ PROCEDURES FOR SAMPLING AND ANALYSIS

Any food inspector can enter and inspect any place where any article of food is manufactured or stored for sale, or stored for the manufacture of any other article of food for sale or exposed or exhibited for sale or where any adulterant is manufactured or kept and take samples of such article of food or adulterant for analysis:

SECTION 1: Nutrition

1. Notice will be issued by the inspector in writing then and there to the seller indicating his/her intention.
2. Three samples are taken and the signature of the seller is affixed to them.
3. One sample is sent for analysis to public analyst under intimation to the local health authority.
4. The other two samples are sent to the local health authority for further reference.

▶ PENALTIES

Guilt will be punished with imprisonment for a term, which shall not be less than 6 months and up to 3 years and with fine up to ₹ 1,000.

▶ IMPORTANT MISCELLANEOUS PROVISIONS

1. If any extraneous additions of coloring matter, the same should be indicated on the labels.
2. From the labels the blending composition of ingredients should be clear to the customer.
3. Sale of khesari gram individually or as an admixture is prohibited.
4. Prohibition of use of carbide (acetylene) gas in ripening is prohibited.
5. Sale of ghee with Reichert value less than the permitted level.
6. Sale of admixture of ghee or butter is prohibited.
7. Addition of artificial sweetener should be mentioned on the label.
8. Sale of food colors without license prohibited.
9. Sale of insect damaged dry fruits and nuts prohibited.
10. Food prepared in rusted containers, chipped enamel containers and untinned copper/brass utensils are treated as unfit for human consumption.
11. Containers not made of plastic material, which is not according to the standards are not to be used.

CHAPTER 6: Food Adulteration

12. Selling sal seed for or any other purpose except for bakery and confectionery is prohibited.
13. Store of insecticides in the same premises where food articles are stored is prohibited.
14. Milk powder or condensed milk can be sold only with ISI mark.
15. Use of more than one type of preservative is prohibited.
16. Crop contaminants beyond certain specified level is treated as adulterant.
17. Naturally occurring toxic substances in the food material beyond certain level is considered as unfit for human consumption.
18. No antioxidant, emulsifiers and stabilizing agent is permitted beyond the prescribed level.
19. No insecticides should be sprayed on the food items.
20. Oils can be manufactured only in factories licensed for such purpose.

▶ CONCLUSION

Food adulteration, act of intentionally debasing the quality of food offered for sale either by the admixture or substitution of inferior substances, or by the removal of some valuable ingredient. Adulteration in food is normally present in its most crude form; prohibited substances are either added, or partly or wholly substituted. In India normally the contamination/adulteration in food is done either for financial gain or due to carelessness and lack in proper hygienic condition of processing, storing, transportation and marketing. This ultimately results that the consumer is either cheated or often become victim of diseases. Such types of adulteration are quite common in developing countries or backward countries. However, adequate precautions taken by the consumer at the time of purchase of such produce can make them alert to avoid procurement of such food. It is equally important for the consumer to know the common adulterants and their effect on health.

Chapter 7

Cooking Methods

▶ INTRODUCTION

Food preparation is an important step in meeting the nutritional needs of the family. Food has to be pleasing in appearance and tasty in order to be consumed. Foods like fruits, vegetables and nuts can be eaten raw, but most foods are cooked to bring about desirable changes. The process of subjecting food to the action of heat is termed as cooking. In cooking, there are some basic methods of cooking that are used. These commonly used basic cooking methods are divided into two general groups. The groups are:

1. Dry heat cookery methods.
2. Moist heat cookery methods.

The methods of cooking are divided into these two groups because of the way food is cooked and the type of heat that is used. Different types of kitchen appliances shown in Figure 7.1.

▶ OBJECTIVES OF COOKING

1. Cooking sterilizes food: Above 40°C the growth of bacteria decreases rapidly. Hence food is made safe for consumption.

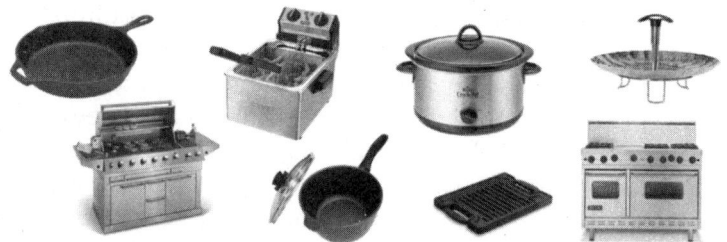

Fig. 7.1: Different types of kitchen appliances

2. Cooking softens the connective tissues of meat and the coarse fiber of cereals, pulses and vegetables. So that, the digestive period is shortened and the gastrointestinal tract is less subjected to irritation.
3. Palatability and food quality is improved by cooking: Appearance, flavor, texture and taste of food are enhanced while cooking.
4. Introduces variety: Different dishes can be prepared with the same ingredients, for example, rice can be made into biryani and kheer.
5. Increases food consumption: Cooking brings about improvement in texture and flavor, thereby increasing consumption of food.
6. Increases availability of nutrients: For example, in raw egg, avidin binds biotin making it unavailable to the body. By cooking, avidin gets denatured and biotin is made available.

▶ DIFFERENT METHODS OF COOKING

Heat is transferred to the food during cooking by conduction, convection, radiation or microwave energy. Cooking takes place by moist and dry heat. Moist heat involves water and steam. Air or fat are used in dry heat.

Moist Heat Methods

Boiling

Boiling is the most common method of cooking and is also the simplest. With this method of cooking, enough water is added to food and it is then cooked over the fire. The action of the heated water makes the food to get cooked. The liquid is usually thrown away after the food is cooked. In the case of cooking rice, all the water is absorbed by the rice grains to make it get cooked. During the heating process, the nutrients can get lost or destroyed and the flavor can be reduced with this method of cooking. If cabbage is overcooked, all the nutrients can get lost. Boiling is a method of cooking foods by just immersing them in water at 100°C and maintaining the water at that temperature till the food is tender. Rice, egg, dal, meat, roots and tubers are cooked by boiling.

Merits: The following are the merits of boiling:
1. Simple method: It does not require special skill and equipment.
2. Uniform cooking can be achieved.

Demerits: The following are the demerits of boiling:
1. Continuous excessive boiling leads to damage in the structure and texture of food.
2. Loss of heat-labile nutrients such as B and C vitamins, if the water is discarded.
3. Time consuming: Boiling takes more time to cook food and fuel may be wasted.
4. Loss of color: Water-soluble pigments may be lost.

Stewing

In stewing process of cooking, food is cooked using a lot of liquid. Different kinds of vegetables are chopped, diced or cubed and added to the pot. Sometimes pieces of selected meat, fish or chicken is also chopped and added to the stew. The liquid is slightly thickened and stewed food is served in that manner. This method is also used, when preparing fruits that are going to be served as desserts. With this cooking method, every food is cooked together at the same time in one pot. The flavor, colors, shapes and textures of the different vegetables that are used, makes stewing a handy method of cooking. The only disadvantage is that some of the vegetables might be overcooked and thus, the nutrient content becomes much less. It is therefore important that vegetables, which take the longest time to cook, to be put into the pot first and the ones that need least cooking time to be put in last. In this way, much of the nutrient contents of the food do not get lost.

It refers to the simmering of food in a pan with a tight-fitting lid using small quantities of liquid to cover only half the food. This is a slow method of cooking. The liquid is brought to boiling point and the heat is reduced to maintain simmering temperatures (82°C–90°C). The food above the liquid is cooked by the steam generated within the pan. Apple, meat along with roots, vegetables and legumes are usually stewed.

Merits: The following are the merits:
1. Loss of nutrients is avoided as water used for cooking is not discarded.
2. Flavor is retained.

Demerits: The process is time consuming and there is wastage of fuel.

Steaming

To steam food, water is added to a pot and then a stand is placed inside the pot. The water level should be under the stand and not above it. There is no contact between the food and the water that is added to the pot. Food is then placed on the stand and heat is applied. The hot steam rising from the boiling water acts on the food and the food gets cooked. It is the hot steam that cooks the food, as there is no contact between the food and the water inside the pot. This method of cooking vegetables is very good as the food does not lose its flavor and much of the nutrients are not lost during the cooking.

It is a method of cooking food in steam generated from vigorously boiling water in a pan. The food to be steamed is placed in a container and is not in direct contact with the water or liquid. Idli, custard and idiyappam are made by steaming. Vegetables can also be steamed.

Merits: As follows:
1. Less chance of burning and scorching.
2. Texture of food is better as it becomes light and fluffy, e.g. idli.
3. Cooking time is less and fuel wastage is less.

4. Steamed foods like idli and idiyappam contain less fat and are easily digested and are good for children, aged and for therapeutic diets.
5. Nutrient loss is minimized.

Demerits: The following are the demerits of steaming:
1. Steaming equipment is required.
2. This method is limited to the preparation of selected foods.

Pressure Cooking

When steam, under pressure is used, the method is known as pressure cooking and the equipment used is the pressure cooker. In this method, the temperature of boiling water can be raised above 100°C. Rice, dal, meat, roots and tubers are usually pressure cooked.

Merits: As follows:
1. Cooking time is less compared to other methods.
2. Nutrient and flavor loss is minimized.
3. Conserves fuel and time, as different items can be cooked at the same time.
4. Less chance for burning and scorching.
5. Constant attention is not necessary.

Demerits: As follows:
1. The initial investment may not be affordable to everybody.
2. Knowledge of the usage, care and maintenance of cooker is required to prevent accidents.
3. Careful watch on the cooking time is required to prevent overcooking.

Poaching

Poaching is an incredibly versatile cooking method; just about everything from fruits to meats can be cooked using this technique. Poaching is merely simmering food in liquid, until it is cooked thoroughly.

As with baking, the density of the food will determine the cooking duration time. Fish is cooked for a short amount of time in liquid that is gradually heated, while denser meats cook longer starting with a cold liquid. The key to poaching meats and proteins is to make sure that the stove temperature is not too high, as this will cause the meat to breakdown, resulting in a greasy meal. Because eggs cook quickly, the liquid is first brought to a boil then turned off. Then, the eggs are added and covered until cooked to the desired doneness. This involves cooking in the minimum amount of liquid at temperatures of 80°C–85°C that is below the boiling point, egg and fish can be poached.

Merits: As follows:
1. No special equipment is needed.
2. Quick method of cooking and therefore saves fuel.
3. Poached foods are easily digested, since no fat is added.

Demerits: These are as follows:
1. Poached foods may not appeal to everybody as they are bland in taste.
2. Food can get scorched, if water evaporates due to careless monitoring.
3. Water-soluble nutrients may be leached into the water.

Blanching

In meal preparation, it is often necessary only to peel off the skin of fruits and vegetables without making them tender. This can be achieved by blanching. In this method, food is dipped in boiling water for 5 seconds to 2 minutes depending on the texture of the food. This helps to remove the skin or peel without softening food.

Blanching can also be done by pouring enough boiling water on the food to immerse it for some time or subjecting food to boiling temperatures for short period and then immediately immersing in cold water. The process causes the skin to become loose and can be peeled off easily.

SECTION 1: Nutrition

Merits: The following are the merits of blanching:
1. Peels can easily be removed to improve digestibility.
2. Destroys enzymes that bring about spoilage.
3. Texture can be maintained, while improving the color and flavor of food.

Demerit: Loss of nutrients, if cooking water is discarded.

Dry Heat Methods

In dry heat cooking methods, the food being cooked does not use water to cook the food. The food is left dry and heat is applied to cook the food. Such methods of cooking are baking, steaming, grilling and roasting. When heat is applied to the food, the food cooks in its own juice or the water added to the food during its preparation evaporates during the heating process and this cooks the food. Heat is applied directly to the food by way of convection thus making the food to get cooked. The action or movement of air around the food cooks it.

Roasting

With roasting, direct heat is applied to the food. The heat seals the outside part of the food and the juice inside the food cooks the food. Roasting is mainly used when cooking fleshy food like fish, meat or chicken. When heat is applied to the outer covering of the food, it seals it up thereby trapping all the juices inside the food. The action of direct heating, heats up the juices inside the food, which then cooks the food. Again there is very little nutrient lost and the flavor is not spoiled. Food is frequently rotated over the spit so that there is even heating applied to all parts of the food. This is so that heat is applied evenly to the food to make it get cooked properly. In this method, food is cooked in a heated metal or frying pan without covering it, e.g. groundnut.

Merits: These are as follows:
1. Quick method of cooking

2. It improves the appearance, flavor and texture of the food.
3. Spices are easily powdered, if they are first roasted.

Demerits: These are as follows:
1. Food can get scorched due to carelessness.
2. Roasting denatures proteins reducing their availability.

Grilling

There are two methods of grilling that are used these days. One type of grilling is the one that is commonly used by the people in the village. This is when food is cooked over hot charcoal on an open fire. The food is placed on top of the burning charcoal. Sometimes people improvise by using wire mesh and place it over the open fire to grill fish or vegetables. The other method is using grills that are inbuilt in stoves. In this method, the griller, which has a tray, is heated up and the food is placed on the grill tray to cook. The heat can be gas generated or electric generated depending on the type of stove used. The food is again left to cook on the grill with the doors of the grill open. People who can afford to buy a stove would use the grilling part to grill their food. What happens in this type of cooking, the heat seals the outside part of the food and the juice inside the food cooks it. The flavor of the food is not lost and much of the nutrients are not lost either. Food is frequently turned over to prevent it from burning and to ensure that equal heating and cooking time is applied to both sides of the food. By doing this, the food is cooked evenly and thoroughly. Grilling or broiling refers to the cooking of food by exposing it to direct heat. In this method food is placed above or in between a red-hot surface. Papads, corn, phulkas, chicken can be prepared by this method.

Merits: These are as follows:
1. Enhances flavor, appearance and taste of the product.
2. It requires less time to cook.
3. Minimum fat is used.

Demerit: Constant attention is required to prevent charring.

SECTION 1: Nutrition

Toasting

Toasting is a method, where food is kept between two heated elements to facilitate browning on both sides. Bread slices are cooked by toasting.

Merits: The following are the merits of toasting:
1. Easy and quick method.
2. Flavor improved.

Demerits: The following are the demerits of toasting:
1. Special equipment required.
2. Careful monitoring is needed to prevent charring.

Baking

In baking method of cooking, the food is cooked using convection heating. The food is put into an enclosed area where heat is then applied and the movement of heat within the confined space, acts on the food that make it get cooked. In this method, the food gets cooked in an oven or oven like appliance by dry heat. The temperature range maintained in an oven is 120°C–260°C.

The food is usually kept uncovered in a container greased with a fat-coated paper. Bread, cake, biscuits, pastries and meat are prepared by this method.

Merits: These are as follows:
1. Baking lends a unique-baked flavor to foods.
2. Foods become light and fluffy, e.g. cakes, custards, bread.
3. Certain foods can be prepared only by this method, e.g. bread, cakes.
4. Uniform and bulk cooking can be achieved, e.g. bun, bread.
5. Flavor and texture are improved.
6. Variety of dishes can be made.

Demerits: These are as follows:
1. Special equipment like oven is required.

2. Baking skills are necessary to obtain a product with ideal texture, flavor and color characteristics.
3. Careful monitoring needed to prevent scorching.

Sautéing

Sautéing is a method in which food is lightly tossed in little oil just enough to cover the base of the pan. The pan is covered with a lid and the flame or intensity of heat is reduced. The food is allowed to cook till tender in its own steam. The food is tossed occasionally or turned with a spatula to enable all the pieces to come in contact with the oil and get cooked evenly.

The product obtained by this method is slightly moist and tender, but without any liquid or gravy. Foods cooked by sautéing are generally vegetables, which are used as side dishes in a menu. Sautéing can be combined with other methods to produce variety in meals.

Merits: These are as follows:
1. It takes less time.
2. It is a simple technique.
3. Minimum oil is used.

Demerit: Constant attention is needed as there is chance of scorching or burning.

Frying

In this method, the food to be cooked is brought into contact with larger amount of hot fat. When food is totally immersed in hot oil, it is called deep-fat frying. Samosa, chips, pakora are examples of deep-fat fried foods. In shallow-fat frying, only a little fat is used and the food is turned in order that both sides are browned, e.g. omelette, cutlets, parathas.

When food is fried using oil or solid fat, it is important that you observe some rules in handling oil or fat. Simple rules to follow when frying:
1. Make sure there is enough oil or fat put in the frying pan or a deep frying pan.

SECTION 1: Nutrition

2. The food to be cooked must not have water dripping from it. This is because, when water comes into contact with hot oil or fat, one will find the oil sizzling and spitting out of the pan, which could burn the skin, if one is not careful.
3. Put the food into the hot oil carefully. Try not to make a big splash as the oil could burn the skin.
4. The oil or fat should be heated at the right temperature before putting food into the pan to be fried. If the food is put in when the oil or fat is not heated to the right temperature, the food will soak up the oil and the food is all oily or greasy. If the oil or fat is over heated, one will end up with food that is burnt. Sometimes, the food especially doughnuts will turn brown on the outside, but the dough inside is uncooked. To cook food using the frying method, there are two ways of doing it. That is the shallow, frying and the deep frying methods.

Shallow frying: In this method, food is cooked in a frying pan with a little amount of oil or fat. The oil or fat is heated to the correct amount and the food is put into the heated oil. The food is turned over a few minutes or is stirred around a couple of times before it is cooked and dished out. If patties, potato chips or coated foods are fried, it is best to put a piece of brown paper or paper napkin inside the tray to soak up any oil from the food before serving it.

Deep frying: This is when a lot of oil or fat is used in cooking the food. The oil or fat is usually put into a deep pan and is heated to boiling point. Food is then put into the hot boiling oil and is cooked in that way. Such food as fish fingers, potato chips, meat balls and doughnuts to name a few, are cooked using the deep-frying method.

Merits: These are as follows:
1. Very quick method of cooking.
2. The calorific values of food are increased, since fat is used as the cooking media.
3. Frying lends a delicious flavor and attractive appearance to foods.
4. Taste and textures are improved.

Demerits: These are as follows:
1. Careful monitoring is required as food easily gets charred, when the smoking temperature is not properly maintained.
2. The food may become soggy due to too much oil absorption.
3. Fried foods are not easily digested.
4. Repeated use of heated oils will have ill effects on health.

▶ COMBINATION OF COOKING METHODS

Braising

Braising is a combined method of roasting and stewing in a pan with a tight-fitting lid. Flavorings and seasonings are added, and food is allowed to cook gently. Food preparations prepared by combination methods are:

1. Upma: Roasting and boiling.
2. Cutlet: Boiling and deep frying.
3. Vermicelli payasam: Roasting and simmering.

Microwave Cooking

Microwaves are electromagnetic waves of radiant energy with wavelengths in the range of $250 \times 10^6 – 7.5 \times 10^9$ Å.

The most commonly used type of microwave generator is an electronic device called magnetron, which generates radiant energy of high frequency. A simple microwave oven consists of a metal cabinet into which the magnetron is inserted. The cabinet is equipped with a metal fan that distributes the microwave throughout the cabinet. Food placed in the oven is heated by microwaves from all directions.

Moist foods and liquid foods can be rapidly heated in such ovens. Food should be kept in containers made of plastic, glass or chinaware, which do not contain metallic substances. These containers are used because they transmit the microwaves, but do not absorb or reflect them.

SECTION 1: Nutrition

Merits

1. Quick method, 10 times faster than conventional method. So loss of nutrients can be minimized.
2. Only the food gets heated and the oven does not get heated.
3. Food gets cooked uniformly.
4. Leftovers can be reheated without changing the flavor and texture of the product.
5. Microwave cooking enhances the flavor of food because it cooks quickly with little or no water.

Demerits

1. Baked products do not get a brown surface.
2. Microwave cooking cannot be used for simmering, stewing or deep frying.
3. Flavors of all ingredients do not blend well as the cooking time is too short.

Solar Cooking

Solar cooking is a very simple technique that makes use of sunlight or solar energy, which is a non-conventional source of energy. Solar cooker consists of a well-insulated box, which is painted black on the inside and covered with one or more transparent covers.

The purpose of these transparent covers is to trap heat inside the solar cooker. These covers allow the radiation from the sun to come inside the box, but do not allow the heat from the hot black absorbing plate to come out of the box. Because of this, temperature up to 140°C can be obtained, which is adequate for cooking.

Merits

1. Simple technique; requires no special skill.
2. Cost-effective, as natural sunlight is the form of energy.

3. Original flavor of food is retained.
4. There is no danger of scorching or burning.
5. Loss of nutrients is minimum as only little amounts of water is used in cooking.

Demerits
1. Special equipment is needed.
2. Slow cooking process.
3. Cannot be used in the absence of sunlight—rainy season, late evening and night.

▶ CONCLUSION

There are many ways to cook food. The outcome of a dish varies nearly as much through cooking methods as it does through the ingredients. Different cultures tend to have their own unique ways of cooking. These differences often come from historical necessities. In cooking, there are some basic methods of cooking that are used. These commonly used basic cooking methods are divided into two general groups. The groups are such as dry heat cookery methods and moist heat cookery methods. The methods of cooking are divided into these two groups because of the way food is cooked and the type of heat that is used. As a rule, rapid cooking techniques are better for retaining nutrients than slower methods. For healthiest results, most experts recommend cooking food thoroughly, but rapidly.

Chapter 8

Food Preservation

▶ INTRODUCTION

Food is the basic necessity of man and is invaluable for healthy existence. However, most foods fit for consumption undergo deterioration and spoilage. In order to combat this problem foods have to be preserved.

Food preservation can be defined as the science that deals with the process of prevention of decay or spoilage of food; thus allowing it to be stored in a fit condition for future use. Preservation of food increases the shelf life of foods, and thus ultimately ensures its supply during times of scarcity and natural drought.

▶ FOOD SPOILAGE

Food spoilage is a state in which food is deprived of its good or effective qualities. Deterioration or spoilage starts from the time, food is harvested, slaughtered or manufactured, and results in undesirable changes in the physical and chemical characteristics of food.

Causes of Food Spoilage

1. Growth and activity of microorganisms such as bacteria, yeast and molds.
2. Activities of food enzymes and other chemical reactions within the food.
3. Inappropriate temperatures for a given food.
4. Gain or loss of moisture.
5. Reaction with oxygen and light.

CHAPTER 8: Food Preservation 213

6. Physical stress or abuse.
7. Insects and rodents.
8. Non-enzymatic reactions in food such as oxidation and mechanical damage.

▶ PRINCIPLES OF FOOD PRESERVATION

Prevention or Delay of Microbial Decomposition

1. By keeping out microorganisms (asepsis).
2. By removal of microorganisms (filtration).
3. By hindering the growth and activity of microorganisms, e.g. refrigeration, dehydration, addition of chemical preservatives.
4. By killing microorganisms, e.g. boiling, irradiation.

Prevention or Delay of Self-decomposition of Food

1. By destruction or inactivation of enzymes, e.g. by blanching. Steaming or boiling of fruits or vegetables in water for few minutes to inactivate natural enzymes, and facilitate removal of skin is known as blanching.
2. By prevention or delay of purely chemical reactions, e.g. prevention of oxidation by the use of antioxidants.
3. Prevention of damage caused by insects, animals and mechanical causes.

▶ METHODS OF FOOD PRESERVATION

A perusal of the history of food preservation reveals that food preservation had its beginning from time immemorial and could be traced to nearly a thousand years ago. Salting of meat, fish and vegetables was the oldest method of preservation, and could be traced back to the ancient Egypt and Greek civilizations.

Pickling in salt and vinegar, sun drying and preservation of fruits and vegetables in sugar and honey were among the other methods used. Storage of food in frozen conditions was also practiced for centuries in places where freezing temperatures were recorded. The discovery of canning as a standard technique of preserving foods in sealed containers subject to high temperature was established in 1810 by Nicolas Appert. Around 1860, Louis Pasteur discovered that microbes were the main cause of spoilage and introduced a heat treatment known as pasteurization to the world.

All methods used for food preservation are based on preventing or retarding the cause of spoilage. When growth of microorganism is retarded, preservation is temporary, but when spoilage organisms are completely destroyed, a more permanent preservation is achieved.

Commercial Methods of Preservation

Commercially, the food preservation technique depicts the following processes.

Canning and Bottling

Canning involves the process of preserving food in sealed containers by the application of heat. Primarily, it is based on the principle of sterilization. Firstly, all the microorganisms present in the food are killed by the application of heat at 275°F–350°F and then sealed in simultaneously sterilized airtight containers to prevent any further attack of microorganism. Fruits, vegetables, fruit juices, pickles, cheese, butter, meat, fish, etc. are generally canned or bottled.

The details of canning procedures vary with the nature of the food to be canned, but there are certain important operations common to canning of all foods:

1. Cleaning.
2. Blanching.
3. Exhausting.
4. Sealing the container.
5. Sterilizing the sealed container.
6. Cooling the container.

Cleaning: The first step in canning, whether done in the home or on a large scale in factories, is the thorough cleaning of the raw food to be preserved. By this means, most of the spoilage organisms are removed. On a large scale, cleaning is done with the help of various kinds of washers. The raw materials may be subjected to high-pressure sprays or strong-flowing streams of water, while passing along a moving belt.

Blanching: It consists of the immersion of raw food materials, especially vegetables and fruits into hot water or exposure to live steam. Blanching serves as an additional hot water wash. It softens fibrous plant tissues, inhibits the action of enzymes and fixes the natural color of certain products, making them more attractive in appearance.

Exhausting: Gases are expelled by passing the open can, containing the food through an exhaust box in which hot water or steam is used to expand the food, and expel air and other gases from the contents and the headspace area. After the gases are expelled, the can is immediately sealed, heat processed and cooled. In the case of certain products, exhausting is done by mechanical means, rather than by the use of heat. There are special machines, which withdraw the air from the cans and they seal them at the same time—'vacuum packing'.

Sealing the container: Each container must be sealed properly before it is subjected to the heat process, since recontamination of the contents must be prevented.

Sterilizing the sealed container: With its contents is done by heat processing. This is meant to bring about complete sterilization to prevent spoilage of the food by microorganisms. This is usually done by the application of steam under pressure.

The temperature and time used for heat processing depend on the kind of food, on the pH of the medium and other factors. It should however be remembered that an excessive period of heating at higher temperatures than necessary, will spoil the product. A longer exposure to a relatively low temperature should be preferred to a short exposure at a higher temperature.

SECTION 1: Nutrition

Cooling the container: The containers should be cooled rapidly to check the action of heat and prevent unnecessary softening of the food or change in color of the contents. Cooling can be done by means of air or water.

Machine Drying

Dehydration in sunlight is an ancient and the lengthiest process of preserving food, practiced at every home. Understanding the difficulties of this process of preserving food, scientists have invented different machines to be used for different foodstuffs, where are dried at different temperatures. Commercially, special types of steamrollers are used for drying milk for reducing it to powder. Similarly, special ovens are used for drying vegetables at a specific temperature. It is found that this method of preservation is better than those of the traditional method of drying food in sunlight.

Freeze-drying

Freeze-drying method of preserving food is adapted to overcome the difficulties of machine or sunlight drying. During drying vegetables or fruits by sunlight or by machine, food are too much squeezed and do not take the original shape when it is in use. In order to overcome this defect, the process of freeze-drying was invented. In this process, foodstuffs is kept at a temperature of -20°C for about 12 hours, so that the water content of the foodstuffs are converted to ice particles. Then it is dried up by machine under low pressure. When it is to be used, it is dipped in hot water. This method retains the shape of the foodstuffs, which is damaged by machine-drying process.

Cold Storage

Cold storage system has become one of the most popular methods of preserving foodstuffs in rural and urban areas of today. Many seasonal fruits and vegetables are stored in cold storages, and according to the demand of the market; they are carried to the place of requirement. This method is based on the principle of refrigeration. Mostly, vegetables, fruits, eggs, meat and fish are kept in cold storages.

Pasteurization

Pasteurization process is applicable to milk only. In this method, milk is boiled at 160°F and then immediately cooled at 55°F. Normally, milk is pasteurized on a large scale to safeguard against any bacterial infection. The process aims at destroying the bacteria and inactivating the rest ones. The pasteurized milk is filled in sterilized bottles, which are sealed. It could be preserved for 5–6 days, and the color and flavor of pasteurized milk does not change in the process, as what happens with the boiled milk.

Irradiation

Irradiation is a new technique of preservation, which is at the stage of experimentation. The WHO has advised the use of this process, only in the case of wheat, onions and potatoes. In this process, γ-rays or high-speed electrons are used to destroy microorganism. These radiations are termed as ionizing radiations. The best advantage of this process is that the food can be stored without refrigeration.

Use of Antibiotics

Use of antibiotics is another method of preservation now under study. Uses of antibiotics in foodstuffs have considerably increased during these days. When fish and poultry are treated with antibiotics, their self-life increases two to three times, because of the reduced growth of the microorganisms. Similarly antibiotics are used in the ice crush, which is used for packing raw fish and shellfish.

Uses of Low and High Temperatures

Use of Low Temperatures

Microbial growth and enzyme reaction are retarded in food stored at low temperature. The lower the temperature is greater the retardation. The low temperature can be employed that are:

SECTION 1: Nutrition

1. Cellar storage temperature (about 15°C).
2. Refrigerator or chilling temperature (0°C–5°C).
3. Freezing temperature (-18°C to 40°C).

Cellar storage temperatures (about 15°C): Temperature in cellars (underground rooms) where surplus food is stored in many villages are usually not much below that of the outside air and is seldom lower than 15°C. The temperature is not low enough to prevent the action of many spoilage organisms or of the plant enzymes. Decomposition is however, slowed down considerably. Root crops, potatoes, onions, apples and similar foods can be stored for limited periods during the winter months.

Refrigerator or chilling temperature (0°C–5°C): This (refrigerator) temperature is obtained and maintained by means of ice or mechanical refrigeration. Fruits and vegetables, meats, poultry, fresh milk and milk products, fish and eggs can be preserved from 2 days to week, when held at this temperature. In addition to the foods mentioned above, foods prepared for serving or leftover may also be stored in the household refrigerator. The best storage temperature for many foods, eggs, etc. is slightly above 0°C.

The optimum temperature of storage varies with the product and is fairly specific for any given food. Besides temperature, the relative humidity and the composition of the atmosphere can affect the preservation of the food. Commercial cold storages with proper ventilation and automatic control of temperatures are now used throughout the country (mostly in cities) and for the storage of semiperishable products such as potatoes and apples. This has made such food available throughout the year and has also stabilized their prices in these cities. Low temperatures chiefly inhibit the growth of microorganisms; although freezing may result in the destruction of some microorganisms.

Freezing temperature (-18°C to 40°C): It may preserve food for long period of time provided the quality of the food is good to begin with and the temperature of storage is far below the actual freezing temperature of food.

CHAPTER 8: Food Preservation

Some microorganisms are destroyed during freezing preservation. The chief preservative effect of freezing temperatures lies in the inability of microorganisms to grow at freezing temperature. In vegetables, enzyme action may still produce undesirable effects on flavor and texture during freezing. The enzymes, therefore, must be destroyed by heating before the vegetables are frozen.

Slow-freezing process: It is also known as sharp freezing. In this method, the foods are placed in refrigerated cabinets at temperatures ranging from -4°C to -29°C. This method is adopted in home freezers. Freezing may require from 3 to 72 hours under such conditions.

Quick-freezing process: The lower temperatures is used to -32°C to -40°C, freezes food so rapidly that fine crystals are formed and the time of freezing is greatly reduced over that required in sharp freezing. The fine crystals formed by quick freezing have a lesser effect on breaking up plant and animal cells than methods of slow freezing that produce coarse ice crystals. In quick freezing, large quantity of food can be frozen in a short period of time.

Dehydrofreezing: Fruits and vegetables consist of drying the food to about 50% of its original weight and volume, and then freezing the food to preserve it. The quality of dehydrofrozen fruits and vegetables is equal to that of fruits and vegetables frozen without preliminary drying. The cost in packing, freezing, storing and shipping of such foods is less, because of the reduction in weight and volume of foods during dehydrofreezing. The following figure depicts the relationship between bacterial growth and temperature. The rapid growth of bacteria occurs in the temperature zone of 60°F–120°F.

Uses of High Temperature

The destruction of microorganisms by heat is due to the coagulation of the protoplasm. The temperature and time used in heat processing a food depend upon the nature of the food and what other methods are combined with heat.

The various degrees of heating used in preservation of food can be classified into three:
1. Pasteurization.
2. Heating up to 100°C or 212°F.
3. Heating above 100°C.

Pasteurization: The time and temperature used in the pasteurization process depend upon the product treated and the method used. In pasteurization, most of the spoilage organisms are killed, but a few survive and hence must be inhibited by low temperatures or some other method, if spoilage is to be prevented. There are two methods of pasteurization—flash method and holder method. In flash method, otherwise called high-temperature short-time method, a high temperature for a short time is used, while in the holder method or low-temperature long-time method, a lower temperature for a longer time is used.

There are slight variations in the time and temperature used for pasteurizing different food, like, milk, cream, ice cream mix and wines.

Heating up to 100°C or 212°F: Most methods of cooking come under this. It temperature can be obtained by boiling any liquid food, by immersing a container in boiling water or by exposure to steam. Before the use of pressure cookers and autoclaves, canning was done at 100°C and this killed all bacteria except spores.

Heating above 100°C: Temperature above 100°C is obtained by means of steam under pressure, as in a pressure cooker or autoclave. Sterilization of foods can be brought about at 121°C for 15 minutes under moist conditions.

Drying Method of Preservation

Microorganisms need moisture to grow. When exposed to sunlight or subjected to dehydration, the moisture in the food is removed and the concentration of water is brought below a certain level. This prevents the growth of microorganisms

CHAPTER 8: Food Preservation

and thereby spoilage of food. Food preservation by drying is one of the oldest methods practiced from ancient times. This method consists of exposing food to sunlight and air until the product is dry.

Factors to be Considered in Drying Food

1. The temperature employed, which will vary with the food and the method of drying.
2. The relative humidity of the air. It is usually higher at the start of drying than later.
3. The velocity of the air.
4. The duration of drying.

Treatments of Food Before Drying

1. Selection and sorting for size, maturity and wholesomeness.
2. Washing, especially of fruits and vegetables.
3. Peeling of fruits and vegetables by hand, machine or abrasion.
4. Subdivision into halves, slices, shreds or cubes.
5. Blanching or scalding of vegetables and some fruits like apricots and peaches.
6. Sulfuring of light-colored fruits and vegetables. Fruits are sulfured by exposure to sulfur dioxide gas produced by the burning of sulfur to a level of 1,000–3,000 ppm.

Types of Drying

Sun drying: It is limited to regions with hot climates and a dry atmosphere and to certain fruits such as raisins, prunes, figs, apricots, pears and peaches. It is a slow process. Many Indian foods are preserved by sun drying. Papads and vathals are made using this principle. Vegetables like cluster beans and curd chili, and fruits like jackfruit are preserved by this method. Fish and meat are also sun dried.

Drying by mechanical dryers: Most methods of artificial drying involve the passage of heated air with controlled relative humidity over the food to be dried or the passing of the food, through such air.

Fruits, vegetables, nuts, fish and meat can be successfully preserved by this method. In the dehydration process, artificial drying methods (e.g. spray dryer) are used for drying foods. Although it is expensive when compared to natural sun-drying procedures, it is very advantageous because the temperature and relative humidity can be manipulated.

Spray drying: Milk and egg are dried to a powder in spray dryers in which the liquid is atomized and sprayed into a hot air stream for almost instant drying.

Foam-mat drying: It may be used commercially with orange and tomato juice. In this process, a small amount of edible foam stabilizer such as monoglycerides or a modified soybean protein with methylcellulose is added to the liquid and stiff foam is produced by whipping. The foam is spread in a thin layer and dried in a stream of hot air. The product separates easily into small particles on cooling.

Drying by osmosis: Drying also results, when fish is heavily salted. In this case, the moisture is drawn out from all cell tissues. The water is then bound with the solute, making it unavailable to the microorganisms.

In osmotic dehydration of fruits, the method involves the partial dehydration of fruits by osmosis in a concentrated sugar solution or syrup.

Freeze-drying: Removal of water from a product, while it is frozen by sublimations is called freeze-drying.

Preservation by High Concentration of Sugar and Salt

Sugar and salt aid in the preservation of products in which it is used due to their ability to bind water and make it unavailable for microbial growth. Salt is an effective preservative because, it also ionizes to yield chlorine ion, which is harmful to organisms and reduces the solubility of oxygen in moisture, which are essential for the growth and multiplication of microorganisms.

Jams, jellies and fruit juices are an important class of fruit products preserved using high concentration of sugar. Pickles are preserved using high concentration of salt.

Jam

Jams are prepared by boiling fruit pulp with sufficient amount of sugar to a reasonably thick consistency, firm enough to hold the fruit tissue in position. In preparing jam, the fruit is crushed or finely cut and measured quantity of sugar and preservatives are added so that when cooked, the mass is fairly uniform throughout. Jams can be prepared from all varieties of pulpy fruits such as grapes, mango, sapota, banana, guava, etc.

Jelly

Jellies are prepared by boiling fruits in water. The extract obtained is strained and measured quantity of sugar is added to it. The mixture is then boiled to a stage at which it will set to a clear gel. A perfect jelly should be transparent, well-set, but not too stiff and should have the original flavor of the fruit. It should retain its shape when removed from the mold.

Usually fruits such as guava, pineapple, apple, grape and a mixture of fruits rich in pectin can be used for the preparation of jellies.

Fruit Juices

Fruit beverages are prepared from different fruits such as apple, mango, grapes, lime, pineapple and sapota and in different forms such as pure juices, crushes, squashes and cordials. The ratio of sugar and fruit juice in the preparation of various beverages is as follows:
1. Crushes: 25% fruit juice and 55% sugar.
2. Squashes: 25% fruit juice and 45% sugar.
3. Cordial: Clarified juice 1 L and 250 g sugar.

In the preparation of fruit juices, citric acid is usually added to clarify the sugar syrup. Preservatives such as sodium benzoate are added to tomato and grape juices while potassium metabisulfite (KMS) is added to all other fruit beverages.

Pickling

The preservation of fruits and vegetables in common salt, vinegar, oil and spices is referred to as pickling. Salt binds the moisture in the food and thereby prevents the growth of microorganisms. The layer of oil that floats on the top of pickles prevents the entry and growth of microorganisms like molds and yeast.

Spices, like turmeric, pepper, chili powder and asafetida retard the growth of bacteria. Vinegar lowers the pH of the product thereby providing an unfavorable acidic environment for microbial growth.

Mango, lime, ginger, garlic, tomato, chili, mixed vegetables such as beans, carrot, cauliflower and peas are used widely in the preparation of pickles.

Preservation by Chemical Preservatives

Preservatives are defined as chemical agents, which serve to retard, hinder or mask the undesirable changes in food. These changes may be caused by microorganisms, by enzymes of food or by purely chemical reactions. Certain chemicals, when added in small quantities can hinder undesirable chemical reaction in food by:

1. Interfering with the cell membrane of the microorganism, their enzyme activity or their genetic mechanism.
2. Acting as antioxidants. Maximum amounts allowed to be added to each type of food are regulated by law because higher concentrations can be a health hazard. Benzoic acid in the form of its sodium salt is an effective inhibitor of molds and is used extensively for the preservation of jams and jellies.

Some of the other chemical preservatives used are:
a. Potassium metabisulfite.
b. Sorbic acid.
c. Calcium propionate.
d. Sodium benzoate.

The development of off-flavors (rancidity) in edible oils is prevented by the use of butylated hydroxyanisole (BHA), butylated hydroxytoluene (BHT), lecithin that is some of the approved antioxidants.

Preservation by Radiation

Radiant energy can be used to preserve food. γ-rays and β-particles produced by special electronic machines are sources of energy used to preserve food.

These waves penetrate throughout the food. As the waves and particles pass through the food, they collide with molecules in the food and in microorganisms. These result in chemical alterations. The goal of irradiation is to kills the microorganism and inactivates the enzymes without altering the food.

Changes in the food are minimized, if it is done in a vacuum and if ascorbic acid is present. Berries and meat are preserved in this way.

▶ CONCLUSION

Food preservation usually involves preventing the growth of bacteria, fungi (such as yeasts), or any other microorganisms (although some methods work by introducing benign bacteria or fungi to the food), as well as retarding the oxidation of fats that cause rancidity. Food preservation can also include processes that inhibit visual deterioration, such as the enzymatic browning reaction in apples after they are cut, which can occur during food preparation. Many processes designed to preserve food will involve a number of food preservation methods. Preserving fruit by turning it into jam, for example, involves boiling

SECTION 1: Nutrition

(to reduce the fruit's moisture content and to kill bacteria, yeasts, etc.), sugaring (to prevent their regrowth) and sealing within an airtight jar (to prevent recontamination). There are many traditional methods of preserving food that limit the energy inputs and reduce carbon footprint. Maintaining or creating nutritional value, texture and flavor is an important aspect of food preservation, although, historically, some methods drastically altered the character of the food being preserved. In many cases these changes have come to be seen as desirable qualities-cheese, yoghurt and pickled onions being common examples.

SECTION 2

Dietetics

Chapter 9

Introduction to Dietetics

▶ INTRODUCTION

The term 'diet therapy' refers to a modification in food intake for the purpose of improving health. Balanced nutrition is essential to overall wellness, but medical nutrition therapy (MNT) describes an intervention that adjusts both the quantity and quality of food to treat a disease or its symptoms. Diet therapy is devised and monitored by a certified healthcare provider, such as a physician or a registered dietitian. Dietetics is concerned with planning of diets in maintaining health, and in prevention and treatment of disease. It is a science as it uses the rudiments of principles of nutrition and it is an art as it is concerned with the aesthetics of food service.

When designing a diet therapy menu, a dietitian will take into consideration a number of factors. These include the age of the patient, the specific illnesses to be treated and the functional ability of the patient to achieve success with a therapeutic diet. The type of diet therapy prescribed will include modifications of three general factors such as texture, nutrients to minimize and nutrients to maximize. Certain medical conditions require a modification in the texture of a diet because of swallowing or chewing difficulties. For example, a liquid diet would be prescribed for a postsurgical patient who needs easily digested nutrition or a person who has had oral surgery and is unable to consume larger chunks of food. A pureed or blended diet would be provided for an elderly patient who is unable to chew food to a safe consistency for swallowing. When a soft diet is prescribed, tough meats are either chopped or ground and served with a sauce or gravy for easier chewing and swallowing. Foods such as corn on the cob or nuts are eliminated from a soft diet.

SECTION 2: Dietetics

▶ DEFINITION

Dietetics is the branch of science that deals with the practical application of the principles of nutrition in health, which is required to the human body.

▶ DIET AS A THERAPEUTIC AGENT

Diet therapy is concerned with the modification of normal diet to meet the requirements of the sick individual. Diet therapy means use of diet (food and drink) not only in the care of the sick but also in the prevention of disease and maintenance of health. Diet therapy in most instances is not a remedy in itself, but is a measure, which supplements or makes the medical or surgical treatment more effective. Therapeutic nutrition begins with the normal diet.

Advantages

Advantages of using normal diet as the basis for therapeutic diets are as following:

1. It emphasizes the similarity of psychological and social needs of those who are ill and those who are well, even though there are quantitative and qualitative differences in requirements.
2. Food preparation is simplified when the modified diet is based upon the family diet pattern and the number of items required is reduced to a minimum.
3. The calculated values for the basic plan are useful in finding out the effects of addition or omission of certain foods, for example, if vegetables are restricted vitamin A and C deficiency can occur.

To correct nutrient deficiencies this may have occurred due to the disease. The following has to be done:

1. Plan and provide a diet that is most suited to the disease condition.
2. Adjust the food intake to the body's ability to metabolize the nutrients in sickness.

CHAPTER 9: Introduction to Dietetics

▶ GENERAL OBJECTIVES OF DIET THERAPY

General objectives of diet therapy are:
1. To maintain a good nutritional status.
2. To bring about changes in body weight whenever necessary.

▶ MEANING OF DIET THERAPY

Diet therapy also refers to nutrient modification for therapeutic purposes. A diet type described as 'low' would minimize a certain nutrient or nutrients. For example, a low-fiber diet might be prescribed for a patient after stomach or intestinal surgery to reduce the amount of digestion taking place after a meal. Other diet therapy types that minimize nutrients include a low-cholesterol diet, a low-sodium diet or a low-oxalate diet.

Certain conditions require an increase in nutrient intake. Pregnancy diets are prescribed to supply the mother and fetus with extra calories, protein, iron and folate. A high-fiber diet might be recommended for patients suffering from constipation, which is a side effect of many pain medications.

A comprehensive diet plan, prescribed for patients with multiple issues, might increase certain nutrients and minimize others. Patients who suffer from heart disease, diabetes or obesity might be prescribed a plan that reduces the amount of calories, fats and sugars in the diet, but increases fiber and protein intake for satiety. For a person to ensure that a diet therapy regimen is sound and appropriate for a particular medical condition, it is important for discuss nutritional intake including the use of alternative therapies such as dietary supplements with a licensed healthcare provider.

▶ PRINCIPLES OF DIET THERAPY

Diet therapy is concerned with the modification of the normal diet to meet the requirements of the sick individual. Its purposes are:

1. To maintain good nutritional status.
2. To correct deficiencies those may have occurred.
3. To afford rest to the whole body or to ascertain body's ability to metabolize the nutrients.
4. To bring about changes in body weight whenever necessary. Therapeutic nutrition begins with the normal diet.

▶ FACTORS TO CONSIDER IN PLANNING THERAPEUTIC DIETS

The alteration of the normal diet requires an appreciation of:
1. The underlying disease conditions, which require a change in the diet.
2. The possible duration of the disease.
3. The factors in the dietary, which must be observed.
4. The patient's tolerance for food by mouth.

In planning meals for a patient economic status, food preferences, occupation and time of meals should also be considered.

▶ MODIFICATION OF NUTRIENTS IN THERAPEUTIC DIETS

The normal diet may be modified:
1. To provide change in consistency as in fluid and soft diets.
2. To increase or decrease the energy value.
3. To include greater or lesser amount of one or more nutrients, e.g. high protein, low sodium, etc.
4. To increase or decrease high bulk and low-fiber diets.
5. To provide foods bland in flavor.

▶ TEAM APPROACH

In order to meet the nutritional needs of the patient, a team approach of physician, nurse and dietitian is necessary (Fig. 9.1).

These health professionals are primarily involved in the nutritional care. However, at times, the services of other health professionals such as social worker, physiotherapist, etc. may also be directly involved. The physician, while prescribing the diet, should also explain to the patient why modified diet has been prescribed.

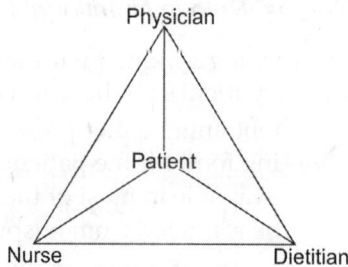

Fig. 9.1: Team approach to meet the nutritional needs

Responsibilities of a Dietitian

1. The dietitian, after receiving the written diet prescription translates it to practicality in terms of food.
2. The dietitian assesses and formulates the nutritional status of the patient.
3. Dietitian formulates nutrition care plan.
4. Dietitian plans individualized meal pattern according to the patient's food habits and modification needed.
5. If patient is on enteral formula, dietitian recommends appropriate proprietary formulas, if needed.
6. Dietitian counsels the patients and their family regarding the therapeutic diet prescribed and its importance.

Role of a Nurse

Nutrition not only deals with food and its components, but it is also a multidisciplinary field, which deals with social, economic, cultural, psychological implications of foods. Nutrition is a discipline intimately related with medicine. It is also closely related with physiology and biochemistry. As nurses should have a thorough understanding of these fields of studies in order to give better care to the patients.

As nurses may choose to work in large hospital, community health centers, nursing homes or irrespective of place of work, and have a crucial role to play in ensuring the medical and nutrition success of therapy.

SECTION 2: Dietetics

Nurses' Role in Nutritional Care in Hospital Setup

1. Keeping in touch with the doctor and dietitian regarding the patient's medical and dietary needs:
   a. Obtaining a diet prescription if there is one and arranging food for the patient. Nowadays, dietary facilities are available in most of the hospitals. In such cases food can be arranged from hospital itself.
   b. Communicate with the dietitians regarding the patient's response to the diet.
   c. Serve as a mediator between the patient, physician and the dietitian.
2. Assisting the patient at mealtime:
   a. To prepare the patient for the meals and educate about the importance of nutrition.
   b. Assist the patient in feeding especially, if the patient is unconscious or unable to feed. Tube feeding, may it be enteral or parenteral, must be done by the nurses.
   c. Teach and encourage the handicapped patients to feed themselves.
   d. Encourage and support the patient at mealtime.
   e. Must make the mealtime a pleasant and relaxed affair.
3. Help the dietitians in special tasks:
   a. Interpret the diet to the patient. A nurse should explain why the modified diet is being given. The patient should also be told what to expect with reference to diet therapy.
   b. Observe, record and report the patient's response to diet and should communicate with the patient regarding food habits, likes and dislikes, and attitude towards the diet or specific foods.
   c. Note the intake of foods according to the diet prescription.
   d. Reporting patient's response to dietitian and physician for any weight loss or gain.
4. Plan for home care:
   a. Before patient leaves the hospital, it is the duty of a nurse to arrange for diet counseling to be followed at home.

b. Along with the patients, members of the family must also be counseled for home care

A nurse can be of great help in community set up can perform the duties of a dietitian in health centers and also can give nutrition education through various methods to prevent nutritional deficiency diseases. The Government of India has launched various nutritional programs to eradicate malnutrition, where a nurse plays a crucial role.

▶ CONCLUSION

Dietetics is the science of applying knowledge in food and nutrition to improving and maintaining good health. Scientific studies are proving that the food we eat has a significant impact on our health. Changes in diet can help prevent or control many health problems, including obesity, diabetes and certain risk factors for cancer and heart disease. Dietetics is the health field that focuses on the interaction between nutrition and health. Dietitians and dietetic technicians design 'nutrition therapies' that help the body use the natural nutrients and properties in food to protect against disease and promote health. The field of dietetics has a strong emphasis on public health and a commitment to educating about the importance of making proper dietary choices. Dietitians who work in facilities preparing food strive to develop menus and recipes that are healthful, tasty and cost-effective.

Chapter 10

Diet in Sickness

▶ INTRODUCTION

Diet is as important as medicine in the treatment of diseases. A modification in the diet or in the nutrients can cure certain diseases. Nutrition during illness should be adequate to prevent weight loss and weakness (Fig. 10.1). An acutely ill or injured patient is in danger of malnutrition.

▶ PURPOSES

1. To meet the metabolic needs of human body.
2. To prevent dehydration.
3. To improve the appetite.
4. To provide adequate nutrition.
5. It is necessary for the growth and maintenance of bones and other tissues.

▶ GENERAL RULES OF TREATMENT

1. The diet must be planned in relation to changes in metabolism occurring as a result of the disease.
2. The diet must be planned to agree as nearly as possible with the patient's food habits, likes and dislikes, and the amount of exercise he/she takes.
3. Changes should be made gradually adequate explanation must be given when it is necessary to make dietary changes gradually.
4. There should be plenty or variety in the diet, hot food should be served hot and cold foods should be served cold.

CHAPTER 10: Diet in Sickness

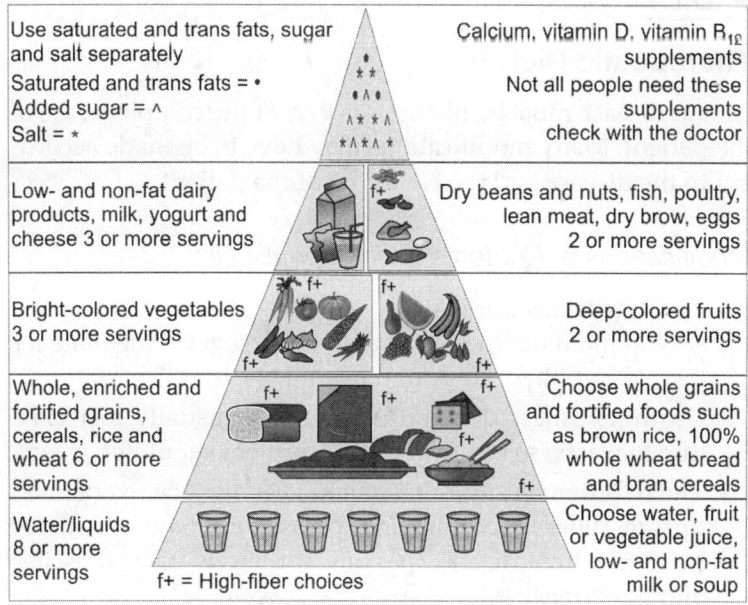

Fig. 10.1: Food guide pyramid

▶ PROBLEMS DURING SICKNESS

1. There will be disturbance of gastrointestinal (GI) function.
2. Anorexia (loss of appetite).
3. Defective digestion and absorption.
4. Lack of exercise decreases need for energy.
5. The process of anabolism and catabolism are not normal in sickness.
6. Vomiting and diarrhea are problems in which intravenous fluid administration is required.
7. In some kinds of illness, protein requirements are more while in some others both protein and carbohydrate are needed in large amounts.

SECTION 2: Dietetics

▶ DIET

Therapeutic Diet

Diet in disease must be planned as part of the complete care of the patient. Many modifications may have to be made according to the disease and the condition of the patient.

Modifications of Nutrients in Therapeutic Diet

1. Carbohydrates are usually well-tolerated and are necessary to maintain the stores of liver glycogen. Adequate intake of carbohydrates can prevent ketosis.
2. During sickness demand of protein is usually increased due to waste, so easily digestible protein should be given.
3. The requirements of calcium and iron must be maintained during illness, sodium and potassium may sometimes need to be restricted especially if there is edema, ascites and hypertension.
4. Fat-soluble vitamin, e.g. vitamin A and D need to be added if the patient is on fat-restricted diet for a long time.
5. Vitamin B complex may not be adequately absorbed in pathological conditions of the GI tract.
6. Requirement of vitamin C is greatly increased in fevers and is especially necessary for the healing of wounds after surgery.
7. Fluids are very important to prevent dehydration especially in conditions such as high fevers, diarrhea and vomiting, in such conditions the fluid intake within 24 hours should be 2,500 mL–3,000 mL.
8. If adequate fluids cannot be given by mouth, they must be given intravenous maintain fluid balance by maintaining accurate intake output chart.
9. Infants require a higher amount of fluid compared to adult requirements they need 150 mL of fluid per kg of body weight.

CHAPTER 10: Diet in Sickness

Objective

1. To improve the general health.
2. To meet the metabolic needs.
3. To promote healing.
4. To prevent dehydration.
5. To facilitate tissue repair and growth.

Principles Involved in Diet Therapy

1. The diet must be planned in relation to changes in metabolism occurring as a result of disease.
2. The diet must be planned according to the habits of the patient based on culture, religion, socioeconomic status, personal preferences, physiological and psychological conditions.
3. As far as possible, changes in the diet should be brought gradually and adequate explanations are given with the changes made, if any.
4. In short and acute illness, the food should not be forced his/her appetite is very poor, but may soon recover the normal appetite.
5. Whatever the diet prescribed, there should be variety of for selection.
6. Small and frequent feeds are preferred to the usual three meals.
7. Hot foods should be served hot and cold foods should be served cold.

Regular Diet

1. **Full diet:** It is a regular well-balanced diet. It is vegetarian or non-vegetarian, this is for patients who do not need any special modification.
2. **Soft light diet:** It is given to provide light and easily digestible food with minimum residue. It contains food, which requires little chewing and contains no fiber or no seasoning.
3. **Bland diet:** The foods are easily digestible, free from substances, which might cause irritation of the GI tract and

generally or low roughage content, used mainly for patients with GI conditions.

Liquid Diet

1. **Liquid diets:** Must be used for patients, who are unable to take or tolerate solid food this diet is given usually to patient having hyperpyrexia, postoperative patients and patients having GI disturbances.
2. **Clean fluids:** Used when there is a marked intolerance to food and roughage, these include clear tea, weak black coffee, clear soups, whey water, strained fruit juices and clear fluid diet should be used only for a short time.
3. **Full liquid diet:** It is given as a total nutrition of the patient and has to be maintained by fluids for considerable time. This is necessary when the patient is unable to swallow solid food or if the patient is fed by intragastric or gastrostomy tubes.

Low-calorie Diet

1. The total calorie intake is reduced to less than the body's requirements so that the remainder of the calories required can be derived from the stored fat.
2. The aim of this diet is to slow steady loss of weight over a period of several weeks or even months. This diet is advised obese patients.
3. Foodstuffs such as ghee, butter, sugar, sweets bread, rice and potatoes are omitted from the diet. Use salads fruits and boiled vegetables. The patient must have plenty of bulk in the diet by using high-fiber foods and low-calorie beverages.

Low-protein Diet

1. Low-protein diet is advised in kidney diseases such as nephritis, uremia. In these diseases, the protein is avoided or given in low moderate type.

CHAPTER 10: Diet in Sickness

2. This type of diet is given to give the rest to kidneys because excessive protein intake acts as an additional load to the kidneys.
3. Foodstuffs such as milk, eggs, meat, etc. are omitted or restricted according to the prescribed protein intake.

Low-fat Diet

1. Low-fat diet is restricted from the diet patients with liver diseases and gallbladder diseases. Carbohydrates in the diet should be increased to supply the liver with glycogen to prevent the ketosis.
2. No fried food ghee, butter or other fat is allowed in the diet, only rice chapatis bread, fruits, dal and vegetables.

Salt-free Diet

1. Sodium is totally or partially restricted the restriction of sodium depends on the severity of the condition of the patient.
2. The patients with heart diseases, hypertension, kidney diseases, etc. are given salt-restricted diet or low-salt diet. The necessity of the restriction should be carefully explained to the patient and relatives.
3. The following foods are totally avoided—salt, baking powder, papads, canned foods, cheese and pickles, salted chips and biscuits, etc.

High-protein Diet

1. In high-protein diet, the protein intake should be average from 75 to 100 g/day for adult. In protein energy malnutrition cases, easily digestible and high nutritive value protein, e.g. milk protein should be given.
2. High-protein diet is given to the patients such as operated cases, tuberculosis accident, burns and nephrotic syndrome and emaciated cases.

3. The foodstuffs contains rich protein are milk and milk proteins, eggs, fish meat, broth, dals, dahi, beans, soybean and groundnuts.

Diabetic Diet

1. In diabetes mellitus, the metabolism of carbohydrate, fat and protein are affected. Diabetes is lifelong disease, which can be treated, but not cured. The dietary treatment depends upon the severity of the condition.
2. The purpose of diabetic diet is to keep the patient in good health to keep the blood sugar level within normal level and to keep urine free from sugar.
3. The diet should be balanced, but there should be restriction of carbohydrates, e.g. rice, biscuits, sugar, jams, sweets, honey, carrots and sweet potatoes. The patient should have egg, milk raw salads all types of green leafy vegetables.
4. The total calories required 20%–25% should be from protein 40% from carbohydrates and 40% from fat.

Diet in Anemia

1. Anemia type of patient requires the diet, which is high in protein, iron and vitamins. The diet should provide necessary nutrients for the formation of new red blood cells or hemoglobin.
2. The main purposes are to provide necessary nutrients for blood cell formation and to remove the cause of anemia.
3. The foodstuffs recommended are liver, meat, eggs, spinach drumstick leaves, ragi, jaggery, etc.

Types of Diet Used in Hospitals

1. Clear fluid diet.
2. Full fluid diet.
3. Soft diet.
4. Normal diet.

Clear Fluid Diet

Whenever an acute illness or surgery produces a marked intolerance for food as may be evident by nausea. Vomiting, anorexia, distention and diarrhea, it is advisable to restrict the intake of food. In acute infection, in acute inflammatory conditions of the intestinal tract, following operations upon the colon or rectum, when it is desirable to prevent evacuation from the bowel, clear fluid diet is suggested. This diet is also given to relieve thirst, to supply the tissues with water, to aid in the removal of gas.

The diet is made up of clear liquids that leave no residue and it is non-gas forming action. This diet is entirely inadequate from a nutritional standpoint. Since, it is deficient in protein, minerals, vitamins and calories. It should not be continued for more than 24–48 hours. The amount of fluid is usually restricted to 30–60 mL/h at first, with gradually increasing amounts being given as the patients tolerance improves. This diet can meet the requirement of fluids and some minerals and can be given in 1–2 hour intervals.

Conditions necessitating the use of clear fluid diet

1. Preoperative period, e.g. as a preparation for bowel surgery.
2. Prior to colonoscopic examination.
3. Postoperative phase, e.g. in the initial recovery phase after abdominal surgery or after a period of intravenous therapy.
4. Acute illness and infections as in acute GI disturbances such as acute gastroenteritis, when fluid and electrolyte replacement is desired to compensate for losses from diarrhea.
5. As the first step in oral alimentation of a nutritionally debilitated person.
6. In temporary food intolerance.

Full Fluid Diet

Full fluid diet bridges the gap between the clear fluid and soft diet. It is used following operations in acute gastritis, acute infections and in diarrhea. This diet is also suggested when milk is permitted and for patients not requiring special diet, but too ill to eat solid or semisolid foods. In this diet, foods which are liquid or which readily become liquid on reaching the stomach are given. This diet may be made entirely adequate and may be used over an extended time without fear of deficiencies developing, provided it is carefully planned. This diet is given at 2–4 hours interval.

Conditions necessitating the use of full fluid diet
1. Postoperative phase when progressing from clear liquids to solid foods.
2. Acute gastritis and infections.
3. Following oral surgery or plastic surgery of face or neck area.
4. In chewing and swallowing dysfunction.
5. In esophageal or stomach disorders causing intolerance to solid food intake.

Soft Diet

Soft diet bridges the gap between acute illness and convalescence. It may be used in acute infections, following surgery and for patients who are unable to chew. The soft diet is made up of simple, easily digestible food and contains no harsh fiber. Patients with dental problems are given mechanically soft diet. It is often modified further for certain pathologic conditions as bland and low-residue diets. In this diet, three meals with intermediate feedings should be given.

Conditions necessitating the use of soft diet
1. While progressing from full fluid diet to general diet.
2. During postoperative phase when a patient is unable to tolerate normal diet.
3. Gastrointestinal problems, e.g. diarrhea.
4. General debilitation and inadequate dentition.
5. Convalescence.
6. Transition from acute phase of illness to convalescence.
7. Acute infections.

A soft diet can be modified as mechanical soft diet.

Mechanical soft diet

Many people require a soft diet simply because they have no teeth and such a diet is known as mechanical or a dental soft diet. It is not desirable to restrict the patient to the food selection of the customary soft diet and the following modifications to the normal diet may be made:

1. Vegetables may be chopped or diced before cooking.
2. Hard raw fruits and vegetables are to be avoided; tough skins and seeds to be removed.
3. Nuts and dried fruits may be used in chopped or powdered forms.
4. Meat to be finely minced or ground.

Normal Diet

Normal diet is used for ambulatory and bed patients whose conditions do not necessitate a special diet as one of the routine diets. Many special diets progress ultimately to a regular diet. The regular hospital diet is simple in character and preparation, easy of digestion and calculated to afford maximum nourishment with minimum effort to the body. The diet is well-balanced, adequate in nutritional value and attractively served to stimulate a possible poor appetite.

A normal diet is defined as one which consists of any and all foods eaten by a person in health. It is planned keeping the basic food groups in mind, so that optimum amounts of all nutrients are provided. As there is no restriction of any kind of food, this diet is well-balanced and nutritionally adequate.

Since, the patient is hospitalized and/or is at bed rest, a reduction of 10% in energy intake should be made, and too many fatty foods and fried foods be avoided as they are difficult to digest. The proteins are slightly increased (+10%) to counteract a negative nitrogen balance. All other nutrients are supplied in normal amounts.

▶ SPECIAL FEEDING METHODS (MANAGEMENT OF SPECIAL DIETS)

Oral feeding is the best for the nourishment of a patient. But in the following conditions it is not possible to give the feeding orally:

1. Those who cannot swallow due to paralysis of the muscles of swallowing (diphtheria, poliomyelitis), etc. or cancer of the oral cavity or larynx.
2. Those who cannot be persuaded to eat.
3. Those with persistent anorexia requiring forced feeding.
4. Semiconscious or unconscious patients.
5. Severe malabsorption requiring administration of unpalatable formula.
6. Short bowel syndrome.
7. Those who are undernourished or at risk of becoming so.
8. Those that cannot digest and absorb.
9. After surgery.
10. Patients with neurological and renal disorders or have continued fevers or diabetes.
11. Babies of very low birth weight.

Tube Feeding

Tube feeding is done by passing a tube into the stomach or duodenum through the nose, which is called nasogastric feeding or directly by surgical operation known as gastrostomy and jejunostomy feeding. A satisfactory tube feeding must be:

1. Nutritionally adequate.
2. Well-tolerated by the patient so that vomiting is not induced.
3. Easily digested with no unfavorable reactions such as distension, diarrhea or constipation.
4. Easily prepared.
5. Inexpensive.

Nutrition Supplied Through the Tube

The nutrition supplied through the tube may be:

CHAPTER 10: Diet in Sickness   247

1. Natural liquid foods.
2. Blenderized to make liquid food.
3. Commercially supplied polymeric mixtures or elemental diet (predigested diet).

Feeding Requirements

A concentration of about 1 kcal/mL is satisfactory. Lesser concentration increases the volume, which must be given to meet the nutrient and energy needs and greater concentration are more likely to produce diarrhea, and may be too thick to pass through a nasogastric tube. The feeding is started through a continuous drip at a rate of 50 mL/h. The rate is increased by 20 mL every 24 hours until the required volume is achieved, usually with 100–120 mL/h. The concentration or rate of flow may have to be reducing, if there is vomiting, abdominal cramps or diarrhea.

Feeding requirements are based on previous nutritional status and other feeds given to the patient:

- Fluids: 30 mL/kg
- Energy: 32 kcal/kg
- Protein: 1 g/kg body weight
- Sodium: 30–40 mmol (provided there are no external losses)
- Potassium: 1 mmol/g of protein.

Vitamins and minerals supplementation should be given.

Care of the Solution

Feeding solutions have to be treated with full hygienic precautions during the preparation, storage and administration. Feeds should be stored in a refrigerator to avoid bacterial growth and taken out before admin in time to reach room temperature; very cold feeds are not tolerated. A feed should be discarded when it has been more than 2 hours out of storage.

Documentation

Nursing staff should accurately record:
1. The time when a feed is started and completed.

2. The volume administered.
3. Water used to irrigate the tubing.
4. The patients output of urine. Careful monitoring is needed to see that the patient is in fluid balance.

Parenteral Feeding

In parenteral feeding, here the nutrient preparations are given directly into a vein. This method may be used to supplement normal feeding by mouth, but can provide all the nutrients necessary to meet patient's requirements. Then, it is known as total parenteral nutrition (TPN). The same process is called hyperalimentation when at least 150% of the daily requirements are provided to produce a positive nitrogen balance for gain in weight. Partial parenteral nutrition provides 30%–50% of daily requirements.

▶ CONCLUSION

Healthy diets and physical activity are key to good nutrition, and necessary for a long and healthy life. Eating nutrient dense foods and balancing energy intake with the necessary physical activity to maintain a healthy weight is essential at all stages of life. Unbalanced consumption of foods high in energy (sugar, starch and/or fat) and low in essential nutrients contributes to energy excess, overweight and obesity. The amount of the energy consumed in relation to physical activity and the quality of food are the key determinants of nutrition related chronic disease.

Chapter 11

Dietary Modifications

▶ INTRODUCTION

Meal frequency modifications often especially in gastrointestinal (GI) related disorders; small frequent meals will be used rather than three larger meals. Perhaps as many as 6–8 small meals or snacks may be consumed daily. By eating smaller meals, the workload placed on the GI tract and cardiovascular system is less than that with a large meal. Small frequent meals may be used for GI disorders, such as hiatal hernia and epigastric distress, during periods of nausea or indigestion, for esophageal reflux and in pancreatitis. They may also be prescribed after myocardial infarction (MI) and in congestive heart failure (CHF).

▶ IMPORTANT FACTORS INVOLVED

Ordinarily, meal is a pleasant experience for every person. But under diseased condition, the digestion mechanism is affected. The hunger may be reduced or may end. Patient has no interest toward meals. Absence from eating or refusal to eat is a common behavior of the patients during illness. Refusal to eat becomes a problem. Hence, it is necessary for the nurse to know the factors under which the patient refuses to eat. Some of these factors are explained below.

Environmental Factors

1. Change in the place of meals or unsuitable dining place or not according to the liking of the patient.
2. Dirty dining environment, presence of undesirable articles or scene, unattractive or unpleasant environment.

SECTION 2: Dietetics

3. Lack of ventilation and lighting.
4. Shouting, excessive noise, disorder, confusion, crying, etc. during meals.
5. Inappropriate temperature and excessive humidity during meals.
6. Bad dress of the patient and of those serving food.

Cultural Factors

1. Unsuitable utensils or to be unfamiliar with their usage.
2. Exchange in style of eating (use of dining table or floor for sitting).
3. Abstinence by vegetarians from meat, eggs, etc. and fearing of mixing with their food.
4. Non-vegetarians disliking about vegetarian or modified diet.
5. To condemn some vegetables, fruits or diets.
6. Timing of meals not suitable with religious beliefs (jams do not eat during night).
7. Irregular timing or excessive punctuality.
8. Not getting food cooked or prepared by desired persons as per religious beliefs or the method of cooking not according to their religious belief.
9. Not getting an opportunity to pray before meals or to follow some religious practices.

Psychological Factors

1. Meals not according to the liking or taste of the patient.
2. Physical and mental exhaustion.
3. Unattractive flavor and color of meals.
4. Feeling fear, worries or confusion, while eating or serving food.
5. Personal experience of the patient not favorable, while eating.
6. Unfavorable behavior of doctor, nurse or those serving meals with the patient.

7. The patient being in a state of worry, anger, emotion or remembering his/her household affairs during eating.
8. Unclean or unprotected serving utensils.

Other Factors

1. Physical weakness of patient.
2. Full rejection of diet by patient.

In this manner, the patient can create problems or non-cooperation in accepting diet for various reasons. Sometimes it becomes difficult to find that due to what unknown fear, doubt or event the patient is not accepting diet. Hence, the nurse, based on the knowledge and previous experience, should skillfully motivate and encourage the patient for accepting food, by removing all the hurdles.

▶ KILOCALORIE MODIFICATIONS

The body requires a specific amount of energy each day to carry out its tasks. Energy intake includes foods and beverages consumed daily. Energy output includes energy used for:

1. Basal metabolic rate (BMR).
2. Physical activities.
3. Digestion of food.

Energy balance is achieved when energy intake equals to output. During energy balance, weight should remain constant if energy intake is greater than output, positive energy balance results causing weight gain. On the other hand if intake is less than output, negative energy balance occurs leading to weight loss.

High-calorie and High-protein Diets

During times of physiological stress, such as after surgery, bone fractures, sepsis, burns, cancer and some other disease states, the body's energy and protein needs are increased. Medical trauma can greatly increase the BMR, so that if energy needs are not met by diet, negative energy balance will result. The patient will lose protein stored and weight.

SECTION 2: Dietetics

Many trauma and cancer patients suffer from anorexia or lack of appetite, and may also have difficulty with the eating process. This further complicates the problem of nutritional inadequacies. Dietary treatment should aim at restoring energy balance in the normal weight patient or creating a positive energy balance in the underweight patient. High-calorie and high-protein diets should provide increased amounts of kilocalorie and problem in a small volume. Commercially prepared liquid supplements may be used.

Suggestions to Increase Kilocalorie and Protein

1. Add milk powder to milkshakes, beverages, soups, puddings and cooked cereals.
2. Spread peanut butter on crackers, fruits or celery.
3. Add cheese to casseroles, soups and sauces.
4. Use extra meat, chicken or fish in casseroles and soups.
5. Add sugar to foods, where reasonable (this only adds kilocalorie).
6. Use generous amounts of dense foods such as butter, margarine, mayonnaise, cream cheese, sour cream and cream in recipes, as spreads or as dips, which are rich in kilocalorie.
7. Have snacks available at all times.
8. Encourage the patient to eat high-calorie foods first and eat the low-calorie foods, if still hungry.

Of course, the diet should still provide a balance of foods from all the food groups. It should be kept in mind that the appearance of the food and how it is served may determine, whether it is eaten or not. That serving foods should do so with a positive attitude and encouragement. The meals should be as attractive as possible. Beverages, especially liquid supplements should be served in glasses, not in cans. Foods should be served at the correct temperature, meals should be served promptly, and snacks and supplements should be refrigerated, if necessary.

If a patient is not able to consume adequate kilocalorie or refuses to eat, then nutritional support in the form of tube feedings or intravenous (IV) feedings may be considered.

CHAPTER 11: Dietary Modifications

Kilocalorie Control and Low-calorie Diets

Obesity is the condition of having an abnormally large amount of fat on the body. Ideally obesity should be determined by using measures of body composition. Methods of measuring body composition includes hydrostatic weighing (submerging the body in a tank of water and measuring displacement), skinfold thickness measures (measuring the pinch of skin using skinfold calipers) and electrical impedance tests (a small electrical current is transmitted through the body and its resistance is measured). These methods measure percent of body fat and are better suited for determining obesity; however, they are not always available and nor are they as simple as using a weight scale.

The cause of obesity is difficult to explain. Many factors may contribute to the positive energy balance that leads to obesity. Most experts agree that both heredity and lifestyle contribute to obesity. Regardless of cause, obesity is a major health problem, particularly in well-developed countries. Obese people have a higher incidence of non-insulin-dependent diabetes mellitus (NIDDM), high blood lipid levels, hypertension, coronary heart disease, postsurgical complications, gynecological irregularities, pregnancy-induced hypertension and gout. Excess weight exacerbates arthritis and some respiratory problems. It can lead to varicose veins and abdominal hernia.

Obesity is resistant to treatment. Some studies have shown that if 'cure' from obesity is defined as reduction to ideal weight and maintenance of that weight for 5 years, a person is more likely to recover from many forms of cancer than from obesity. Treatment of obesity has ranged from diets, medications and psychotherapy to surgery. The goal of any treatment is to cause a negative energy balance resulting in weight loss. The most common treatment and probably the safest is a low-calorie diet and exercise. Low-calorie diet must be based on the exchange lists for meal planning discussed later on under

the heading of diabetes mellitus. A successful weight reduction program should incorporate three major components. They are:
1. A low-calorie diet.
2. Exercise and physical activity.
3. Behavior modification and other lifestyle changes.

The program should help and prepare patients to control weight throughout life and not just on a temporary basis. Diet should be not less than 1,200 kcal/day and weight loss should occur at the rate of approximately 1–2 lb/week. Diets that require the purchase of specially prepared foods, supplements or magic diet aids should be avoided. Person who is trying to lose weight must learn to take change of their own life and not rely on expensive products for weight control. Individuals consuming less than 1,500 kcal/day may need to take a multivitamin/minor supplement providing approximately 100% of the recommended dietary allowance (RDA).

Very-low-calorie Diets

Very-low-calorie diet (VLCD) programs, sometimes called liquid fasts, are being used increasingly in many hospital outpatients, clinics and doctor's offices. These diets consist of a low calorie and nutritionally balanced. Liquid diet provides 300–500 kcal/day. Throughout the liquid fast, patients are monitored by their physician and other health professionals. They should receive dietary and behavioral counseling, and should be involved in an exercise program. The patient continues on the liquid fast for a given period, eating the other foods and then begins a gradual refeeding program, and is instructed on a diet for weight maintenance.

Long-term results of VLCDs prove disappointing, showing a higher percentage of dieters regaining over half of the weight lost on the program. With VLCDs as with any weight reduction regimen, the principles of weight management still apply. Unless exercise continues, food intake is controlled and dietary habits are changed, weight loss will be only temporary.

Carbohydrate-modified Diets

Diabetes Mellitus

Probably the most common type of carbohydrate-modified diet is the diabetic diet used for that person with diabetes mellitus. In diabetes mellitus, β-cells in the pancreas do not produce enough insulin or cannot use it properly. Insulin is the hormone, which is necessary to move glucose from the bloodstream into the cells, where it is used for energy. Without insulin, glucose builds up in the bloodstream, leading to hyperglycemia (elevated blood glucose). Diabetes also may affect fat metabolism and increase levels of blood lipids (cholesterol and triglycerides) over time, elevated blood glucose and lipid levels may cause serious long-term complications.

Perhaps not enough emphasis has been placed on the role of diet in the management of diabetes. Proper diet is essential for blood glucose control and may help to reduce insulin needs, if strictly followed. By keeping blood glucose levels relatively constant and in an appropriate range, the risk of diabetic complications may be lessened. Persons with diabetes should continually be encouraged to follow their individualized meal plan. Dietary goals differ somewhat depending on the type of diabetes being treated.

Insulin-dependent diabetes mellitus

Insulin-dependent diabetes mellitus (IDDM) occurs most often in children and adolescents. Those with IDDM do not produce insulin; their body cannot use glucose for energy and begins to burn the fat. When fat is burned for energy in the absence of glucose with the production of waste called ketones. Ketone builds up in the blood and lead to a life-threatening condition called ketoacidosis. People with IDDM must take insulin to avoid this condition.

The most important principle for those with IDDM is consistency. Meals and snacks should be eaten at about the same time each day. The types and amounts of foods eaten should be similar from day to day. This is necessary because the carbohydrate eaten must balance the insulin administered each day.

Carbohydrate intake should be distributed evenly throughout the day to provide adequate amounts of glucose for the available insulin to move from the bloodstream to the cells. This is called carbohydrate distribution.

The patient should be given a meal plan to follow that specified number of food choices (exchanges) to be consumed at each meal and snack. Carbohydrate is distributed among the meals to correspond with insulin dosage.

If a person taking insulin fails to consume adequate carbohydrate, blood glucose levels may drop, causing hypoglycemia (low blood glucose). Symptoms of hypoglycemia may include headache, confusion, weakness, perspiration, shallow breathing, nervousness, visual disturbances and vertigo, and also may lead to unconsciousness. Sometime the person experiencing hypoglycemia may be mistakenly judged to be intoxicated. Proper medical identification should be worked to prevent such a mistake. Hypoglycemia should be treated with immediate administration of glucose in a readily available form, such as orange juice, followed by food containing both carbohydrate and protein. If juice is not available, sugar or hard candy may be eaten. In the event of unconsciousness, glucose should be administered intravenously.

In times of illness, the patient with diabetes may not want to eat the usual foods on the meal plan. In such cases, it is essential to provide carbohydrates in the diet to correspond with insulin dosage. Carbohydrate containing beverages, such as juices and punch, should be offered. Popsicles, flavored gelatin, crackers, puddings and ice milk provide carbohydrate and may be better accepted during illness.

Non-insulin-dependent diabetes mellitus

Non-insulin-dependent diabetes mellitus usually occurs in adults, many of whom are overweight. People with NIDDM produces insulin, but either there is not enough insulin or the body is unable to use it properly. This type of diabetes often may be controlled by diet and exercise. Some people with NIDDM use oral hypoglycemic agents, medications that stimulate

CHAPTER 11: Dietary Modifications

insulin production and use. In some instances, insulin injections may be needed to help to regulate blood glucose levels. Whenever insulin is administered, the dietary principles for NIDDM should be used.

Many people with NIDDM are overweight and one of the major dietary goals with this type of diabetes is weight control. For the obese person with NIDDM, weight reduction can help to control blood glucose level and reduce the need for medication. Kilocalorie control is more important than carbohydrate distribution in this type of diabetes. A diet using the exchange lists is an ideal method of weight control. As with NIDDM, simple sugar should be restricted and adequate fiber intake emphasized.

Exercise reduces blood glucose levels. This is helpful in the control of blood glucose and is also important or weight control. People with either type of the diabetes may be able to reduce insulin or medication needs with regular exercise. Diet can also be adjusted to compensate for exercise. If a patient with NIDDM is to be involved in a physical activity that he/she is not accustomed to some carbohydrate containing food (milk, fruits, vegetables or starches) may be added to the meal just before engaging in the activity. In this way, the extra carbohydrate will provide more glucose to satisfy the demands of exercise.

Dumping Syndrome

Dumping syndrome may occur after surgery, where a portion of all of the stomach is removed (partial or total gastrectomy). After partial or total gastrectomy, the stomach contents may empty too rapidly into the jejunum. The body reacts by sending water to the intestinal tract, thus blood pressure is reduced. The load on the intestinal tract increases peristalsis (contractions that move food through the GI tract), leading to diarrhea. Symptoms occur 15–30 minutes after meals and include cramping, weakness, diaphoresis, vertigo, nausea and possibly vomiting.

Diet therapy involves giving small, frequent meals that are higher in protein and fat, but lower in carbohydrates. Concentrated sweets should be avoided and fluids should be taken

30–60 minutes before or after a meal. The dumping syndrome diet may be needed only temporarily until the body adjusts to the changes caused by surgery.

Lactose Intolerance

Lactose intolerance occurs as a result of lack of the digestive enzyme, lactase. Because of this, the GI tract is unable to breakdown lactose (milk sugar). Symptoms occur after ingestion of milk products and include nausea, cramps, bloated feeling, flatulence and diarrhea.

Diet for lactose intolerance excludes milk and milk products, such as ice cream, puddings cheese and powdered milk. Food with milk added such as biscuit or muffin mixes, some soups and other prepared foods, are needs to be avoided.

Some individuals have a deficiency rather than a total absence of lactase. These individuals may be able to tolerate small amount of milk products. Yogurt and cheese are often well-tolerated. Lactase enzyme-containing preparations are available and can be added to milk before drinking.

Fat-modified Diets

Dietary fat intake may also be modified in the treatment of disease.

Fat-controlled Diets

A fat-controlled diet is desirable for the treatment of atherosclerosis, heart disease and hyperlipidemias. Diabetic diets also incorporate fat control. A fat-controlled diet limits both total fat and saturated fat intake. Usually when saturated fat intake is reduced, cholesterol intake also drops, since it is often found in foods containing saturated fat. The individual, who is reducing saturated fat in the diet, should choose low-fat dairy products, lean meats, skinless poultry and fish. Eggs should be limited to three per week and organ meats such as liver, limited to one serving per week or less. Visible fats, such as butter, margarine, mayonnaise, cream, sour cream, nuts and rich desserts should be limited. Cooking methods may need to be altered as well. Patients should be encouraged to bake, boil or poach the food, rather than to fry and add bread or butter to it. Foods should be eaten without the addition of sauces, gravies or dips that are high in fat.

When fat is necessary in food preparation, unsaturated fats (monounsaturated and polyunsaturated) should be used in place of saturated fats.

Low-fat Diets

Some medical conditions warrant the use of a low-fat diet. It differs from fat-controlled diets in which all fat is limited, regardless of saturation. Any time fat malabsorption occurs, dietary fat should be limited. GI diseases that involve malabsorption of fat include cystic fibrosis, inflammatory bowel disease, pancreatitis and short bowel syndrome secondary to bowel resection. Gallbladder disease often requires a low-fat diet. The gallbladder stores bile and contracts whenever fat is present in the intestinal tract. If gallstones are present or inflammation of the gallbladder exists, contraction may be painful. A low-fat diet may alleviate some discomfort. After the gallbladder is removed (cholecystectomy), as low-fat diet is no longer required. Some patients with gallbladder disease may be overweight or obese. Weight reduction is indicated for these individuals and may reduce symptoms of gallbladder disease.

Protein-restricted Diets

In disease states, increased protein needs are often considered to facilitate healing. However, in the presence of defects in protein metabolism or excretion, protein intake should be reduced or controlled. One such case is during renal failure or may progress slowly (end-stage renal disease). Acute renal failure is often temporary, whereas end-stage renal disease is irreversible.

The kidney normally functions to excrete wastes, concentrate urine and conserve needed electrolytes. During renal failure, the

SECTION 2: Dietetics

nephrons (working units of the kidney) fail to maintain normal function so that oliguria (decreased urine output) or anuria (no urine output) may result. Urea and other nitrogenous wastes, the end products of protein metabolism, build up in the bloodstream, leading to a condition known as azotemia. Many electrolytes, particularly potassium, sodium and phosphorus are retained and increased blood levels of these nutrients may occur.

Because of the buildup of protein waste products, dietary protein should be restricted. A therapeutic diet for renal failure limits the amount of protein consumed; the degree of limitation depends on extend of the renal failure. Patients are encouraged to consume moderate amounts of only high quality or complete proteins found in milk, meat, fish, poultry and eggs. Incomplete proteins, those found in plant products, contribute to uremia, so that it should be restricted. Other dietary modification in renal failure includes the restriction of potassium, sodium, phosphorus and fluids. Vitamin and mineral supplements are generally prescribed.

Cirrhosis is a chronic, degenerative disease of the liver. It is most often seen secondary to alcoholism, but may also be seen as a result of hepatitis A and B or other infection. Scar tissue develops in the liver, hampering its effectiveness in removing waste products from the bloodstream. In this case, ammonia, which is a waste product of protein metabolism, builds up in the bloodstream. If not controlled, high ammonia levels may contribute to hepatic coma (coma secondary to liver disease), brain damage and death. Ascites, a condition characterized by an accumulation of fluid in the abdominal cavity, may occur. If the liver is unable to produce bile, fat malabsorption also may take place.

In the presence of cirrhosis, protein intake should initially be at or above the RDA to facilitate healing and tissue regeneration. However, if blood ammonia levels become elevated and signs of impending coma are present, such as confusion, apathy and drowsiness, a strict low-protein diet should be followed. The low-protein diets for cirrhosis restrict milk and milk products, meats, fish, poultry, cheese, eggs, legumes and nuts.

Special nutritional support formulates with modified protein content have also been developed for hepatic coma.

The veins at the lower end of the esophagus may become enlarged and tortuous during cirrhosis, this condition known as esophageal varices. Esophageal varices are painful and the use of a soft or liquid diet may is beneficial in this case. Other dietary modifications for cirrhosis include total abstinence from alcohol and may require restriction if malabsorption is present. Vitamin and mineral supplements are also given.

Sodium-restricted Diets

Sodium restrictions may be used to treat a number of medical conditions. Hypertension is often responsive to a lowered sodium intake. It is estimated that 20% of the population is 'sodium sensitive', i.e. they have a genetic sensitivity to sodium that leads to hypertension. In such individuals, sodium reduction appears beneficial in controlling blood pressure.

Sodium is also restricted when water retention or edema is present. In the presence of CHF, sodium intake should be decreased to alleviate pulmonary and peripheral edema. Directly after a MI, sodium fluid, high-calorie foods (kcal) and fat restrictions may be implemented. These restrictions are to minimize the workload on the heart. As recovery progresses, the diet will be liberalized as individual condition permits. If cirrhosis is accompanied by ascites, sodium intake should be reduced and in renal failure, if anuria or oliguria exists, sodium should be restricted.

Sodium-restricted diets vary in degree of restriction. The no-added-salt diet is the least restrictive, allowing 2,000–3,000 mg of sodium/day. This diet allows the use of most foods with the exception of highly salted snack foods and prepared foods. Patients following this diet should read nutrition labels to assess the sodium content of food products and determine, which would be appropriate for their diet. No salt should be added in cooking or at the table. Other sodium restricted diets range from 2,000 mg (2 g) sodium to as little as 250 mg of sodium/day. In the presence of cystic fibrosis, the sweat glands produce excessive amounts of sodium and chloride. In uses special condition, sodium intake is not restricted, but generous amounts of sodium and salt are encouraged to compensate for the excess losses of sodium.

Potassium-modified Diets

Potassium is considered to play a role in blood pressure control. Evidence indicates that populations with higher potassium intakes have less incidence of hypertension. Increased potassium intake from foods may be beneficial for blood pressure control. Many patients with hypertension or other conditions that cause water retention may get potassium-wasting diuretics. An increased intake of potassium is needed to counteract the loss of potassium caused by the diuretic. In end-stage renal diseases and other kidney diseases, potassium intake may need to be restricted to as little as 1,500–2,000 mg/day.

Fluid-modified Diets

Fluid is found in the diet in a number of forms of course, all beverages, milk, juices, coffee and tea add fluid to the diet. Other dietary fluid sources include gelatins, ice cream, sherbet, puddings, popsicles, fruit ices and soups.

During end-stage renal disease and other kidney disease with oliguria and anuria fluid is restricted to 400–500 mL/day plus an amount equal to daily urine output, if any. Fluid restrictions may also be implemented during CHF, directly after MI or in hepatic coma or ascites.

During fluid restrictions, patients may experience excessive thirst. Some suggestions to help alleviate thirst include rinsing the mouth with cold mouthwash, putting lemon into cold water to make it more refreshing, freezing fluid so it takes longer time to consume, eating cold fruits and raw vegetables, chewing gum, sucking, breath mints or hard candies (in moderation) and brushing teeth often can helps to alleviate thirst.

Increased fluid intake is a common dietary treatment for renal calculi (kidney stones) a urinary tract infection. Additional fluid helps to dilute the urine and increases urinary output. Fluid needs are also increased during periods of diarrhea, vomiting or malabsorption such as in inflammatory bowel disease. Care should be taken to replace fluids that are lost, to prevent dehydration.

The burn victim loses a large volume of fluids from the wounds, immediately after a severe burn, fluids, electrolytes and protein are given intravenously rather than orally, because burn patients experience a temporary loss of bowel function. Once bowel activity resumes, adequate fluids should be a part of dietary treatment. Most conditions requiring diet therapy involve combinations of therapeutic diets.

▶ NURSE'S RESPONSIBLITIES IN FOOD SERVING

It is necessary to plan different diets for different patients considering the physical and mental condition of the patient, his/her social and cultural background, the treatment requirements, availability of food and the economic aspects.

Preparing Environment for Meals

The nurse's responsibilities in serving food to the patient are as follows:

1. Dressing and other such painful procedures should be ended 1 hour before serving meal.
2. Keep the dining place clean (while serving food on bed, dining table/cardiac table/small stool should be used).
3. Provide privacy to the patient (if no separate room is available, curtains can be used).
4. The meal hours should be fixed. Avoid the rounds, treatment formalities and visitors during mealtime.
5. The articles disliked by the patient or causing nausea, e.g. appliances like bedpan, urine pot, dirty dressing, dreadful equipment, dirty substances, refuse, etc. should be removed before serving meal.
6. Try to save the patient from the cry of other patients, noise and confusion, etc. at the time of meals.

7. Arrange for proper lighting and temperature.
8. Keep the patient clean (if necessary, the clothes are changed before meals).
9. Attempts should be made to reduce the patient's physical and mental fatigue. Diversional technique, soft melodious music and flower arrangement give pleasant environment for meals.

Serving Food

1. Keep the patient in Fowler's or comfortable position (as far as possible the patient should be encouraged to eat in sitting posture).
2. Mouth and hands of the patients should be washed.
3. Serve the food in an attractive manner through covered and cleaned utensils.
4. Motivate the patient to eat meals.
5. Direct the patient to use spoons or take small morsels (weak patient should be fed by nurse himself/herself).
6. Engage the patient in entertaining conversation during meals.
7. Give sufficient time to patient for mastication.
8. Give water whenever required.

Aftercare and Other Precautions

1. The patient should be provided comfortable position after washing their hands and mouth, following meals.
2. Food hygiene should be followed right from cooking to consumption.
3. The quality of food consumed by the patient and any abnormality if observed should be noted.
4. The cooperation offered by the patient, while consuming food should be appreciated, so that the morale goes up.
5. The opportunity of serving food should be fully utilized for giving nutrition education.

Feeding a Helpless Patient

It is the responsibility of the nurse, to feed or meet the nutritional requirements of the patient, when patient is too weak to accept food by himself/herself or is unconscious. Weak patients also include those, who are fully conscious yet unable to take diet orally because of physical weakness. While feeding the helpless patient, the following things should be kept in mind:

1. The patient's inability or weakness should be assessed. It is necessary to give full attention to the patient's requirement of diet, likes and dislikes, and the instructions about diet.
2. All instruments and appliances required in connection with diet and feeding, e.g. tray, plate, jug, drinking tube, thali, spoon, fork, knife, glass for drinking water, napkin, kidney tray, Mackintosh towel, etc. should be ready and placed near the patient.
3. The patient's surroundings should be made pleasant before serving food.
4. The patient should be fed with small pieces or morsels by sitting in a convenient position near the patient.
5. Sufficient time should be given to the patient for mastication.
6. While spoon feeding, the diet should not be spilled on the bed. Dry food can be consumed by the patient himself/herself.
7. The patient should be engaged in interesting conversation, while eating.
8. Anger or regret should not be expressed over the weakness of the patient.
9. The patient should be encouraged to consume all the food served. The importance of the proposed diet, in the disease should be explained to them.
10. The patient should not be forced to overeat after he/she is satisfied. Do not make patient eat against their wishes.
11. The mouth and hands of the patient should be washed, as after a normal meal. Water can be served with glass or tube.

12. The weak patient should be encouraged and motivated to eat with their own hands, as far as possible.
13. Nutrition education should be given, while feeding.
14. All the articles should be removed after feeding and the patient should be placed properly. The quantity and the type of food consumed should be entered in the patient's chart. Any abnormality, if observed should be noted.
15. It is necessary to observe the other instructions about nutrition and serving food. Semiconscious, unconscious or mental patients are given nutrition through nasal tube feeding/gastric gavage.

▶ CONCLUSION

All therapeutic diets are modifications of the normal diet made in order to meet the altered needs resulting from disease. Therapeutic diet is planned to meet or exceed the dietary allowances of a normal person as the aim of diet therapy is to maintain health and help the patient to regain nutritional well-being. A modified diet is any diet altered to include or exclude certain components, such as calories, fat, vitamins and minerals. Diets are typically modified for therapeutic reasons, including treatment of high blood pressure, low body weight or vitamin and mineral deficiencies. A modified therapeutic diet is designed to be part of an overall treatment regimen to combat a potentially serious condition. Diets low in fat and cholesterol, for example, may help avoid clogged arteries that can lead to heart attack or stroke. Several studies performed by Dr John Freeman and Dr Eileen Vining during the mid-1990s at John Hopkins University found that a less restrictive modified Atkins diet reduces the occurrence of seizures in adults with epilepsy.

Chapter 12

Diet Therapy for Perioperative Conditions

▶ INTRODUCTION

Malnutrition has long been recognized as a risk factor for postoperative morbidity and mortality. Traditional metabolic and nutritional care of patients undergoing major elective surgery has emphasized preoperative fasting and reintroduction of oral nutrition 3–5 days after surgery. Attempts to attenuate the consequent nutritional deficit and to influence postoperative morbidity and mortality have included parenteral, enteral and oral-sip feeding. Recent studies have emphasized that an enhanced rate of recovery can be achieved by a multimodal approach focused on modulating the metabolic status of the patient before (e.g. carbohydrate and fluid loading), during (e.g. epidural anesthesia) and after (e.g. early oral feeding) surgery.

▶ PREOPERATIVE DIET

Good nutrition prior to and following surgery ensures fewer postoperative complications for better wound healing. Short convalescence, lower mortality and chronic diseases increase the nutritional requirements. Malnutrition can lead to weight loss, poor wound healing, decreased intestinal motility, anemia, edema or dehydration and ulcers. The circulating blood volume and the concentration of the serum proteins, hemoglobin and electrolytes may be reduced.

Preoperative Nutritional Assessment

The objectives in the dietary management of surgical conditions are:

SECTION 2: Dietetics

1. To improve the perioperative nutrition whenever the operation is not of an emergency nature.
2. To maintain correct nutrition after operation or injury as far as possible.
3. To avoid harm from injudicious choice of foods.

Proteins

A satisfactory state of protein nutrition ensures:
1. Rapid wound healing.
2. Increases the resistance to infection.
3. Exerts a protective action upon the liver against the toxic effects of anesthesia.
4. Reduces the possibility of edema at the site of the wound. The level of protein to be used in preoperative and postoperative diets depends on the previous state of nutrition, the nature of the operation and the extent of the postoperative losses. Intake of 1.0–1.5/kg of body weight or about 100 g of protein is necessary as a rule.

Energy

With 2,500–3,000 kcal patients make progress. Obesity constitutes a hazard in surgery. Whenever possible it should be corrected. Rapid weight loss results in loss of lean body mass and should be avoided.

Minerals

A liberal intake of protein and ascorbic acid, and administration of iron salt is necessary.

Fluids

A patient should not go to operation in a stage of dehydration since the subsequent dangers of acidosis are great. If the patient is unable to ingest sufficient liquid by mouth, parental fluids are administered.

CHAPTER 12: Diet Therapy for Perioperative Conditions

Vitamins

Vitamin C is important for wound healing. Loss of vitamin K results in bleeding. Hemorrhage is especially likely to occur in patients who have diseases of the liver.

▶ POSTOPERATIVE DIET

Following minor surgery, liquids are often tolerated within a few hours and rapid progression to a normal diet is made after major surgery, oral intake may be delayed for days. Complete nutritional support is provided by conventional intravenous feedings, catheter jejunostomy, total parenteral nutrition (TPN), tube feedings or semisynthetic fiber-free diets.

The success of the surgery depends on following a modified textured diet for the next 8–10 weeks. Below is an idea of the timescale for this:

1. Weeks 1–3: Liquid diet only.
2. Weeks 4–6: Pureed diet.
3. Weeks 7–8: Soft, mashable diet.
4. Weeks 8 and onward: Resume solid food.

Step 1: For the first 3 weeks consume a liquid diet only

To ensure an adequate intake of protein, calcium and other nutrients to help in healing, the liquid diet must be based on milk, ideally low-fat milk, which can be flavored with milkshake powder or low-calorie hot chocolate. If the patient is diabetic, then a milkshake may not be appropriate.

Aim to have two pints of milk per day. If the patient does not like milk choose an alternative, such as soya milk, but make sure it is enriched with calcium. If the patient finds very hot or very cold drinks difficult to tolerate then can drink fluids at room temperature. Other fluids allowed:

1. Slimming drinks, e.g. slim fast or chemists/supermarket own brands.
2. Complan or 'Build up' soups and shakes.
3. Yogurt drinks and smoothies.
4. Still mineral water and still low-calorie fruit squash.

5. Clear low-calorie soups.
6. Smooth soups, e.g. cream of tomato or cream of chicken.
7. Tea and coffee without sugar.
8. Unsweetened fruit juice.
9. Marmite or Bovril drinks.

Be cautious with the quantities of fluid patients drink over the first few days until establish how much liquid patient can tolerate. Do not drink fizzy drinks at any time as they will cause bloating and increase stomach size.

Some people experience constipation in the first few weeks. This is due to the low intake of fiber in the diet. Weetabix in the meal plan may help, but make sure it is liquidized to a thin smooth liquid.

Step 2: For weeks 4–6 progress to a pureed diet

Gradually introduce pureed foods. These should be high in protein and low in fats and sugars:

1. A pureed diet means patients food should be like the consistency of baby food or applesauce; many people find a handheld blender most suited to pureeing small quantities of food.
2. Eat 4–5 small meals per day (about 1–2 tablespoons at each).
3. Eat slowly and stop as soon as you feel full.
4. If a food makes patient feel nauseous avoid it for a few days and then try again.

Step 3: For weeks 7–8 progresses to a moist, soft, mashed diet

This is similar to the pureed diet, but food simply needs to be soft and moist, and mashed with a fork. Adding sauces and gravies can be helpful.

Step 4: For 8 weeks and lifelong (returning to a normal diet)

Patient will now begin to include normal texture foods. Crispy textures may be better tolerated at first. For example, crisp breads and breadsticks rather than bread.

Aim for three meals per day. You can include healthy snacks between meals, but try to avoid high fat and sugary foods, such as chocolate. These foods can still be included as treats, but not as meal replacements.

CHAPTER 12: Diet Therapy for Perioperative Conditions

▶ DIET PLAN FOR PRE- AND POST-OPERATIVE SURGERY

Start with a Healthy Liver

In the case of operations involving a general anesthetic, the liver is the organ that takes the hardest knock from the drugs used. A good form of preparation for an operation would, therefore, involve restoring the liver to optimum health prior to undergoing surgery. Avoid alcohol and saturated fats. Wake up to a cup of hot water with the juice of half a lemon squeezed into it. Eat grapefruit with breakfast and plenty of fresh fruit with lemon juice squeezed over it. Eat lots of fresh, raw or lightly steamed vegetables, especially the colorful varieties. Drink plenty of juiced carrots, beetroot or any other vegetable juices can tolerate. These will very effectively detoxify the liver.

Sulfur-containing Foods

To prevent the after effects of anesthetics, such as hepatitis, eat foods rich in the sulfur-containing amino acid, methionine, such as free-range eggs, Brazil nuts, fish and meat. St Mary's Thistle, which contains the active ingredient, silymarin, is excellent in protecting the liver against anesthetics and so is dandelion root. These also help to regenerate liver cells, if there is damage to the liver.

Antioxidants

Plenty of antioxidants are needed to neutralize the free radicals, which result from all the chemicals in anesthetics and other drugs that may be prescribed. Mopping up of these free radicals depend upon the levels of beta carotene, vitamin A, C and E as well as zinc, manganese and copper levels. Take a good plant-based green leaf multivitamin and mineral supplement, such as AIM BarleyLife for a few weeks before the operation. Surgeon may insist patient to stop all vitamin supplements just prior to and immediately after the surgery. This is fine however;

do try to get back onto them as soon as possible to give the body a fighting chance against infection. Prior to surgery eat plenty of paw paw, beetroot, carrots, broccoli, apricots, all citrus, even the pith and green, yellow and red peppers.

Preventing Blood Clots

For at least a month before the operation, take a pharmaceutical grade fish oil capsule daily to keep patient's blood thin and prevent clotting after surgery. The patient need to inform the surgeon about this as the surgeon may wish to put the patient on a blood thinning drug, such as warfarin and the two should not be taken together as this may cause excessive bleeding during surgery. Continue with the fish oil capsules as soon as possible after surgery.

Healing of Wounds

Build up the liver stocks of beta carotene a week prior to surgery with carrot and beetroot juice, which will also detox the liver. Beta carotene converts to vitamin A in the body and will improve wound tensile strength, thus preventing possible tearing. Eat lots of apricots and watermelon, if in season. Vitamin E promotes healing of ulcerated tissue and helps prevent hard scar formation. Use it mainly as an ointment rubbed on the scar after the wound has closed, but the vitamin E in the plant-based multivitamin supplement will also be of great benefit.

Vitamin C

Vitamin C promotes elastogen and collagen formation and prevents pressure sores. Mouth ulcers common after surgery or chemotherapy; heal faster with 250 g vitamin C at meals and 500 mg at bedtime. Eat broccoli, paw paw, kiwifruit and oranges pre- and post-surgery. Throw in bioflavonoids to strengthen the integrity of mucous membranes and zinc for the correct formation of collagen and elastogen, particularly for leg ulcers.

Cancer Patients

Cancer patients should try to avoid infections after any surgery as infections will hinder recovery. Supplement with buffered vitamin C (2 g per day in divided doses, 20 mg zinc, 2 g bioflavonoids). This same program may be used by all patients going for surgery.

Bromelain

Bromelain, an enzyme found in pineapple, reduces edema and inflammation. Either eat lots of pineapple or take bromelain in supplement form. If undergoing plastic surgery, the patients could minimize bruising by using vitamin C, bioflavonoids and zinc before surgery and bromelain after surgery.

▶ CONCLUSION

The stress of surgery or trauma creates a hypermetabolic state, increasing protein and energy requirements. Macronutrients (fat, protein and glycogen) from the labile reserves of fat tissue and skeletal muscle are redistributed to more metabolically active tissues such as the liver and visceral organs. This response can lead to the onset of protein calorie malnutrition (defined as a negative balance of 100 g of nitrogen and 10,000 kcal) within a few days. The rate of development of post-operative malnutrition in a given individual depends upon their pre-existing nutritional status, nature and complexity of the surgical procedure, and the degree of hypermetabolism. Reduced food intake results in loss of fat, muscle, skin, and ultimately bone and viscera, with subsequent weight loss, and expansion of the extracellular fluid compartment. Nutritional requirements fall as an individual's body mass decreases, probably reflecting more efficient utilization of ingested food and a reduction in work capacity at the cellular level. However, the combination of decreased tissue mass and reduced work capacity impedes normal homeostatic responses to stressors such as surgery or critical illness.

Chapter 13

Diet Therapy in Fevers

▶ INTRODUCTION

Fever is a common symptom, which is associated with a host of infectious and chronic conditions. Fever is a natural response of the body, to destroy virus or pathogens in the blood, by raising the body's natural metabolic rate. There are various dietary measures that have been suggested to improve and hasten recovery after a fever. Though the dietary modalities will differ depending upon the cause of the fever, however, there are certain basic guidelines that have been found to be highly beneficial fever is an elevation in body temperature above the normal, which may occur due to exogenous and endogenous factors.

▶ DIET FOR COMMON FEVERS

There are certain simple dietary recommendations that can help hasten the recovery from fever. Eating right and getting enough rest is essential when trying to avoid illnesses and this includes the prevention of fevers:

1. To begin with the patient should be put on a juice and water diet for a couple of days. A glass full of orange juice every 3 hours is considered beneficial for health. Orange juice is a great source of energy and is also loaded with vitamin C, which helps enhance immunity and natural ability of the body to fight infection.
2. Following the juice diet, an all fruit diet is recommended. Fruits are easier to digest and loaded with essential vitamins and minerals, which hasten the process of recovery.
3. Fresh fruits including grapes, apple, oranges, peach, pineapple, lemons, etc. should be included in the diet. Fresh fruit juices are also recommended. Avoid tinned or canned

fruit juices as they are loaded with preservatives and can delay the recovery process.
4. Always ensure that you consume about 3 L of water each day, especially during fever. Water helps flush the toxins out of the body system and hastens recovery.
5. Once the fever subsidizes, opt for a soft diet. A soft diet may comprise of boiled eggs, steamed vegetables, vegetable soups, porridge and yogurt. These foods are easier to digest and supply with loads of energy, which is essential to hasten the recovery process.
6. Rice porridge with ginger and made with vegetable both is good to have when have a fever. This diet is easy to digest. Further ginger has strong anti-inflammatory properties, which are beneficial in resolving the fever at the earliest.

A healthy lifestyle practice is considered to be beneficial in reducing the incidence of fevers. Increase the intake of water, green vegetables, fresh fruits and low-fat dairy products. These foods are loaded with essential vitamins and enhance the overall immunity of the body. These dietary measures can help improve the body's natural immune system and can also help in preventing the occurrence of infections.

▶ DIET THERAPY IN DIFFERENT TYPES OF FEVER

Acute Fever of Short Duration

Acute fevers of short duration, such as influenza, typhoid, chickenpox, pneumonia. In such cases, the diet should be planned with the objective of eliminating any exertion on the part of the patient in taking their food. For the first 2–3 days, the diet should be fluid or semifluid and small feeds given at frequent intervals of 2–3 hours. Sufficient intake of fluids and salt is essential. If the illness continues for more than a few days, high-protein and high-calorie food should be provided. Milk should be the main sustaining item of the diet and nearly 1 L should be given daily. This will provide easily digestible proteins. Diet could include daily, more than one egg and plenty of fresh fruit juice. At least 2–3 L of fluids should be taken daily. As soon as the temperature comes down a bland diet containing plenty of protein and energy should be given. In case of typhoid fever, low-fiber foods such as white bread, refined cooked and dry cereals, egg, cheese, tender meat, fish, potatoes and simple desserts may be given.

Long-continued Fever

Long-continued fever, as in tuberculosis (pulmonary tuberculosis, in inflammatory disease of the lungs), followed by a wasting of the tissues, exhaustion, cough and fever. It is necessary to take care of the dietary intake, particularly of proteins and to ensure that the energy is sufficient to meet the extra requirements caused by the fever. This minimizes weight loss, which is quite common in such continued fevers.

It is very important to include calcium in the diet to promote the healing of the tuberculosis lesions. At least a liter of milk should be included daily. Iron supplementation may be necessary, if one suffers from hemorrhage. In case of vitamins, since the conversion of carotene to vitamin A is poor, it should be supplied in the form of retinol through the diet. In addition vitamin A supplement may be necessary. Ascorbic acid deficiency is normally found and therefore, an additional amount of citrus fruits or ascorbic acid supplementation is essential.

Intermittent Fever

Intermittent fevers, as in malaria during this type of fever there is an increased rate of metabolism, increased restlessness and hence the demand for calories increases. There is a decrease in the glycogen and adipose tissue stores. There is also an increase in the catabolic processes. Loss of body water increases due to excessive perspiration and excretion from the body.

▶ CAUSES OF FEVER

1. Some of the illnesses that almost always have fevers as part of the list of symptoms they have include colds, flu,

CHAPTER 13: Diet Therapy in Fevers

chickenpox, measles, mumps, bronchitis, tetanus, tonsillitis and other ailments that are brought about by viruses and bacteria.

2. Other causes for fevers that have nothing to do with bacteria or viruses include overexposure to the sun or heat. Also called sunstroke, people can develop fevers from staying in the sun too long.
3. Fatigue and overexertion can also cause people to have fevers. When a person is stretching their body's limits beyond what it can manage, a fever may signal them that it is time to get some rest.
4. Sometimes staying out too long in the rain can also cause fevers to happen.
5. People who live in rather unhygienic conditions as well as those who do not take care of their health may be prone to fevers.

Causes of Fever in Children

Fever in children causes due to any kind of infection like bacterial or viral infection, or through use of medications, illicit drug and heat illnesses, etc.

Low-grade Fever

Causes of low-grade fever can be mumps, chickenpox, wound infection, scarlet fever, hepatitis, mononucleosis and others. Autoimmune and viral diseases can also cause low-grade fever.

Recurrent Fever

Possible causes of recurrent fever are typhoid, brucellosis, malaria, cholera, etc.

High Fever

Common medical conditions resulting in high fever are measles, roseola, scarlet fever, glandular fever, sinusitis, etc.

SECTION 2: Dietetics

▶ GENERAL DIETARY MANAGEMENT

Energy

The caloric requirement may be increased as much as 50%, if the temperature is high and the tissue destruction is great. The patient may be able to ingest only 600–1,200 kcal daily, but this should be increased as rapidly as possible.

Proteins

About 100 g protein or more is prescribed for the adult when a fever is prolonged. High-protein beverages may be used as supplements to the regular meals.

Carbohydrates

Glycogen stores are replenished by a liberal intake of carbohydrates. Glucose, which readily absorbed is preferred.

Fats

The energy intake may be rapidly increased through the judicious use of fats, but fried foods and rich pastries are to be avoided.

Minerals

A sufficient intake of NaCl is accomplished by the use of salty broth and soups, and by liberal sprinklings of salt on food. Fruit juices and milk are relatively good sources of minerals.

Vitamins

Fevers apparently increase the requirement for vitamin A and vitamin C just as the B complex vitamins are needed at increased levels.

Fluids

Daily 2,500–5,000 mL is necessary including beverages, soups, fruit juices and water.

CHAPTER 13: Diet Therapy in Fevers

Ease of Digestion

Bland readily digested food should be used to facilitate digestion and rapid absorption. The food may be soft or of regular consistency. Fluid diets can be used initially.

Intervals of Feeding

Small quantities of food at interval of 2–3 hours will permit adequate nutrition without overtaking the digestive system at anytime. During an acute fever the patient's appetite is often very poor and small feedings of soft or liquid foods as desired should be offered at frequent intervals. Sufficient intake of fluids and salt is essential. If the illness persists for more than a few days high-protein and high-calorie foods will be needed.

▶ TYPHOID FEVER

Typhoid is an infectious disease with an acute fever of short duration and occurs only in human. *Salmonella typhi* causes typhoid. Feces and urine of the patients or carriers of the disease are the source of infection. Drinking water or milk and food contaminated by intestinal contents of the patients or carriers or by flies often transmit the disease. The disease is characterized by a continued and high inflammation of the intestine. Formation of intestinal ulcers, hemorrhage and enlargement of spleen can occur. The patient may complain of diarrhea or constipation and severe stomach ache. Abdominal absorption of nutrients can cause headache.

Definition

Typhoid fever is the result of systemic infection mainly by the bacteria *S. typhi* found only in man. The disease is clinically characterized by a typical continuous fever for 3–4 weeks. The primary sources of infection are feces and urine of cases or carriers.

Symptoms

Typhoid fever, medically also called enteric fever, can be a serious illness and needs good medical care. It is an infectious disease and can last for any number of days. Some of the causes of typhoid fever are drinking impure water contaminated by human waste-like excreta and eating unhygienic food among others. Typhoid fever shows symptoms like high fever, headache, stomach pain, skin rashes, exhaustion, poor appetite, constipation and diarrhea. Unhygienic habits like not washing hands after using the toilet and being in close contact with people suffering from typhoid fever can result in the condition. The fact that typhoid fever is most common in places and society where surroundings are not kept clean proves the fact that this disease breeds in unhygienic environment.

Principles of Dietary Therapy

A high calorie, high protein, high carbohydrates, low fat, high fluid, low fiber and bland diet is suggested for typhoid patients. At first clear-fluid diet is given followed by full fluid and soft diet is suggested because of the intestinal inflammation. Great care must be exercised to eliminate all irritating fibers and spices in the diet. Refined cereals, bread, eggs, boiled potato and simple desserts-like custards, porridges can be given. Adequate nutrition reduces convalescence period.

Guidelines for Dietary Treatment

1. High-calorie diet is prescribed to maintain the weight or to gain weight. Caloric requirement may be as high as 2,500–3,000 k/day.
2. Daily requirement of protein ranges from 80 to 120 g to make up for tissue wasting. Good quality proteins like egg and milk should be incorporated.
3. Minerals especially calcium, iron and phosphorus is to be provided liberally as they help in regeneration of cells, blood and body fluids.

4. Diet must be planned judiciously to provide good dose of vitamins especially vitamin A and vitamin C as these are essential for the regenerative purpose.
5. High fluid and soft diet in small frequency is recommended.
6. Food must be appetizing, and made after considering the likes and dislikes of the patient.
7. Fatty, highly fibrous and very spicy foods should be avoided as they are hard to digest.

Treatment Through Diet

Treatment is essential to have a healthy, hygienic diet, if someone suffers from typhoid fever. There is a need to keep the body hydrated enough in this condition. So please drink plenty of fluids like unsweetened lime water, clear soups, fresh juices (which you are sure is safe and uncontaminated) and especially boiled and filtered water. As for food, must eat food items that provide plenty of calories, protein and carbohydrates. When a person gets fever, their metabolic rate becomes high, hence calorie intake has to be increased. Protein is also essential in curing a fever, so consume plenty of eggs and milk to fulfill the requirement. Carbohydrates also meet the new needs that your body develops due to typhoid fever. These elements are known to be effective to this disease.

Care-digestible Diet

Care-digestible is absolutely necessary for food to be thoroughly cooked and easily digestible for a typhoid fever patient. Avoid raw food in any form. You will also have to control the urge to eat outside food, as it is likely to be unhygienic. You also have to steer clear of alcohol, canned or carbonated drinks as well as too much of caffeine. As for eating rice in this condition, it will be better, if you avoid rice in the initial stages and focus on a liquid based diet instead. Rice is solid food, which is not recommended in this condition. However, after a few days, you can eat unpolished rice, if you still crave for rice. It is healthy to eat that along with fruits that are easily digestible such as banana, apples and watermelon as it has a high content of water in it. In addition to these dietary tips, you need to maintain proper hygiene to avoid typhoid fever.

Foods to be included: Fruit juices with glucose, coconut water, barley water, milk, milkshakes, if there is no diarrhea, custards, thin dal curries, eggs, baked fish, minced meat, curds, cottage cheese, cereals, gruels, steamed vegetable juices, milk puddings and vegetable puree.

Foods to be avoided: Butter, ghee, vegetable oil, no irritating fibrous food, chili's and other spices, rich pastries, fried foods, heavy puddings and cream soups.

▶ CONCLUSION

Fever increases the requirement for vitamin A, ascorbic acid, calcium, phosphorous, sodium and B complex vitamins. Liberal intake of milk, fruits, fruit juices and two or three eggs will take care of the above requirement. As soon as the temperature comes down readily digestible bland food should be given to the patient for better digestion and rapid absorption depending on the patient's need of the food can be soft or normal consistency. Initially the interval of feeding should be 2 hours. Later on improvement it can be made into 4 hours interval or 4 meals a day. Typhoid fever is an infectious disease with a characteristic pattern of acute fever. The disease is usually transmitted by contaminated food. A high calorie, high protein, high carbohydrate, low fat, high fluid, low fiber, and bland diet are advisable for typhoid patients. Since typhoid fever is associated with intestinal inflammation, diet should preferably be free of spices and fibers. Refined cereals, eggs, boiled potato, simple desserts like custard, and porridge should be given.

Mineral and calcium should be provided liberally since it is essential for the healing of tuberculosis lesions. At least a liter of milk should be consumed daily. Iron supplementation may be necessary if one suffers from hemorrhage. The vitamin A metabolism is adversely affected in tuberculosis so vitamin A rich foods such as carrot, tomato, papaya, mango, green leafy should be included in the diet. Another important vitamin deficiency associated with this condition is that of vitamin C. Vitamin C is essential for many regenerative purposes. An additional amount of citrus fruits such as orange, sweet lime, lemon, gooseberry or ascorbic acid supplementation is essential.

Chapter 14

Diet Therapy for Gastrointestinal Disorders

▶ INTRODUCTION

Diet therapy is an important factor in overall care of most gastrointestinal (GI) patients. Historically, diets have been used unscientifically in many of these patients without positive results. Nutritional care and diet therapy are critical for two reasons. First, malnutrition is expected sequelae to most, if not all, GI diseases or disorders. Failure to eat, digest or assimilate nutrients can provoke malnutrition in just a few weeks, although, careful assessment of anthropometric, clinical, biochemical and nutritional history by a trained professional can protect against this. Diet therapy through the elimination of offending foods, such as wheat gluten or lactose, or inclusion of specialized products such as medium chain triglycerides or elemental formulas, can sustain nutritional status. Dietary components, such as insoluble fiber appear to have physiologic effects, while soluble fibers may have metabolic effects important to diabetes and cardiovascular disease. There is a high potential for malnutrition in Crohn's disease during active and remittent phases. Elemental enteral formulas or total parenteral nutrition (TPN) are used during the active phase to ensure optimal nutritional status and bowel rest. Hyperalimentation using the GI tract during remittent stage maintains this. Avoiding offending foods by Crohn's patients is an acceptable practice as long as entire categories of foods are not deleted. Avoiding all foods containing gluten from wheat, rye, barley and oats, however, is a crucial prerequisite to recovery from celiac disease. Gluten is commonly used as a stabilizer, emulsifier and extender in the food industry and is not always shown on food labels. Careful consultation with a registered dietitian can identify hidden sources of gluten in the diet.

CHAPTER 14: Diet Therapy for Gastrointestinal Disorders

▶ DIARRHEA

Diarrhea is the passage of stools with increased frequency, fluidity or volume compared to the usual for a given individual. Diarrhea is a symptom of underlying functional or organic disease and is acute or chronic in nature:

1. **Chemical toxins:** Such as arsenic, lead, mercury or cadmium.
2. **Bacterial toxins:** Such as *Salmonella* or staphylococcal food poisoning.
3. **Bacterial infections:** Such as *Streptococcus, Escherichia coli.*
4. **Drugs:** Such as quinidine, neomycin.
5. **Psychogenic factors:** Such as emotional instability.
6. **Dietary factors:** Such as food sensitivity or allergy.

Chronic Type

1. Malabsorptive lesions of anatomic, mucosal or enzymatic origin.
2. Metabolic diseases, such as diabetic neuropathy, uremia or Addison's disease.
3. Alcoholism.
4. Carcinoma of small bowel or colon.
5. Postirradiation to small bowel or colon.
6. Cirrhosis.
7. Laxative abuse.

Nutritional Considerations in Diarrhea

Fluid electrolyte and tissue protein losses are usually severe, if diarrhea is prolonged.

Fluids

Losses of fluids should be replaced by a liberal intake to prevent dehydration, especially in susceptible age groups.

Electrolytes

Losses of sodium, potassium and others with severe diarrhea; potassium loss is detrimental, as potassium is necessary for normal muscle tone of the gastrointestinal tract. Losses can be replaced by liberal fluids, such as fruit juices that are high in potassium.

Nutrient Malabsorption

Long continued diarrhea may result in depletion of tissue, proteins and decreased serum protein levels. Fat losses are considerable in certain disorders with consequent loss of calories and fat-soluble vitamins. Intake of calories as high as 3,000, which includes 100–150 g protein, 100–120 g fat and the remainder as carbohydrates.

Vitamin deficiencies frequently seen in chronic diarrhea are related to the decreased intake of vitamins and the increased requirements because of losses in the stools.

Iron deficiency owing to the increased losses of iron in the feces, the occasional blood losses and the reduced intake of iron rich foods because of fear that some foods might aggravate an existing lesion.

Dietary Considerations

In acute diarrhea, current recommendations include oral intake of glucose electrolyte solutions for those able to drink with progression to foods as tolerated in small frequent feedings as appetite improves. Many patients with chronic diarrhea do not tolerate milk or foods high in fat or fiber content. Generally speaking, however the need is for a diet high in protein and calories with adequate amounts of vitamins and minerals and liberal amounts of fluids.

▶ CONSTIPATION

In this condition, there is the duodenum and intervention or difficult evacuation of feces from the intestine. Insufficient or infrequent emptying of the bowel may lead to malaise, headache,

CHAPTER 14: Diet Therapy for Gastrointestinal Disorders 287

coated tongue, foul breath and lack of appetite. These symptoms usually disappear after satisfactory evacuation has taken place. Correction of constipation depends in large measure on establishing regularity in habits, eating, rest, exercise and elimination.

Requirements for Normal Defecation

1. Moist bulky fecal bolus.
2. Stimulus capable of transporting bolus to distal colon.
3. Normal colon.
4. Rectum capable of reasonable degree of distension.
5. Normal internal and external sphincters.
6. Normal peripheral nervous system to send afferent impulses.
7. Normal central nervous system response to send efferent impulses.
8. Conducive physical and psychological environment.
9. Appropriate posture, Valsalva maneuver.
10. Desire and ability to evacuate bolus.

Causes of Constipation

1. Dietary:
    a. Low-fiber intake.
    b. Reduced food intake.
    c. Reduced fluid intake.
2. Functional:
    a. Reduced physical inactivity.
    b. Weakness.
    c. Immobility.
    d. Depression.
    e. Disorientation.
    f. Physical disability.
    g. Repeated suppression of urge to defecate.

3. Secondary causes:
    a. Metabolic, endocrine disorders.
    b. Neuromuscular disorders.
    c. Colonic obstruction.

Medication

1. Aluminum/Calcium antacids.
2. Anticholinergics.
3. Antidepressants.
4. Antihypertensives.
5. Antiparkinsonian drugs.
6. Antispasmodics.
7. Bismuth-containing drugs.
8. Diuretics.
9. Narcotic analgesics.
10. Opiates.

Dietary Considerations

The diet should contain sufficient fiber to induce peristalsis and to contribute bulk to the intestine. A regular diet with an abundance of both raw and cooked fruits and vegetables is suitable for such patients. Whole grain cereals should be substituted for refined ones. Bran is useful, but excesses are to be avoided since it may act as an irritant to sensitive intestinal tracts. Fat containing foods are useful because of the stimulating effect of the fatty acids on the mucous membranes. Excesses may cause diarrhea and should be avoided. Mineral oil, if used should not be taken at mealtime because of its interference with the absorption of fat-soluble vitamins. A fluid intake of 8–10 glasses a day is useful in keeping the intestinal contents in a semisolid state for easier passage along the tract. Some individuals find that one or two glasses of hot or cold water plain or with lemon are helpful in initiating peristalsis when taken before breakfast.

CHAPTER 14: Diet Therapy for Gastrointestinal Disorders

Dietary Management

Energy
Normal calories according to age, sex and occupation.

Proteins
About 60–80 grams of proteins per day.

Fats
Fats stimulate the flow of bile and lubricate the bowel. Fried foods should be avoided.

Carbohydrates
Adequate bulk should be supplied in the form of bran, vegetables and whole fruits, which are rich in unabsorbable cellulose. Bran is made more palatable by adding cooked fruits and vegetables.

Vitamins
The B group vitamins help to regulate the bowel function.

Minerals
Acutely ill or bedridden patients require potassium in the form of vegetable soup and fruit juice to prevent constipation.

Fluids
A liberal amount of fluids, about 10 glasses per day is advised. Warm fluid taken early morning on an empty stomach helps in the evacuation of bowel.

Fiber
The intake of dietary fiber should be increased by eating whole cereals and increasing consumption of fruits and vegetables. The most important factor is the water holding capacity of the fiber.

SECTION 2: Dietetics

Oranges, carrots and cabbage fibers hold more water effectively. Whole grain breads and cereals should be used instead of refined cereals, e.g. whole wheat flour instead of maids.

▶ PEPTIC ULCER

The term peptic ulcer is used to describe any localized erosion of the mucosal lining of those portions of the alimentary tract that come in contact with gastric juice. The majority of ulcers are found in the stomach, although they also occur in the duodenum, jejunum or any other part of the GI tract exposed to the gastric juice.

Dietary Management

It was customary to suggest a bland diet for ulcer patients. Bland diet is a diet, which is mechanically, chemically and thermally non-irritating.

Milk and Protein Foods

Milk and protein foods do have some buffering effect, but they also evoke gastric secretions more than carbohydrates and fats. Milk should be included as a source of nutrients factors for healing purposes. Protein provides the necessary amino acids for synthesis of tissue proteins, which helps in healing ulcer.

Fats

Moderate amounts of the fat help to suppress gastric secretion and motility through the enterogastrone mechanism.

Foods believed to be chemically irritating because of their stimulatory effect on gastric secretion include meat extractives, caffeine, alcohol, citrus fruits and juices and some spicy foods. Mechanically irritating foods include those with indigestible carbohydrates, such as whole grains and most raw fruits and vegetables. Foods believed to be thermally irritating are those ordinarily served at extremes of temperatures such as very hot or iced liquids. In addition, certain foods traditionally forbidden

CHAPTER 14: Diet Therapy for Gastrointestinal Disorders

include strongly flavored vegetables, such as cabbage, cauliflower, onions and turnips and fried foods. Restriction of these foods is based on subjective evidence from patients who experience distress following ingestion of these items including good food.

Food to be Included

Dairy products such as milk, cream, butter, milk cheese and eggs (not fried), steamed fish, rice, rice flakes, puffed rice, margarine, well-cooked cereal, semolina, cooked green leafy vegetables, custards, malted drinks.

Food to be Avoided

Alcohol, strong tea, coffee, cola, beverages, gravies, soups, pickles, spices, curries, condiments, all fried foods, pastries, cakes, heavy sweets such as halva, barfi, raw unripe fruits, raw vegetables such as cucumber, onions, radish and tomatoes.

Dietary Guidelines

1. Whether a patient is on bland diet or regular diet, the patient and the family need to know, which foods are needed for a nutritionally adequate diet and the importance of including these daily.
2. The patient should select foods from the basic five food groups, omitting those foods known to irritate the mucosa.
3. Small and frequent meals at regular intervals are essential.
4. Patient should consume moderate quantities of food, as heavy foods tend to exert antral pressure against the stomach wall stimulating gastric secretion through the gastrin mechanism.
5. The cultural pattern, economic status, preferences of the patient and effect on the family has to be taken into consideration, while planning the diet.
6. Meals should be eaten in a relaxed atmosphere.
7. A short rest before and after meals may be conducive to greater benefit of meals.

8. Food should be eaten slowly and chewed well as fast eating provokes gastric feeding reflex.

Modification of Diet in Bleeding Ulcer

The degree of dietary modification in bleeding ulcer depends on the peculiarities of the individual case. The severe hemorrhage, it is customary to give no food until the bleeding has been controlled and the patient's condition is stabilized. If hemorrhage is not severe, and if nausea and vomiting are not a problem, the patient may desire food and tolerate it well. Initial dietary treatment consists of mild alternated at 2 hours interval with small feedings of easily puddings toast and tender cooked fruits and vegetables. Gradual progression in amounts and types of foods is made as the patient improves.

▶ CONCLUSION

Diet therapy is an important factor in overall care of most GI patients. Historically, diets have been used unscientifically in many of these patients without positive results. Nutritional care and diet therapy are critical for two reasons. First, malnutrition is expected sequelae to most, if not all, GI diseases or disorders. Failure to eat, digest, or assimilate nutrients can provoke malnutrition in just a few weeks, although careful assessment of anthropometric, clinical, biochemical and nutritional history by a trained professional can protect against this. Diet therapy through the elimination of offending foods such as wheat gluten or lactose, or inclusion of specialized products such as medium-chain triglycerides or elemental formulas, can sustain nutritional status. Dietary components such as insoluble fiber appear to have physiologic effects, while soluble fibers may have metabolic effects important to diabetes and cardiovascular disease. There is a high potential for malnutrition in Crohn's disease during active and remittent phases. Elemental enteral formulas or TPN are used during the active phase to ensure optimal nutritional status and bowel rest. Hyperalimentation using the GI tract during remittent stage maintains

CHAPTER 14: Diet Therapy for Gastrointestinal Disorders

this. Avoiding offending foods by Crohn's patients is an acceptable practice as long as entire categories of foods are not deleted. Avoiding all foods containing gluten from wheat, rye, barley and oats, however, is a crucial prerequisite to recovery from celiac disease. Gluten is commonly used as a stabilizer, emulsifier, and extender in the food industry and is not always shown on food labels.

Chapter 15

Diet Therapy for Liver Diseases

▶ INTRODUCTION

The liver is one of the main organs of nutritional metabolism, including protein synthesis, glycogen storage and detoxification. These functions become damaged to a greater or lesser extent in patients with liver diseases, resulting in various metabolic disorders and their disturbed nutritional condition is associated with disease progression. Therefore, dietary counseling and nutritional intervention can support other medical treatments in some liver diseases.

It is vitally important that patients with liver disease maintain a balanced diet, which ensures adequate calories, carbohydrates, fats and proteins. Such a diet will aid the liver in the regeneration of liver cells. Nutrition that supports this regeneration is a means of treatment of some liver disorders.

Patients with cirrhosis, who are malnourished, require a diet rich in protein and providing 2,000–3,000 calories per day to help the liver rebuild itself. However, some cirrhotic patients have protein intolerance. Too much protein will result in an increased amount of ammonia in the blood, while too little protein can reduce healing of the liver. Doctors must carefully prescribe a specific amount of protein that will not elevate the blood ammonia. Lactulose and neomycin are two drugs that help keep the ammonia down.

It is believed that the risk of gallbladder disorders can be reduced by avoiding high fat and cholesterol food, and preventing obesity. The gallbladder is a storage sac for the bile produced by the liver. During digestion, the gallbladder releases bile into the small intestine through the common bile duct. Most gallbladder problems are caused by gallstones and

CHAPTER 15: Diet Therapy for Liver Diseases

80%–90% of all gallstones are produced from excessive cholesterol, which crystallizes and forms stones. By maintaining a well-balanced diet and avoiding high cholesterol intake, the incidence of gallstone formation may be lowered.

▶ INFECTIVE HEPATITIS (JAUNDICE)

Infective hepatitis is otherwise known as viral hepatitis. This is the common cause of jaundice. The two viruses responsible are hepatitis A and B virus. The former enters the body through oral fecal route like through food or water, while the latter is passed through by using infected blood products from carriers, use of unsterilized needles and through sexual contact. Jaundice may be produced due to the following factors/reasons:

1. Obstructive jaundice results from the interference of the flow of bile by the formation of stone and tumors.
2. Hemolytic jaundice results from an abnormally large destruction of red blood cells as in hemolytic anemia.
3. Toxic jaundice originates from poisons, drugs or viral infection.

Symptoms

Anorexia, fever, headache, rapid weight loss, loss of muscle tone and abdominal discomfort.

Dietary Management

Energy

In nasogastric feeding stage about 1,000 kcal are supplied. In severe cases, 1,600–2,000 kcal are suggested.

Proteins

For the liver cells to regenerate an adequate supply of proteins are needed. Protein requirements vary according to the severity of the disease with severe jaundice 40 g, while in mild jaundice 60–80 g of protein is permitted with hepatic precoma and coma, protein containing foods are withheld and only high carbohydrate containing foods are given.

Fats

During hepatic precoma and coma due to severe liver failure, fats are not metabolized by the liver and so fat is restricted, in severe jaundice 30 g and in moderate jaundice 50–60 g. A high protein, high carbohydrate, moderate fat diet is recommended. Small attractive meals at regular intervals are better tolerated.

Carbohydrates

High carbohydrate content in the diet is essential to supply enough calories, so that tissue proteins are not broken down for energy.

Vitamins

They are essential to regenerate liver cells; 500 mg of vitamin C along with 10 mg vitamin K and supplements of vitamin B.

Minerals

Oral feeds of fruit juice, vegetable and meat soups with added salt, given orally or through a nasogastric tube help in maintaining the electrolyte balance.

Food to be Included

Cereal porridge, soft chapatis, bread, rice, skimmed milk, tapioca, potato, yam, fruit, fruit juices, sugar, jaggery, honey, biscuits, soft custards without butter cream and non-stimulant beverages.

Foods to be Avoided

Pulses, beans, meat, fish, chicken, egg, soups, sweet preparations where ghee, butter or oil are used, bakery products, dried fruits, nuts, spices, papads, chutney, alcoholic beverages, fried preparations and whole milk creams.

CHAPTER 15: Diet Therapy for Liver Diseases

▶ CIRRHOSIS OF LIVER

Cirrhosis is a condition in which there is destruction of the liver cell due to necrosis, fatty infiltration and fibrosis. The cirrhotic process may commence many years before it becomes clinically obvious and usually the patient when first seen is at a very late stage with complications, such as ascites, ruptured esophageal varices or hepatic coma. Almost 85%–90% of liver damage also does not produce symptoms. The initial change in cirrhosis is widespread liver cell necrosis due to viral hepatic, alcohol, etc.

Causes

- Viral infection by hepatitis A and B viruses
- Alcohol
- Toxins of food, aflatoxin, bush tea.

Symptoms

The onset of cirrhosis may be gradual with gastrointestinal disturbances such as anorexia, nausea, vomiting, pain and distension. As the disease progresses jaundice and other serious changes occur. Ascites is the accumulation of abnormal amounts of fluids in the abdomen.

Principles of Diet

A high calorie, high protein, high carbohydrate, moderate or restricted fat and high-vitamin diet helps in regeneration of liver and helps to prevent the formation of ascites. Low fat with supplements of fat-soluble vitamin and minerals should be given. Sodium should be restricted only when there is ascites. When there is danger of esophageal varices or portal hypertension, fiber should be restricted.

SECTION 2: Dietetics

Dietary Management

Energy

Consumption of food is difficult because of anorexia and ascites. The patients are usually emaciated and require highly nutritious food, i.e. high-calorie diet is necessary because of prolonged undernourishment. The calorie requirement should be between 2,000 and 2,500 kcal.

Proteins

A high-protein diet is helpful for regeneration of the liver. In the absence of hepatic coma a high intake of proteins about 1.2 g/kg of body weight can be given. If the patient is in precoma or coma, proteins should be withheld till the patient tides over the crisis. Vegetable proteins containing more valine are beneficial in preventing encephalopathy.

Fats

About 1 g of fat/kg of body weight is given. Even if fatty changes are present in the liver, fats should be given provided adequate amounts of protein is supplied. Medium-chain triglycerides (MCTs) containing caprylic acid (C8) and capric acid (C10) fatty acids can be given as these are digested and absorbed in the absence of bile salts. Coconut oil contains medium-chain fatty acids.

Carbohydrates

Carbohydrate should be supplied liberally, so that the liver may store glycogen. Liver function improves when an adequate store of glycogen is present in liver cells. 60% of the calories should come from carbohydrate, so that liver damage is minimized.

CHAPTER 15: Diet Therapy for Liver Diseases

Vitamins

The liver is the major site of storage and conversion of vitamins into their metabolically active form. In cirrhosis, the liver concentration complex of folate, riboflavin, niacin, cobalamin and retinol are decreased. Vitamin supplementation especially of B vitamins is required to prevent anemia.

Minerals

Sodium is restricted in edema and ascites. Potassium salt is administered for ascites and edema to prevent hypokalemia. Anemia is common among cirrhosis patients, so iron supplementation is essential.

Foods to be Included

All cereals in a soft form such as cooked rice, chapati, bread and idli, milk pudding, milkshakes, curds, pureed or cooked vegetables, khichdi and porridge, pulses, beans, meat, fruit and fruit juices.

▶ HEPATIC COMA

Complex syndrome characterized by neurological disturbances, which may develop as a complication of severe liver disease. It results from entrance of certain nitrogen containing substances, such as ammonia into the cerebral circulation without being metabolized by the liver.

Precipitating Factors

Gastrointestinal bleeding, severe infections, surgical procedures and excessive dietary protein and sedatives may precipitate hepatic coma.

Symptoms

Confusion, restlessness, irritability, inappropriate behavior, delirium and drowsiness are present. There may be incoordination, and a flapping tremor of the arms and legs when extended. Electrolyte imbalance occurs. The patient may go into coma and may have convulsions. Breath has a fecal odor. Prompt treatment is imperative or death occurs.

Treatment

1. Dietary protein restriction.
2. Cleansing of the bowel with enemas or laxative to reduce the nitrogenous load or antibiotics to suppress bacterial growth.
3. Administration of lactulose to increase motility. This is a synthetic disaccharide containing galactose and fructose, which is metabolized by colonic bacteria to acetic and lactic acids, which lowers the pH of the colon, thereby favoring diffusion of ammonia from blood to the colon.
4. Oral or intravenous administration of branched-chain amino acids or their ketoanalogues improve both the plasma amino acid pattern and the encephalopathy. Branched-chain amino acids are believed to decrease the transport of aromatic amino acids into the brain and also serve as energy in muscle, thereby lessening efflux of amino acids into the circulation.

Dietary Management

The patients pose problems in feeding because of anorexia and behavioral patterns ranging from apathy and drowsiness and hyperexcitability. The protein-free diet consisting of commercial sugar, fat emulsions, a butter sugar mixture or glucose in beverages or fruit juices may be used initially through oral or tube feeding. With improvements, the diets providing 20, 40 and 60 g protein may be gradually introduced.

Dietary Modifications

Low-protein diet should be given. At the same time, catabolism of tissue proteins must be avoided.

CHAPTER 15: Diet Therapy for Liver Diseases

Energy

About 1,500–2,000 kcal are needed to prevent breakdown of tissue proteins for energy, and are provided chiefly in the form of carbohydrates and fats. Although, anorexia may occur attempts should be made to keep the calorie intake as high as is practical to minimize tissue breakdown.

Proteins

First 2 or 3 days, protein is completely omitted or 20–30 g/day are given. As the patient improves the protein intake is gradually increased to 1 g/kg of body weight. Nitrogen balance can be achieved on protein intake as low as 35 g/day, if high-quality protein is used and calorie intake is adequate.

▶ CHOLELITHIASIS

The function of the gallbladder and bile ducts is to concentrate, store and deliver bile into the duodenum at appropriate times to assist digestion.

Hormonal and nervous factors play a part in this process. The stimulus for this activity is the entry of food into the small intestine. This causes the mucosa of the duodenum and jejunum to secrete a hormone, cholecystokinin (CCK), which is carried in the blood to the gallbladder and causes it to contract. Fats and foods rich in fats are especially effective for this purpose.

The bile is concentrated in the gallbladder and when it is supersaturated gallstones are likely to form. Supersaturation arises when there is insufficient amount of solubilizing agents, such as bile acids and to a lesser extent lecithin to keep cholesterol and bile pigments in solution. By far the most common gallstones are mixed stones composed of cholesterol, bile pigment and various calcium salts including calcium palmitate. Gallstones are more common in women than in men. Advanced age, repeated pregnancies and sedentary life, and use of oral contraceptives are the contributing factors. In man, it has been suggested that high-cholesterol diets, lack of dietary fiber and an insufficiency of polyunsaturated fats predispose to gallstones.

Energy

Excess calorie intake appears to be a risk for development of gallbladder disease. The disease is more common in obese persons.

Fat

The patient receives no food initially during attacks of cholecystitis. Progression to a 20–30 g fat diet is made. If this is tolerated the fat can then be increased to 50–60 g/day.

▶ DIETARY RESTRICTION FOR LIVER DISEASES

Beyond the maintenance of a good, well-balanced diet, several conditions that develop in the later stages of cirrhosis require specific dietary management.

Hepatic Encephalopathy

Hepatic encephalopathy is a condition of impaired mental function due to altered liver function. It is often seen when scar tissue formation (cirrhosis) in the liver prevents the normal flow of blood through the liver. The blood, which contains toxins are 'shunted' or redirected, back to the central circulation and into the brain without first going through the liver for detoxification. Cirrhosis with portal hypertension (an elevation of the portal pressure due to the obstruction of blood flow through the liver) may be treated surgically by shunting some of the blood around the liver, connecting the portal system with the systematic circulation. This 'shunted, blood contains high concentrations of amino acids and ammonia, and probably other as yet unidentified, toxic substances that may cause altered mental function in some patients.

The treatment for hepatic encephalopathy is aimed at reducing toxins that cause this disorder. Just as patients with

CHAPTER 15: Diet Therapy for Liver Diseases

cirrhosis who have protein intolerance must restrict protein intake, so must patients with hepatic encephalopathy reduce the amount of protein in their diet. Severe protein restriction (to 20 g a day or less) is impractical for long-term therapy. Most physicians will encourage their patients to take approximately 40 g of protein a day, and will prescribe lactulose and neomycin to decrease the production of ammonia in the intestines. Certain specific amino acids (hepatamine) may be less likely to cause hepatic encephalopathy and have even been suggested as therapy. Certain foods (vegetables, milk) contain protein, rich in these amino acids and are preferred to meat as a source of protein in affected patients. A dietary supplement rich in these amino acids (hepatic aid) is available and is in use in many liver centers.

Ascites and Edema

Ascites are the accumulation of fluid in the abdominal cavity. Edema is fluid built up in the tissues, usually the feet, legs or back. Both conditions result from abnormal accumulation of sodium associated with portal hypertension and liver disease. Most affected patients will not require strict fluid restriction. Sodium intake is often restricted for patients with cirrhosis to avoid retention of fluids in the body. Such a diet would allow only 2–4 g of sodium, and would exclude canned soups and vegetables, cold cut meats, condiments such as mayonnaise and ketchup, dairy products, cheese and ice cream. Most fresh foods are low in sodium. The best salt substitute is lemon juice (which is salt free).

Cholestasis

Cholestasis is an inability of the liver to excrete bile. This may result in steatorrhea (fat malabsorption due to inadequate amounts of bile, which dissolve fat in the intestines). Steatorrhea may go unnoticed by the patient or can be associated with weight loss due to lost calories. Stools may be foul smelling and float. Fat supplements are available; the most commonly used being MCT oil and safflower oil, which are absorbable with less dependence upon bile. They may be used as a caloric supplement. MCT oil is used like any other cooking oil, in salad dressings or in cooking. Patients with steatorrhea may also have difficulty absorbing fat-soluble vitamins. However, water-soluble vitamins are absorbed normally. Supplementing the diet with fat-soluble vitamins is possible, though it should only be carried out under the guidance of a physician.

Wilson's Disease

There is a defect in copper metabolism when patients affected by this disorder have an abnormal build up of copper in the body due to the inability of the liver to excrete it. This inability allows the copper to accumulate in several organs such as first the liver and then, usually the brain and the cornea of the eye. Treatment involves the use of a decoppering agent, penicillamine, which removes the excess copper from the body. Dietary therapy for this disease includes the avoidance of copper-containing foods like chocolate, nuts, shellfish and mushrooms.

Hemochromatosis

Hemochromatosis is a disease in which there is an inappropriate absorption of iron from the intestine. The excessive iron then accumulates in the liver, pancreas and other organs in the body. Patients with this disease should not be given iron supplements. Aside from this precaution, those with hemochromatosis may follow a normal diet. Treatment is achieved by frequent removal of blood from a large vein.

Fatty Liver

Fatty liver is related to alcohol, obesity, starvation, some drugs and other factors. It is not caused by eating fat and it should be treated with a well-balanced diet or the removal of the responsible chemical substance or drug.

CHAPTER 15: Diet Therapy for Liver Diseases

Finally, patients with liver disease should be wary of supplements to the diet, particularly fad foods or packaged 'nutritional' aids. Such foods can contain a lot of salt, potassium or inappropriate protein mixtures. Those that are safe should be taken only under a physician's guidance.

▶ CONCLUSION

It is vitally important that patients with liver disease maintain a balanced diet, one which ensures adequate calories, carbohydrates, fats and proteins. Such a diet will aid the liver in the regeneration of liver cells. Nutrition that supports this regeneration is a means of treatment of some liver disorders.

Patients with cirrhosis, for example, who are malnourished, require a diet rich in protein and providing 2,000–3,000 calories per day to help the liver rebuild itself. However, some cirrhotic patients have protein intolerance. Too much protein will result in an increased amount of ammonia in the blood, while too little protein can reduce healing of the liver. Doctors must carefully prescribe a specific amount of protein that will not elevate the blood ammonia. Lactulose and neomycin are two drugs that help keep the ammonia down.

It is believed that the risk of gallbladder disorders can be reduced by avoiding high fat and cholesterol foods, and preventing obesity. The gallbladder is a storage sac for the bile produced by the liver. During digestion, the gallbladder releases bile into the small intestine through the common bile duct. Most gallbladder problems are caused by gallstones and 80%–90% of all gallstones are produced from excessive cholesterol, which crystallizes and forms stones. By maintaining a well-balanced diet and avoiding high cholesterol intake, the incidence of gallstone formation may be lowered.

Chapter 16

Diet Therapy for Endocrine and Metabolic Disorders

▶ INTRODUCTION

Metabolism is the word, which describes how the body breaks down the nutrients found in food and how the body uses nutrients for energy, growth, healing and all other body functions. An 'inborn error of metabolism' or metabolic disease occurs when a person inherits abnormal (mutated) genes that stop or change the flow of normal metabolism. There are hundreds of metabolic diseases that vary widely in severity and rarity. In many of these diseases, diet is the primary and often the only treatment. Dietary treatment is successful for many metabolic diseases that could not be treated even 10 years ago and can make it possible for people with metabolic disease to live normal and healthy lives. However, success depends on compliance with significant restrictions that are complicated and often difficult to follow. New products that make these diets easier to live with are continually introduced and research is ongoing to find new therapies. For now, diet is the medical treatment and should be followed with care throughout life.

▶ DIABETES MELLITUS

Diabetes mellitus is a chronic metabolic disorder that prevents the body to utilize glucose completely or partially. It is characterized by raised glucose concentration in the blood and alterations in carbohydrate, protein and fat metabolism. This can be due to failure in the formation of insulin or liberation or action.

Causes

1. Genetic factors: Heredity.
2. Obesity.

3. Sugar intake.
4. Infections.
5. Acute stress: Body releases adrenaline, noradrenaline and cortisol hormones that raise blood glucose levels.
6. Secondary diabetes: Results of diseases, which destroy the pancreas and lead to impaired secretion of insulin, e.g. pancreatitis, hemochromatosis, carcinoma of the pancreas and pancreatectomy.

Symptoms

Initially

- Polydipsia: Increased thirst
- Polyuria: Increased urination
- Polyphagia: Increased hunger
- Weight loss.

Other Possible Symptoms

- Blurred vision
- Skin irritation or infection
- Weakness, loss of strength
- Decreased healing capacity.

Continued Symptoms

- Fluid and electrolysis imbalance
- Acidosis (ketosis, ketonuria)
- Coma.

Types

Type I

Insulin-dependent diabetes mellitus (IDDM) also known as juvenile-onset diabetes and patients depend on insulin. There is usually sudden onset and occur in the younger age group of 10–12 years and there is an inability of pancreas to produce adequate amount of insulin.

Type II

Non-insulin-dependent diabetes mellitus (NIDDM) also known as adult-onset diabetes. In non-insulin dependent form, diabetes develops slowly and is usually wilder and more stable. Insulin may be produced by pancreas, but action is impaired (Table 16.1).

Table 16.1: Insulin and meal distributions of calories and carbohydrates

Sl No	Types of insulin	Breakfast (BF)	Noon	Midafternoon	Evening	Bedtime
1.	None	1/3	1/3	Nil	1/3	Nil
2.	Short acting (before BF and dinner)	2/5	1/5	Nil	2/5	Nil
3.	Intermediate acting neutral protamine Hagedorn (NPH)	1/7	2/7	1/7	2/7	1/7
4.	Long acting	1/5	2/5	Nil	2/5	20–40 g of carbohydrate
5.	Long acting with regular insulin at BF	1/3	1/3	Nil	1/3	20–40 g of carbohydrate

Calculation of Ideal Body Weight

Men

- Allow 100 lb for 5 feet of height
- Add 6 lb for each additional inch over 5 feet
- Subtract 10% for small frame and add 10% for large frame.

Women

- Allow 100 lb for 5 feet of height
- Add 5 lb for each additional inch over 5 feet
- Subtract 10% for small frame and add 10% for large frame.

For example, ideal body weight (IBW) for a 5'4" adult and corresponding dietary requirements are given in Table 16.2.

Table 16.2: Dietary requirement

Group	Body weight (kg)	Particulars	Energy (kcal/day)	Proteins (g/day)	Fats(g/day)
Men	60	Sedentary	2,425	60	20
		Moderate	2,875		
		Heavy	3,800		
Women	50	Sedentary	1,875	50	20
		Moderate	2,225		
		Heavy	2,925		
		Pregnant	+ 300	+15	30
		Lactating			
		0–6 month	+ 550	+25	45
		6–12 month	+ 400	+18	45
Boys	35	10–12 year	2,190	54	22
Girls	31	10–12 year	1,970	57	22

Treatment

The main modes of treatment of diabetes are:
- Diet
- Exercise
- Drugs
- Education.

Dietary Management

The principle of treatment for all the types of diabetes is the same. It aims at amelioration of the key defect, inability to utilize carbohydrate normally, and by the prevention of hyperglycemia and glycosuria by dietary regulation, exercise, drug therapy and avoidance of the symptoms of ketosis. Diet is the sheet anchor of the treatment in obese, elderly diabetics and a useful supplement to insulin therapy in younger ones. Dietary management is a long-term goal. It is essential to ensure that it is individualized considering the following factors:

1. Individual dietary requirements and goal regarding the desirable weight.
2. Past history and food habits.
3. Economic viability.
4. Educational level and ability to understand instructions and weighing all foodstuffs is a formidable task. It is best to express quantities in terms of household.

Principles of Diet

Diabetic diet need not be a complete deviation from the normal diet. The nutrition requirements of a diabetic are the same as in the non-diabetic. Normal Indian diet is generally high in carbohydrate and low in fat, with carbohydrates providing 60%–65% and fat providing 15%–25% of total calories, the rest are derived from proteins. Thus, even a normal Indian diet is ideal for a diabetic. However, the nutrient intake has to be tailor-made to the individual based on the age, sex, weight, height, physical activity and physiological needs of the patient. It is always better to consult a dietitian to prescribe and formulate a suitable individual diet. Eight principles of low-glycemic eating:

1. Eat lot of non-starchy vegetables, beans and fruits such as apples, pears, peaches and berries. Even tropical fruits like bananas, mangoes and papayas tend to have a lower glycemic index than typical desserts.
2. Eat grains in the least-processed state if possible: 'Unbroken', such as whole-kernel bread, brown rice, whole barley, millet and wheat berries; or traditionally processed, such as stone-ground bread, steel-cut oats and natural granola or muesli breakfast cereals.

3. Limit white potatoes and refined grain products such as white breads and white pasta to small side dishes.
4. Limit concentrated sweets including high-calorie foods with a low-glycemic index, such as ice cream, to occasional treats. Reduce fruit juice to no more than one cup a day. Completely eliminate sugar-sweetened drinks.
5. Eat a healthy type of protein at most meals, such as beans, fish or skinless chicken.
6. Choose foods with healthy fats, such as olive oil, nuts (almonds, walnuts, pecans) and avocados. Limit saturated fats from dairy and other animal products. Completely eliminate partially hydrogenated fats (trans fats), which are in fast food and many packaged foods.
7. Have three meals and one or two snacks each day and do not skip breakfast.
8. Eat slowly and stop when full.

Diabetic Diet Prescription

The nutrition and diet prescription is based on:
1. History of both the patient and the family.
2. Sex, age, weight, height and activity of the patient.
3. Type I or type II diabetes.
4. Type of insulin and dosage taken by the patient.

Food Exchange

Lists are groups of measured foods of the same calorific value and similar protein, fat and carbohydrate, and can be substituted one another in a meal plan.

Food Exchange List Helps

1. To restrict the food intake according to the insulin prescription.
2. To have variety in the diet.
3. For easy learning of the principles of diet.

Dietary Fiber

Dietary fiber and complex carbohydrates and restricted fat, benefit type I and type II diabetes. Such diets are:
1. Lower insulin requirements.
2. Increase peripheral tissue insulin sensitivity.
3. Decrease serum cholesterol and triglyceride values.
4. Aid in weight control.
5. Lower blood pressure (BP).

Soluble fibers such as pectin, gums and hemicelluloses (in fruits) increase intestinal transit time, delay gastric, emptying slow glucose absorption and lower serum cholesterol.

Insoluble fibers such as cellulose and lignin (vegetables, grains) decrease the intestinal transit time, increase fecal bulk, delay glucose absorption and slow starch hydrolysis.

Fiber Content of Food

1. 1%–3%: Maize, whole wheat, coriander, mint, carrots, brinjal, cauliflower, French beans, lady's finger, green mango.
2. 3.5%: Ragi, whole legumes, groundnut, cluster beans, double beans, peas, guava.

Nutritional Requirements

- Calories: 1,700–1,800
- Carbohydrate: 180 g
- Fats: 60 g
- Protein: 90 g.

A minimum amount of 100 g of carbohydrate should be given to prevent ketosis. Suggested calories from protein are 15%–20%, from carbohydrate 55%–60% and 20%–25% as fat, cholesterol 100 mg/100 kcal 50 g of fiber. This diet reduces insulin requirements, improves glycemic control, lower lasting serum cholesterol and triglyceride values and promote weight loss.

A diet high in protein is good for the health of diabetic patient. It supplies essential amino acids. It does not raise blood sugar during absorption as carbohydrate.

Excess fat is avoided as diabetics are prone to suffer from atherosclerosis, ketone bodies. The intermediary products of fats are accumulated, when carbohydrate is deficient.

Foods to be Included

Clear soups, lemons, salted pickle, pepper water, plain coffee or tea (without sugar), skimmed buttermilk, unsweetened lime juice, tomato juice, soda water, raw vegetables, salads, soup cubes, salt seasonings like onion, mint, pepper, garlic, curry leaf, coriander, vinegar, mustard and spices.

Foods to be Avoided

Sugar, glucose, honey, syrup, jaggery, sweets, halwas, burfies, nuts, jam, jellies, preserved fruits, dried fruits, aerated drinks, cake, pastries, candy, fried food and alcohol.

Myths and Facts About Diabetes and Diet

Myth: You must avoid sugar at all costs

Fact: The good news is that you can enjoy your favorite treats as long as you plan properly. Dessert does not have to be off limits, as long as it is a part of a healthy meal plan or combined with exercise.

Myth: A high-protein diet is best

Fact: Studies have shown that eating too much protein, especially animal protein, may actually cause insulin resistance, a key factor in diabetes. A healthy diet includes protein, carbohydrates and fats. Our bodies need all three to function properly. The key is a balanced diet.

Myth: You have to cut way down on carbohydrates

Fact: Again, the key is to eat a balanced diet. The serving size and the type of carbohydrates you eat are especially important. Focus on whole-grain carbohydrates since they are a good source of fiber and they are digested slowly, keeping blood sugar levels more even.

Myth: **You will no longer be able to eat normally. You need special diabetic meals**

Fact: The principles of healthy eating are the same—whether or not you are trying to prevent or control diabetes. Expensive diabetic foods generally offer no special benefit. You can easily eat with your family and friends if you eat in moderation.

▶ VARIOUS METABOLIC DISORDERS

Hyperthyroidism

Hyperthyroidism is a disturbance in which there is an excessive secretion of the thyroid gland with a consequent increase in the metabolic rate. It is believed to be an autoimmune disease occurring in genetically predisposed persons. The disease is also known as exophthalmic goiter, thyrotoxicosis, Grave's disease or Basedow's disease.

The chief symptoms are weight loss, sometimes to the point of emaciation, excessive nervousness, prominence of the eyes and a generally enlarged thyroid gland. Increased appetite, weakness and signs of cardiac failure are also present.

The increased level of energy metabolism increases the requirement of B vitamins. The excretion of calcium and phosphorus is greatly increased in hyperthyroidism. Frequent feedings will help satisfy hunger. A liberal calcium intake is desirable and may be provided in addition to the liberal use of milk.

Hypothyroidism

Decreased production or activity of the thyroid hormone or hypothyroidism is a relatively common problem. Obesity is a problem for some patients with hypothyroidism, since they may continue in their earlier patterns of eating even though the energy metabolism has been significantly reduced. In other patients, the appetite may be so poor that undernutrition results. For overweight persons, reduction of calories is necessary. Reduction of dietary cholesterol may be indicated. Adequate fluids and foods high in dietary fiber are needed to overcome constipation.

Joint Diseases

The term arthritis and rheumatism are applied to many joint diseases. The most common form of arthritis is osteoarthritis or degenerative arthritis. The characteristics of this disease is joint stiffness is characteristic. Pain is confined to joints. Joints of the fingers, knees, hip and spine are involved.

Rheumatoid Arthritis

Rheumatoid arthritis is a highly inflammatory and very painful condition having its onset in young women. This is characterized by fatigue, pain, stiffness, deformity, which may be severe and with limited function.

Dietary Counseling

Arthritic patients require the same amount of calories as other persons need.

Obesity is a common problem in osteoarthritis. Weight loss should be brought about in order to bring down the added stress on weight-bearing joints. Many patients with rheumatoid arthritis have lost weight and are in poor nutritional status. A high-calorie and high-protein diet is given.

Gout

Gout, an inherited disease more often occurring in men, is due to abnormal uric acid metabolism. About 5% of patients with gout are women; about 80% of them are postmenopausal at the time of onset.

Excretion of the uric acid precursors hypoxanthine and xanthine by the kidney is reduced. The disturbance of purine metabolism is of similar magnitude in women as in men. Serum uric acid is raised with deposition of urate (uric acid salt) in the cartilages and articular cartilages of the joints. There are recurrent attacks of pain and swelling of the joints, frequently of the metatarsophalangeal joint of the big toe, though other joints may also be affected. Joints vulnerable to injury are most liable to be involved.

Principles of Diet

A low purine, low protein and easy digestible diet with a liberal fluid intake is advised.

Dietary Management

The dietetic treatment of gout has undergone a great deal of reorientation due to changing concepts of the disease. High-purine diet alone used to be implicated at one time. The knowledge that uric acid can be synthesized from endogenous sources and that in some patients an abnormality of excretion of uric acid exists, and has focused attention on the role of heredity. However, in a susceptible person, an attack of gout can be precipitated by purine-rich foods.

Calories: Obese persons may be more prone to gout. The body weight should be reduced to normal not only to prevent recurrence of gout but also to prevent changes in the weight-bearing joints that occur in the obese. A heavy meal supplying high calories should be avoided, as it tends to precipitate an attack.

Proteins and purines: Meats having high purine content such as meat extracts and meat soups, organ meats such as liver, kidney, fish such as herring, salmon and sardines, as well as sweetbread are always excluded. Flesh in the form of meat, fish and fowl is excluded during an acute attack, but allowed as an average helping during quiescent periods. About 60 g of protein a day is adequate, preferably supplied as vegetable or milk proteins.

Fats: Fat consumption is restricted partly, because its ingestion tends to cause retention of urates by the kidney and partly to prevent obesity.

Carbohydrates: During an attack of gout the main source of calories should be carbohydrate, because of its 'protein-sparing effect', which reduces endogenous protein breakdown.

Fluids: Liberal intake of fluid should be advised to ensure a daily excretion of about 2,000 mL of urine.

Beverages: Tea and coffee contain methyl purines, which are not converted by the body into uric acid. About two or three cups a day is permitted.

Alcohol: There appears to be individual susceptibility to an attack of gout after ingestion of alcohol. Stopping alcohol may prevent attack of gout in such people. Otherwise, patients with gout usually tolerate a couple of ounces of white wine or whisky, but not beer, stout or red wines.

Foods to be avoided

1. Organ meat: Liver, heart, kidney, brain.
2. Fatty meats, also sausages, bacon, salami, fatty beef, pork.
3. Shellfish, lobsters, oysters, shrimps, prawns, crabs.
4. Egg yolk.
5. Sauces containing egg yolk, also puddings containing egg custards.
6. Chocolate, cake, pastries, ice cream, honey, sugar, jam, jelly, jaggery.
7. Cream, butter, ghee, fish liver oil, lards.
8. Concentrated milk preparations, khoa, sweets, etc.
9. Alcoholic drinks and sweet soft drinks.
10. Nuts and dry fruits.
11. Root vegetables: Potato, yam, colocassia and beetroot (limited quantities permitted).
12. Fruits: Mangoes, bananas, sapota, sitaphal (limited quantities permitted).

Free foods

1. Green leafy vegetables.
2. Tomato.

3. Cucumber.
4. Radish.
5. All gourds (e.g. ridge gourd, bitter gourd, etc.).
6. Lime.
7. Clear soups.
8. Buttermilk.
9. Vinegar, chutney, spices, pickles without oil.
10. Black tea, coffee, plain soda.

Foods for a patient with gout
Permitted
1. Refined cereals and cereal products; cornflakes, white bread, pasta, flour, arrowroot, sago, tapioca and cakes.
2. Milk, milk foods, cheese and eggs.
3. Lettuce, tomatoes and green vegetables (except all beans, lentils, peas, spinach, asparagus, cauliflower, mushrooms).
4. Vegetables and cream soups made from vegetables.

Excluded
The following foods contain purine and are best avoided during an acute attack:
1. Sugar and sweets, gelatin.
2. Butter, polyunsaturated margarine and fats of any kind.
3. Fruit, nuts, peanut butter.
4. Beverages include fruit juice, cordials, carbonated drinks, tea, coffee and cocoa may be taken if uric acid in the urine is to be measured by uricase method.
5. Beans, peas, lentils, spinach, oatmeal, asparagus, cauliflower, mushrooms.
6. Fish, seafood, sardines, herrings, anchovies.
7. Meats, poultry or other flesh, meat extract, gravies, Marmite.
8. Liver, kidney, heart, sweet bread, brains.
9. Yeast and beer products, beer, alcohol.

▶ CONCLUSION

Diet therapy is the use of appropriate foods as a tool of recovery from illness. In most illness, the rate of recovery thus is determined by the patient's acceptance and the intake of the diet prescribed. In certain ailments such as obesity and diabetes mellitus, modified diet is the most important input to help the patient's recovery.

Chapter 17

Diet Therapy for Urinary Disorders

▶ GLOMERULONEPHRITIS

An inflammatory process affecting the glomeruli and the small blood vessels in the head of the nephron, and most common in its acute form in children 3–10 years of age.

Symptoms

Hematuria, proteinuria, edema, shortness of breath, tachycardia and elevated blood pressure anorexia. There may be oliguria or anuria.

Dietary Management

Fluids

The fluid intake will be adjusted to output including losses in vomiting or diarrhea. Daily fluid replacement should be 1,000 mL plus daily amount excreted in the urine.

Insensible water loss: It is as follows:
- 30 mL/kg body weight for infants
- 20 mL/kg body weight for older children
- 10 mL/kg body weight for adults.

Energy

Sufficient calories are given without increasing the protein intake by means of sugar, honey and glucose.

Proteins

Usually the diet contains 0.5 g of protein per kg body weight for older children and 1–1.5 g/kg per day body weight for younger children. A low-protein diet is recommended so as to give rest to the kidney. An intake of 20–40 g/day is considered sufficient. Out of the recommended protein 50 g/day should be from animal protein.

Sodium

The restriction of sodium varies with the degree of oliguria and hypertension. If renal function is impaired the sodium will be restricted to 500–1,000 mg/day. If edema is present, sodium (Na) is restricted.

Potassium

When the kidneys do not work properly, potassium (K) builds up in the body and causes heart to beat uneven and stop suddenly.

Phosphorus

Eating foods high in phosphorus (P) will raise the phosphorus in the blood and this can cause calcium (Ca) to be pulled from the bones. This will make bones weak and cause them to break easily.

▶ NEPHROSIS (DEGENERATIVE BRIGHT'S DISEASE)

Symptoms

Heavy proteinuria, hypoalbuminemia and peripheral edema.

Principles of Diet

High protein, high calorie, high carbohydrate and salt restricted moderate fat with restricted fluid are recommended. Vitamin supplements especially vitamin C are given.

Dietary Management

To ensure protein use for tissues synthesis, sufficient kilocalories must always be provided. The 200 kcal is suggested. About 100–120 g of protein should be provided. A high-protein diet is required to meet the heavy loss of albumin and protein depletion of the tissues.

Sodium is restricted to prevent accumulation of edema fluid and prevent hypertension.

Special Instructions

1. Since Ca and K deficiency may accompany severe proteinuria, bone refraction and hypokalemia are common.
2. The diet has to be soft.
3. Low quality proteins like pulses should be mixed with cereals or milk to improve quality of protein, high quantity proteins such as egg, meat are preferred.
4. Vitamin supplements especially vitamin C are essential.

▶ ACUTE RENAL FAILURE

There is a sudden shutdown of renal function following metabolic or traumatic injury to normal kidneys.

Symptoms

The symptoms are anuria or oliguria (low urine volume), i.e. 20–200 mL/day. Accumulation of waste products of protein metabolism in blood, excretion of K is diminished. There is also increased phosphate and sulfate with decreased Na, Ca and base bicarbonate. Lethargic, anorexia, nausea, vomiting, blood pressure and uremia are other symptoms.

Dietary Management

Energy

A minimum of 600–100 kcal is necessary. A high calorie intake is desired mainly form carbohydrate and fats.

CHAPTER 17: Diet Therapy for Urinary Disorders

Proteins

All foods containing protein is stopped if the patient is under conservative treatment and if blood urea nitrogen (BUN) is rising. However, 40 g is allowed when patient is on hemodialysis or peritoneal dialysis.

Carbohydrates

A minimum of 100 g/day is essential to minimize tissue protein breakdown.

Fluids

The total fluid permitted is 500 mL plus losses through urine and gastrointestinal tract with visible perspiration an additional 500 mL may be necessary.

Sodium

Sodium loss through urine is measured and replaced. Na restriction is also judged based on Na loss in the urine.

Potassium

Hyperkalemia occurs when the serum potassium increased to 0.7 mEq. It has deleterious effects on heart.

▶ CHRONIC RENAL FAILURE

Chronic renal failure is also known as uremia as the level of urea in blood is very high, when 90% if function renal tissue is destroyed, uremia occurs. It may be the end result of acute glomerulonephritis, pyelonephritis and nephritic syndrome.

Causes

- Progression of acute nephritis or nephrotic syndrome
- Chronic infection of the urinary tract
- Kidney stones

- High blood pressure
- Exposure to toxic substances.

Once chronic renal failure occurs, the normal functions of the kidneys like regulation of body fluids, electrolytes, pH and excretion of metabolites are disrupted.

Symptoms

In chronic renal failure, symptoms appear when the glomerular filtration rate (GFR) is inadequate to excrete nitrogenous wastes. When the GFR is less than 10 mL/min (normal: 120 mL/min) and the BUN is more than 90 mg/dL (normal: 8–18 mg/dL), dietary modification brings about improvement. As GFR falls, daily protein intake is restricted:

1. Gastrointestinal tract: The symptoms are nausea or vomiting. The breath has an ammonia-like odor. Ulcerations of the mouth and hiccups interfere with food intake.
2. Nervous system: Patients are drowsy, irritable and sink to coma.
3. If there is hypertension, headache, dizziness, muscular twitching and failing vision occur.
4. The functioning of the heart is seriously disturbed.
5. Death results when hyperkalemia (elevated serum potassium) blocks the contraction of the heart.
6. Dehydration, sodium depletion, high serum potassium, acidosis and increased susceptibility to infection are the most general manifestations.

Dietary Management

Diet should be palatable, must have varieties, adjusted according to altered biochemistry and physiology (hyperphosphatemia and hypertension) adequate enough for growth in children.

CHAPTER 17: Diet Therapy for Urinary Disorders

Energy

Adequate kilocalories are mandatory. Carbohydrate and fat must supply sufficient non-protein kilocalories to spare protein for tissue protein synthesis and to supply energy.

Requirements: The following are the requirements of energy:
- Infancy: 100–120 kcal/kg/day
- Childhood: 80–110 kcal
- Adults: 35–50 kcal.

Proteins

Failing kidney need to be given rest. Protein intake can be reduced to 0.5 g/kg of body weight per day.

Fluids

The usual fluid permitted is volume of daily urine plus 500 mL.

Sodium

Sodium intake for infants is 1–2 mmol/kg of body weight and 40–60 mmol/day for older children. Strict restriction is necessary only if hypertension and edema are present.

Potassium

Potassium has to be restricted to 1 mmol/kg of body weight. Double boiling and draining excess water reduces potassium content.

Objectives of Treatment

- To maintain optimal nutritional status
- To minimize uremic toxicity
- To prevent protein catabolism
- To improve the patient's well-being
- To delay the progression of renal failure
- To delay the need for dialysis.

▶ UROLITHIASIS OR URINARY CALCULI

Urinary calculi (kidney stones) may be found in the kidney, ureter, bladder or urethra. About 90% of all renal stones contain calcium. The occurrence of kidney stones may be due to an outcome of different nutritional status, dietary habits and environmental factors such as temperature and humidity.

In warm climates, the urine volume is low and concentrated with urates, oxalates and calcium salts. Frequent urinary tract infection may contribute to the formation of stones. In India the most common type of calculi is calcium oxalate.

The diet should be low in oxalic acid and purine. Intake of calcium and phosphates should be reduced. Large amounts of fluid should be taken to increase urine output. Dilute urine prevents the formation of stones. Limit foods are rich in calcium and phosphates. When stones are composed of calcium, magnesium, phosphates and carbonates the urine is alkaline- and acid-ash diet is used. The acid-ash diet should maintain the urine pH between 4.5 and 5 and with an alkaline-ash diet, the urine pH of 7.6–8 is maintained.

Causes

1. Climate: In warm climate the urine volume is low.
2. Occupation: People working under the sun and perspire a lot and pass concentrated urine.
3. Infection of urinary tract: Frequent infection of urinary tract may be contributory in that pus cells and epithelial cells may form a focus around which the stone may be formed.
4. Dietary habits: Foods rich in oxalates, calcium, purines and phosphate may predispose to formation of renal calculi.
5. Heredity.
6. Vitamin A and B complex deficiency.
7. Hyperthyroidism.

Types of Calculi

- Calcium phosphate
- Calcium oxalate—mostly found in India

CHAPTER 17: Diet Therapy for Urinary Disorders

- Uric acid
- Magnesium ammonium phosphate.

Dietary Management

Planning Acid-ash Diet

- A liberal fluid intake
- Salt in moderation
- The fruits and vegetables so selected should not contribute more than 25 mL of base daily.

Planning Alkaline-ash Diet

If stones of uric acid or cystine type occur, the diet should give alkaline-ash. Alkaline producing foods (Table 17.1) such as fruits, vegetables and milk should be used acid producing foods and meat, eggs and cereals are restricted.

Table 17.1: Acid- and alkali-producing foods

Acid producing	Alkali producing	Neutral
Bread, especially whole wheat	Milk	Butter
Cereals	Fruits	Coffee
Cheese	Vegetables	Tea
Corn	Almonds	Fats
Eggs	Dried apricots	Sugar
Lentils	Beans	Tapioca
Macaroni, spaghetti	Beet greens	
Noodles	Dates	
Meat, fish and poultry	Figs	
Peanuts	Dried peas	
Rice	Raisins	
Walnuts	Spinach	
	Foods prepared with baking powder or baking soda	

Planning Low-oxalate Diets

An acid or alkaline reaction of the diet is little value for oxalate urolithiasis. Sources of oxalates should be omitted, which include beans, beet greens, chocolate, cocoa, dried figs, plums, potatoes, spinach, tea and tomatoes.

Fluid: About 0.2–2.5 L should be given. Coconut water and barley water, fruits.

▶ CONCLUSION

Several ailments may cause kidney disorders; these include infection, degenerative changes, chronic diseases, medications, toxic metal consumption, cysts and renal stones or trauma. Chronic renal failure is a condition resulting from slowly progressive destruction of kidneys. The dietary management provides optimal nutritional support.

Chapter 18

Diet Therapy for Cardiovascular Disorders

▶ INTRODUCTION

Cardiovascular diseases are characterized by a thickening of the arterial valves and their loss of elasticity.

▶ TYPES

Types of cardiovascular diseases.

Atherosclerosis

Atherosclerosis is a degenerative disease of arteries and consists of focal accumulation in the intimal lining of arteries of a variable combination of lipids, complex carbohydrates, blood and blood products, fibrous tissue and calcium (Ca) deposits.

Coronary Heart Disease

Coronary heart disease is a syndrome arising from failure of the coronary arteries to supply sufficient blood to the myocardium, also known as ischemic heart disease (IHD).

Myocardial Infarction

Necrosis or destruction of part of the heart muscle due to failure of blood supply and may lead to sudden death.

Angina Pectoris

Pain in the chest, exercise or excitement provokes severe chest pain and so limits patient's physical activities.

▶ DIETARY MANAGEMENT IN CARDIOVASCULAR DISORDERS

Objectives

- Maximum rest for the heart
- Prevention or elimination of edema
- Maintenance of good nutrition
- Acceptability of the program.

Principles of Diet

Low calories, low fat particularly low saturated fat, low cholesterol, high in polyunsaturated fatty acids (PUFAs), low carbohydrate and normal protein, minerals and vitamins, high-fiber diet is also recommended.

Energy

Usually a 1,000–1,200 calorie diet is suitable for an obese patient in bed. Those patients with desirable level are permitted a maintenance level of calories during convalescence and their return to activity.

Fat

The first step involves restriction of fats to no more than 30% of the total calories consumed and levels as low as 20% are tolerated without side effects. Total fat 30% met by saturated 10% monounsaturated vegetable oil.

Normal Allowances

1. **Duration of meal:** Three or four smaller meals are suggested instead of two meals. The evening meals must be 2 hours before doing to bed.
2. **Sodium:** It is restricted when there is hypertension.
3. **Fluid:** The restriction of fluid is not required as long as sodium is not restricted.

CHAPTER 18: Diet Therapy for Cardiovascular Disorders

4. **High-fiber diet:** Increasing fiber will serve to reduce cholesterol.

▶ HYPERTENSION

Elevation of the blood pressure above normal is a symptom, which accompanies many cardiovascular and renal diseases. High blood pressure of unknown cause is known as essential hypertension.

Causes

Cardiovascular diseases, renal diseases, tumors of the brain or adrenal glands, hyperthyroidism or diseases of ovaries and pituitary may cause hypertension.

Types

1. **Mild hypertension:** Diastolic pressure is 90–104 mm Hg.
2. **Moderate hypertension:** Diastolic pressure is 105–119 mm Hg.
3. **Severe hypertension:** Diastolic pressure is 120–30 mm Hg.

Symptoms

Headache, dizziness, impaired vision, failing memory, shortness of breath, pain over the heart and gastrointestinal disturbance, unexplained tiredness.

Dietary Management

Low-calorie, low-fat and low-sodium diet with normal protein intake is prescribed.

Energy

Obese patient must be reduced to normal body weight with low-calorie diet.

SECTION 2: Dietetics

Proteins

A diet of 50 g protein is necessary to maintain proper nutrition.

Fats

About 40 g fat, partly as vegetable oil is permitted.

Sodium

Restrictions for moderate low-sodium diet (1,000 mg).

Sodium-restricted diets: The normal diet contains about 3–6 g of sodium daily. The normal diet is modified for its sodium content:

1. **Extreme sodium restriction (200–300 mg/day):** No salt is used in cooking. Low-sodium foods are selected. This diet is used in cirrhosis of the liver with ascites and congestive heart failure (CHF).
2. **Severe sodium restriction (500–700 mg/day):** No salt is used in cooking. Careful selection of foods is necessary. This level is used for severe CHD.
3. **Moderate restriction (1,000–1,500 mg/day):** No salt is used in cooking. Low-sodium foods are selected. Measured amount of salt is used. This level is suggested for those with a strong family history of hypertension and patients with borderline hypertension.
4. **Mild sodium restriction (2,000–3,000 mg/day):** Some salt is used in cooking, but no salty foods are permitted. No salt is used at the table. This level is used as a maintenance diet in cardiac and renal disease.

Do Not Use

- Salt in cooking or at the table
- Salt-preserved foods, pickles, canned foods
- Highly salted foods, such as potato chips
- Spices and condiments, such as ketchup, sauce

CHAPTER 18: Diet Therapy for Cardiovascular Disorders

- Cheese, peanut butter, salted butter
- Frozen peas
- Shellfish
- Regular baking powder, sodium metabisulfite, ajinomoto
- Prepared mixture.

▶ CONCLUSION

Diseases of cardiovascular system are one of the killer diseases. The common risk factors that can be reduced are cigarette smoking, hyperlipidemia, low levels of high-density lipoproteins (HDL), obesity, hypertension, sedentary lifestyles, hyperglycemia and diabetes, increased thrombosis, stressful situations, changes in behavior, exposure to cold and alcohol consumption. Coronary heart diseases rate have shown a downward trend based on the dietary changes implemented. Risk factors of coronary heart diseases can be controlled to reduce the occurrence of coronary heart diseases. The workload of heart must be reduced; the dietary progression is similar to that given above for myocardial infarction. In addition severe sodium restriction (500–1,000 mg) and fluid restriction may be advised.

Chapter 19

Diet Therapy for Allergy

▶ INTRODUCTION

Food allergy (hypersensitivity) is an exaggerated immune response to a food, involving glycoprotein components in foods. Reactions can vary by the person, the food, the symptoms, the type of response and by biotype. There are five kinds of exaggerated immune responses that cause food allergies. These can be divided into two general groups—immediate IgE allergies and delayed non-IgE hypersensitivities. These reactions can cause a wide variety of physical, mental and emotional symptoms, and some inflammatory and autoimmune diseases.

The treatment of food allergy depends on diagnosis and may seem complex. This syndrome is definitely not a problem that fits the preconceived notions of our 'for every ill there is a pill' society. Food allergies are often treated from several directions at the same time, such as eliminating allergens, strengthening the patient nutritionally and modifying the patient's immune response. Special diets are the most commonly used treatment for food allergies. If the patient is allergic to only one or two foods, eliminating the offending foods may be the only treatment necessary.

▶ FOOD AS ALLERGENS

Description of main food allergies:
1. **Cow's milk:** Proteins in milk may cause reactions, such as intradermal and facial swelling, and respiratory problems. Those allergic to cow's milk are often allergic to goat's milk since it contains similar proteins.

2. **Legumes and nuts:** Peanuts may cause abdominal distress, skin eruptions and asthmatic paroxysm in some individuals; soybean can also be offensive. Reactions include asthma, hives, eczema and anaphylaxis. Nuts such as pistas, macadamia and cashews are common offenders.
3. **Eggs:** Though most of the allergen potential is in the egg white, the yolk may also be offensive to some. Allergic reactions include pruritus and atopic dermatitis, asthma, vomiting, hives, facial swelling, diarrhea and anaphylaxis.
4. **Fish and meat:** The allergic symptoms due to consumption of fish are usually confined to a particular species and the symptoms are urticaria, edema, dermatitis, gastrointestinal (GI) disorders and even asthma.
5. **Milk lactose intolerance:** The individual experiences cramping and diarrhea due to a lack of enzymes needed to digest lactose.
6. **Cereals:** Wheat proteins may cause severe reactions of intestinal problems. Corn is a common allergen and others like rye and buckwheat are also allergenic.
7. **Vegetables and fruits:** The common ones are asparagus, carrot, spinach, onion, garlic, potato, celery and pumpkin. Among fruits such as strawberries, banana, orange, grapes and apples are principal offenders. Citrus fruits cause asthma, hives and eczema. Non-citrus fruits cause swelling and irritation of mouth and lips.
8. **Beverages:** The beverages from rye, corn and yeast in cheap wine and champagnes have some allergic reactions.

Principles

Although the term 'food allergy' is sometimes used to describe all adverse reactions to food, the term is more often used to refer specifically to food reactions that are mediated by the immune system.

To protect us from illness and disease, our immune systems are continuously trying to lessen the danger represented by substances called antigens. Antigens are parts of proteins that our bodies recognize as dangerous and take steps to neutralize. Antigens can be found most anywhere there is protein—in foods, of course, but also in microorganisms like bacteria.

When our immune cells identify a dangerous antigen, they act to neutralize it and prevent it from causing harm in the body. When antigens from bacteria or viruses interact with our cells, we can get the flu or the common cold. We do not get the flu from food antigens, but we can get a wide range of immune-related symptoms that range from sniffles to hives to anaphylactic shock.

▶ IMMEDIATE VERSUS DELAYED HYPERSENSITIVITY

Allergic reactions to food, also called food hypersensitivities, are further classified as either immediate or delayed. Immediate hypersensitivity reactions occur within hours or even a few minutes after a food is eaten, typically causing very obvious physical symptoms such as a rash, the hives, a running nose or a headache.

In rare cases, immediate hypersensitivity reactions can cause anaphylactic shock, a life-threatening condition in which the throat swells and blocks the passage of air. Immediate hypersensitivities affect only a small percentage of the population.

Immediate Reactions to Food

The foods that are most often implicated as the cause of immediate allergic responses include milk, eggs, peanuts, tree nuts (walnuts), soy, strawberries, wheat, fish and shellfish. Many people with immediate food hypersensitivities must completely eliminate the offending food from their diet to avoid the serious symptoms.

Delayed Reactions to Food

Many of the same foods that are known to cause immediate hypersensitivities in a small number of people have been

CHAPTER 19: Diet Therapy for Allergy

implicated as a cause of delayed or 'masked' food allergies in much larger numbers of individuals. Delayed food hypersensitivity reactions are believed to affect millions of people; some physicians have suggested that as many as 60% of all Americans suffer from masked food allergies.

These reactions may be responsible for a variety of symptoms including dark circles or puffiness under the eyes, fluid retention, dermatitis, sinus congestion, fatigue, abdominal pain or discomfort, joint inflammation, mood swings, indigestion, headaches, chronic ear infections, asthma, poor memory, anxiety and depression.

As the name suggests, delayed hypersensitivities do not appear immediately after consuming a particular food. In fact, in most cases the immune response is so delayed that it is difficult to determine, which food is causing the symptoms and many people are unaware that they are sensitive to certain foods.

Only through careful dietary manipulation, such as elimination diet or rotation diet is usually possible to identify these hidden food allergies. The foods most often associated with delayed hypersensitivities include dairy products, eggs, wheat, soy products, peanuts, shellfish and refined sugar.

▶ DIAGNOSIS OF FOOD ALLERGY

The presence of food allergy may be established by:
1. Dietary history.
2. Cutaneous tests.
3. Provocative food tests.
4. Strict elimination diets.

Dietary History

History taking is the most important of all diagnostic procedures and should be completed first. In some cases of food allergy, the symptoms develop so rapidly and dramatically, immediately after eating the offending food that the patient is able to make his/her own diagnosis.

The patient's should be given a diary in which all the food they eat and timing of their meals can be recorded with great care over a period of many days or even weeks. The patient should also note the symptoms and time of their occurrence after the ingestion. If a careful study of the diary suggests a relationship between the intake of a certain food and the onset of allergic manifestations, other tests should be carried out.

A comprehensive investigation of the occurrence of allergic conditions in the patient and the family should be obtained, since the presence of bronchial asthma, hay fever and allergic coryza gives a clue to the inherited nature of sensitivity and suggests that cutaneous tests will be of value.

Cutaneous Tests

A minute quantity of an extract of the suspected food is injected into the skin or rubbed into a scratch. If a wheal develops and there is a surrounding red flare, skin test result is taken as positive. The value of skin tests is limited by the frequency of false-positive and false-negative results. However, if there is a well-marked reaction to one single article of food, while tests of other food extracts are negative, this may be of value in confirming a suspicious history.

Provocative Food Tests

The patient should be given a small quantity of suspected food in a made-up dish. This makes the patient unaware that they are eating the food, which he/she suspects and dreads. The test should be repeated two or three times before either a positive or negative result is accepted. If negative result is obtained on three occasions, it can be concluded that the symptoms are not due to the suspected food. If the tests are positive, appropriate food tests should not be made in patients who develop severely allergic reactions immediately after the ingestion of a recognized item of the food, as it may lead to dangerous anaphylactic shock.

Strict Elimination Diets

In the case of infants and young children, this method is easier than in the case of adults because of the limited variety of foods they eat. It is possible to eliminate from a child's diet foods like milk, egg or wheat, which may cause allergy. In adults the procedures are much more difficult because of the extended range of foods to which the sensitivity may develop.

▶ TREATMENT

1. **Elimination of causative foods:** If a positive food factor is identified and can be eliminated from the diet, then the symptoms will not recur. This is difficult in case of milk, eggs and wheat that are present in many foods—cakes, puddings, bread, etc.

2. **Substitution of alternate foods:** In case of cow's milk allergy in children, substitution of goat's milk can be done. Similarly, a child sensitive to wheat may do well with rice, oats or barley.

3. **Denaturation of protein:** Sometimes, if a protein is denatured by heat it ceases to act as an allergen. Eggs or milk, if boiled for at least 10 minutes may not produce allergic manifestations in a few patients.

4. **Desensitization:** Many attempts have been made to desensitize patients who suffer from food allergy by repeatedly injecting small quantities of the allergen or giving small amounts orally. This method is generally regarded as being of little or no value.

5. **Drugs:**
   a. **Antihistamines:** They are effective in controlling local forms of allergy like urticaria and angioedema.
   b. **Bronchodilator drugs:** Effective in asthma.
   c. **Corticosteroids:** They are effective in prevention of attacks.

6. **General advice:** If the patient is allergic to a particular food, should be advised to avoid it at least for some time

and may try it cautiously some years later, especially if it is an important item of diet. All patients must inform their doctors about the allergy since those sensitive to eggs may react badly to vaccines made of egg medium, e.g. yellow fever, influenza, etc.

As some patients with allergy tend to avoid many kinds of food, they become severely undernourished. It must be stressed that patients with allergy should not be subjected to dietary restrictions without good evidence that their symptoms are due to a food allergen. This can be determined by appropriate tests and following which are the particular food items alone can be avoided.

▶ FOOD INTOLERANCE

As discussed above, immune-mediated food allergies represent one type of adverse food reaction. Another type of adverse food reaction is called food intolerance. Food intolerance is an umbrella term that refers to any abnormal physiological response to a food that is not caused by an antibody/antigen reaction. For example, some food intolerances are caused by enzyme deficiencies, while others are caused by poor function of the digestive tract, or sensitivity to a natural or synthetic chemical.

Role of an Elimination Diet

Food allergies and food intolerances are a major source of undesirable symptoms that negatively impact the quality of life of many people. Many healthcare practitioners believe that the only definitive way to identify and manage adverse food reactions is through the use of an elimination diet followed by carefully organized food challenges.

This process is quite arduous and must be done carefully, if adverse food reactions are to be identified. As a result, it is best to perform an elimination diet with the support of a knowledgeable health practitioner.

In an elimination diet, any food that is suspected to cause an allergy or intolerance is eliminated. Depending on the severity and type of symptoms, the elimination diet may range from moderately restrictive to severely restrictive in the amount of foods allowed.

Food Excluded on an Elimination Diet

Standard elimination diets eliminate the most common allergens, such as wheat, soy, corn, dairy, eggs, gluten, nuts, citrus, fish, chocolate and shellfish, caffeine, alcohol and artificial food additives. More restrictive elimination diets remove all of the foods previously listed plus those foods that contain salicylates and amines.

Challenge Phase of an Elimination Diet

The purpose of the elimination diet is to avoid all problematic foods for a minimum of 4 days or until a person experiences some relief from his/her symptoms. For some people, it takes up to 3 weeks before improvement is seen. Once the body is cleansed, the foods that were eliminated are systematically added back into the diet, one food at a time. This readdition of foods is called the 'challenge' phase of the diet. On the first day of food challenges, a food is eaten one to two times during the day. Over the next few days, the dieter returns to the elimination diet and watches for the return of any symptoms.

If any symptoms develop, it is possible that the dieter is 'allergic' to the recently reintroduced food. If no symptoms develop, it is likely that the reintroduced food is not a problem for the dieter and he/she can move onto the next food challenge. To more accurately determine food allergies and food intolerances, it is extremely helpful during the challenge phase to keep a diary of foods eaten and any emotional, mental or physical reactions.

It can take several months to complete elimination and challenge diet. If a person does not have the time or desire to undertake such a process, a rotation diet may be a more appropriate option for managing the symptoms associated with food allergies.

In a rotation diet, foods are rotated, so that a person eats a food (or food family) only once every 4 days. For example, if you suspect a sensitivity to wheat, you would rotate wheat-containing foods into your diet every 4th day. It is believed that by decreasing the consumption of problematic foods by rotating them, the symptoms associated with these foods can be reduced.

▶ CONCLUSION

Food allergy denotes an adverse immunologic responses to a specific substance with characteristic symptoms whenever food as ingested. It is also called altered reaction of the tissue to foreign protein or antigen. The substance responsible for initiation of the allergic reaction is an allergy or antigen. Allergy can be caused due to ingestion of food or drugs, contact with foods, pesticides, drugs, adhesives, feather and fungi, inhalation of pollen, cosmetics and perfumes and injections of vaccines, serums, antibodies and hormones. Elimination diets have a proper place in the diagnosis and management of food intolerance. In elimination diets, the suspected food is excluded in the daily diet.

Chapter 20

Diet Therapy for Respiratory Disorder

▶ TUBERCULOSIS

Tuberculosis is an infectious disease caused by the *Bacillus, Mycobacterium tuberculosis*. It affects the lungs most often, but may also be localized in other organs such as the lymph nodes or kidneys or it may be generalized. Pulmonary tuberculosis is accompanied by wasting of tissue, exhaustion, cough, expectoration and fever. The acute phase resembles pneumonia with high fever and increased circulation and respiration. As the disease progresses, the patient begins to exhibit loss of appetite, pain in the chest and worsening cough.

Dietary Management

A high-calorie, high-protein, high-vitaminized and mineralized, high fluid and soft diet is recommended.

Energy

Since the metabolic rate is not as high as in other fevers, satisfactory weight can be maintained with 2,500–3,000 kcal.

Proteins

A protein intake somewhat in excess of normal requirements is necessary in tuberculosis. The daily requirement may be from 80 to 120 g.

Minerals

Calcium, especially should be provided liberally, since, it is the essential for the healing of tuberculosis lesion. At least

1 liter of milk should be taken daily. The iron needs may also be increased, if there has been hemorrhage. Calcium, iron and phosphorus help in regeneration of cells, blood and fluids.

Vitamins

The metabolism of vitamin A is adversely affected in tuberculosis. Ascorbic acid deficiency is present with slight tuberculosis. Vitamin C is essential for many regenerative purposes.

Dietary Guidelines

1. Many patients with tuberculosis have very active peristalsis so that the selection of food should be from those bland in flavor, non-stimulating and easily digested.
2. Since patients have poor appetite, food must be appetizing and patient's likes and dislikes must be considered.
3. During the acute stage, a high-calorie fluid and soft diet are prescribed followed by high-calorie soft regular diet.
4. Initially, small quantities of fluid diet should be given once in 3 hours. When the fever comes down, the interval can be increased to every 4 hours.
5. In meeting the protein requirement, good quality protein like eggs should be included.
6. Fatty foods, highly fibrous foods, very spicy foods, which are hard to digest, should be avoided.

▶ CONCLUSION

The invasion of the body by a pathogen results in infections and lung diseases. The nutritional needs of the body are increased to resist the pathogen, to recoup the losses incurred metabolically and rebuild the cells damaged by the invader. Hence a high-protein diet is indicated. Asthma, chronic bronchitis and emphysema are grouped together as chronic obstructive pulmonary disease. The group has common characteristics, which is airflow reduction or obstruction. Breathing

CHAPTER 20: Diet Therapy for Respiratory Disorder

difficulties do not permit normal eating. The sputum formed affects taste adversely. Due to insufficient oxygen supply, peristalsis is reduced resulting in poor appetite. Dust allergy is one of the most common causes of asthma. The first aim of diet therapy is to prevent malnutrition or correct it if it has occurred.

Chapter 21

Nurse's Role in Diet Therapy

▶ INTRODUCTION

Diet therapy is the treatment of disease. It involves modifying diets in such a way as to meet the requirements created by disease or injury. A diet used as a medical treatment is called therapeutic diet. If a patient needs a special diet, the physicians prescribe the diet and write the diet order in a medical record. The therapeutic diet is planned by the dietitian and usually served and monitored by the nurse. Nurses and other health professionals should consult with the physician when conditions may necessitate a change in diet order.

Good nutrition is essential not only to promote health and well-being but also to aid recovery from trauma, surgery or disease. Yet there is growing evidence that malnutrition is common among hospital patients. Many hospital patients do not receive enough food and in some wards up to 60% do not eat enough calories or protein. Poor nutritional status is known to be associated with delayed recovery and adverse outcomes of illness and injury. Nurses have an important role to play in the prevention of malnutrition. Primarily, they should identify those at risk of malnutrition and plan for the care to meet their needs. In addition, they have a role in ensuring those who are initially well-nourished, but do not become malnourished, while in hospital. Appropriate and ongoing assessment is a key factor.

Most hospitals have developed a tool to assist in nutritional assessment and the identification of those at risk. One monitoring tool for patients over 18 years of age is often used in conjunction with a nutritional assessment tool called body mass index (BMI). If the patient is unable to stand, arm span can be used instead for measuring the height. This is measured by extending both arms sideways from the body at shoulder height and measuring the distance between the tips of the middle fingers. BMI is calculated by dividing the weight in kilograms by the height in meters squared, i.e. kg/m^2. The BMI of 20–24.9 indicates an average or desirable weight. The BMI of greater than 30 is classified as obese and greater than 40 as grossly obese. Patients with a BMI of less than 20 may show signs of malnutrition. It is important to note, however, the patients who are overweight or obese can also be malnourished.

▶ FACTORS AFFECTING THE RISK OF MALNUTRITION

In addition to the BMI, most nutritional assessment tools will incorporate consideration of the following factors, which are known to increase the risk of malnutrition.

Mental Condition

Any deterioration in mental state or conscious level is likely to affect the patient's desire, and ability to eat and drink independently and so, it will increase the risk of malnutrition. This includes patients who may become depressed, lethargic or apathetic.

Weight

Weight is important to note, whether there has been any recent weight loss, particularly if it is unintentional. This may be apparent from loose-fitting clothes, rings or dentures. Patient's who appear thin or emaciated are at an increased risk of malnutrition. Less than 5% weight loss in 6 months is not significant. Between 5% and 9% is only significant if the patient is already malnourished. Between 10% and 20% is clinically significant and requires intervention, and more than 20% weight loss may require long-term support.

Appetite

Patients who are able to maintain their usual appetite and eating habits are less likely to be at risk than those who have a poor appetite or refuse meals and drinks. It is important to check, whether the patient has altered their eating habits recently.

Functioning of the Gastrointestinal Tract

The presence of diarrhea or constipation is likely to affect the desire to eat and drink, and may also lead to malabsorption. Nausea and vomiting are also likely to result in a reduced nutritional intake. Patients who are unable to take oral food or fluids following surgery involving the gastrointestinal tract or who have conditions affecting it, such as intestinal obstruction, will be at high risk.

Skin and Pressure Ulcers

Dry and scaling skin may be an indication of dehydration and possibly related malnourishment. The existence of pressure ulcers is significant and is often included on nutritional assessment tools. Pressure ulcers are often associated with poor nutrition and healing pressure ulcers requires increased nutritional intake.

Dexterity

Dexterity is important to assess, whether patients have the manual dexterity to feed themselves.

Other Factors

A number of conditions will affect the ability to eat and so will increase the risk of developing malnutrition. These include:
1. Neurological conditions, especially those affecting coordination or mental state.
2. Difficulty in swallowing the food (e.g. after stroke) and malabsorption.
3. Surgery or major trauma.
4. Malignant disease and chronic conditions such as chronic obstructive pulmonary disease.

CHAPTER 21: Nurse's Role in Diet Therapy

5. Reduced mobility or confinement to bed.
6. Bereavement, depression or other mental illness.

As with tools designed to identify patients at risk of developing pressure ulcers, most nutritional assessment tools involve a scoring system that allocates a score for each of the possible contributing factors. The total score will indicate whether the patient is at risk; appropriate measures can then be taken. Whether a high score indicates, a high or a low risk will vary between different assessment tools. Patients identified as high risk should be referred to a dietitian. Patients must be assessed within 24 hours of admission. The frequency of further assessments should be determined by the result of the initial assessment. For example, if a patient is well-nourished on admission to hospital then weekly reassessment is adequate. However, if the nutritional assessment score indicates at risk, then reassessment may need to be within 48 hour.

Hospital food service must accommodate a wide range of patients from varying backgrounds. Many different therapeutic diets must be planned, and the number and type of meals to be served changes daily. There is no wonder hospital food does not always measure up to home cooking. Nevertheless, hospital menus are planned to be nutritionally adequate and well-balanced, efforts are made to accommodate each individual patient. Sometimes patients have a negative perception of hospital food. If they are on a restricted diet, they may have even less of a desire to eat.

The nurse can make an impact on the patient's nutritional therapy in a number of ways. First, it is imperative for the nursing and dietary department to have a working communication link. For example, if a patient, who has a food allergy is admitted, the nurse should inform the dietary department promptly so as to avoid having that particular food sent to the patient or if a diagnostic test is being performed that requires the patient to omit the breakfast. The nurse could alert dietary the night before and ask them to with hold breakfast, but send a snack at the time the patient will be back from the test. Also, the nurse works closely with the patient on a daily basis and may notice, whether

SECTION 2: Dietetics

inappropriate foods are served or the patient has an inadequate intake or manifest clinical signs of malnutrition. It is essential for the nurse to report these findings to the dietitian and physician so that proper nutrition intervention can be made.

Second thing is the meal trays should be served in a positive manner. Nurses should avoid making negative statements about the food. Meal trays should be served promptly, while foods are at the correct temperature. Some patients may need assistance opening milk cartons, cutting meats or sitting up to eat. The nurse must be sensitive to these needs, for many patients, will leave the food uneaten rather than ask for help.

▶ ASSISTANCE WITH MEALS

Assistance with meals consists of the following steps.

Preparing the Patient

Before taking a meal tray into the patient's room, the nurse must ensure that the patient is ready to eat; face and hands are washed oral hygiene completed and if necessary, the bladder is emptied. The nurse should help the patient into a comfortable eating position; this must be individualized to each patient, as not everyone is allowed or able to sit up to eat a meal.

Preparing the Environment

Nurse should make every effort to see that the physical environment is as conducive to a pleasant mealtime atmosphere as possible. This may necessitate cleaning and clearing the overbed table so that, the tray can be placed on it, tidying the room to remove offensive sights, smells and brightening the room.

Serving the Tray

Nurse should check that the tray contains the diet, ordered for that patient; everything on the tray is appropriate for the diet and that nothing has spilled. For example, if a low-sodium diet tray has a salt packet, the packet should be removed. The nurse

CHAPTER 21: Nurse's Role in Diet Therapy 351

should then check the patient's identification (ID) band against the name (in the tray, it is very important that, the correct meal is served to each patient). The nurse should prepare the food by opening cartons or cutting food, if necessary.

Assisting with Eating

Patient who needs assistance in eating should be served last. This way, the nurse will have ample time and need not have to hurry the patient through the meal.

▶ FEEDING ADULTS

While feeding adults nurse has to:
1. Establish what the patient would like to eat and drink. Check whether there are any dietary restrictions.
2. Ensure the patient is comfortable, i.e. has an empty bladder, clean hands, clean mouth and if applicable, clean dentures.
3. Ask/assist the patient to sit upright, if their condition allows.
4. Check whether the patient is able to swallow; to prevent choking and aspiration into the lungs.
5. Maintain clean environment.
6. Remove any offensive materials from the patient's table or eating area, e.g. sputum pot, urinals, etc.
7. Clear a space for the tray.
8. Position a chair beside the bed for the nurse.
9. Nurse has to wash hands and dry thoroughly.
10. Put on apron (appropriate color if applicable).

Procedure

During Procedure

The nurse should:
1. Ensure to make the mealtime, a pleasant experience for the patient.
2. Obtain the correct food and drink, cutlery and napkins.

3. Set the meal out in a pleasing manner to tempt the appetite.
4. Take the tray to the bedside and if the patient is unable to see the food, describe the meal.
5. Cut up the food, if necessary.
6. Protect the patient's clothing with a napkin or paper towel.
7. Sit down so that a more relaxed approach is conveyed to the patient.
8. Tailor the speed and manner in which food/drink is offered according to the patient's needs/wishes. It should not be hurried.
9. Allow the patient to chew and swallow the food before presenting the next mouthful to suit the patient.
10. Avoid asking questions, while the patient is eating.
11. Respect the patient's dignity and use the napkin to remove dribbles of food or drink that may run down to chin.
12. When giving a drink, tip the cup/glass very gently so that the flow is controlled. Care should be taken with hot drinks, particularly if using polystyrene cup, as it is difficult to judge the temperature of the liquid inside.
13. Encourage the patient to eat and drink if necessary, but do not force patients once they have indicated that they have had sufficient. Small amounts taken more frequently may be more successful.

After Procedure

The nurse has to:
1. Assist the patient to meet hygienic needs (mouth, teeth and hands), as necessary.
2. Remove unwanted food, crockery and cutlery.
3. Wipe up any spillages on the table or locker.
4. Restore the patient's environment, i.e. a glass of water and the patient's belonging back within easy reach.
5. Remove apron and wash hands.
6. The complete relevant documentation, i.e. fluid balance and/or food chart.
7. Report any abnormal occurrence, e.g. vomiting, food refusal:

a. In some hospitals, different-colored aprons are used for activities such as serving meals, washing patients and doing dressings.
   b. If, supervising the patient, rather than feeding them, place all food and drink within easy reach of the patient. If the patient is visually impaired, clock instructions may help them locate different foods, e.g. meat is at 12 o' clock, potatoes are at 5 o'clock, etc.
   c. Always check any particular cultural practices related to eating and drinking. For example, where possible, the Muslim patient should be fed with the right hand because left hand is considered dirty.
   d. If the patient is only able to use one hand, a plate guard and non-slip mat may help. If they are unable to grip ordinary cutlery, large-handled cutlery can usually be obtained from the occupational therapy department.
8. Measuring weight daily or weekly and measuring the amount of food and the fluid intake monitors therapy effectiveness.
9. After the patient has finished eating, the tray should be promptly removed. The amount of food eaten should be recorded, usually as the percentage of the meal eaten. When a patient with diabetes, does not eat all the food on the tray, both the charge nurse and the dietitian must be noticed so that, a supplemental feeding can be sent later. If the patient is on intake and output, the amount of fluids consumed during the meal must be recorded. Any problems or difficulty in eating as well as likes and dislikes should be reported and documented on the patient's medical record.

▶ FEEDING THE HELPLESS PATIENT

Feeding the helpless patient and assisting a dependent patient to take food and fluids (Fig. 21.1).

Purposes

1. To assist the patient to eat meal.
2. To meet the nutritional need.

3. To promote health.
4. To prevent dehydration.
5. To improve appetite.

General Instructions

1. The diet is prescribed by doctor planned by dietitian and served by nurse.
2. Food should be served at correct time in a pleasant manner and in a pleasant atmosphere.

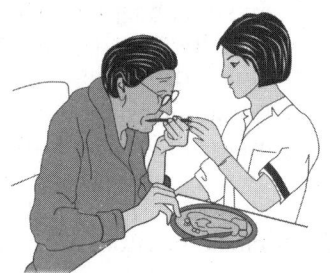

Fig. 21.1: Nurse assisting in feeding

3. Small and frequent meals are preferable for a sick person.
4. Maintain a chart for intake of food and fluids for seriously ill patients.
5. The patient should be free from pain and other discomfort during mealtime.
6. Food should be sewed in an attractive manner so that the sight and smell of food should increase their appetite.
7. Food should not be too hot or too cold.
8. Meals should be served in clean and covered vessels.
9. Give enough time for the patient to enjoy their food.
10. Encourage the patient to develop a taste to their therapeutic regimen of diet.
11. Be careful not to spill food. Wipe the patient's mouth and chin whenever necessary.
12. Wash patient's hands and make them brush their teeth after meals.

Preliminary Assessment

Check

1. Doctors order for any specific precautions.
2. Patient's likes and dislikes and socioeconomic status.
3. The food habits of the patient.
4. General condition and the ability for self-care.
5. Patients ability to follow instructions.

CHAPTER 21: Nurse's Role in Diet Therapy

6. Ensure that the ordered diet is prepared properly and with safety.
7. The articles available in the patient's unit.

Preparation of the Patient and the Environment

1. Create a pleasant environment for the patient by well ventilated, free from noise, odor and unpleasant sight.
2. Send the visitors away tactfully.
3. Give bedpan or urinal to patient, if required before meals.
4. If patient can sit, help them to have Fowler's position with cardiac table or overbed table.
5. Provide handwashing facility to patient and if necessary help them, so that they will feel fresh.
6. Place the towel over the chest and under the chin to protect clothing.

Equipments

A tray containing:
1. A glass of water to give at the end of the meal.
2. Napkin to wipe the face in between.
3. Mackintosh and towel.
4. Feeding cup or spoon.
5. The required amount of feed in a mug at the right temperature.
6. Kidney tray.

Procedure

1. Wash hands thoroughly.
2. Make sure that patient is not starving for any procedure.
3. Explain procedure to patient.
4. Make sure that therapeutic restriction are considered.
5. Cover patient below chin with face towel.
6. Feed the patient either by using spoon or fingers.
7. Offer water as required.

SECTION 2: Dietetics

8. After meal, rinse the mouth with water and spit into k-basin.
9. Complete the feed and wipe the mouth.
10. Record the procedure in the nurse's record sheet and intake output chart.

Aftercare

1. Help the patient to wash their mouth and hands.
2. Remove towel around the neck.
3. Make the patient comfortable.
4. Take all the articles to utility room, discard the waste, clean the articles and replace it.
5. Record the procedure in the nurse's record sheet and intake output chart.

▶ NASOGASTRIC TUBE INSERTION

Nasogastric tube insertion is a method of introducing a tube through nose into stomach.

Purposes

1. To feed patient with fluids when oral intake is not possible.
2. To dilute and remove consumed position.
3. To instill ice-cold solution to control gastric bleeding.
4. To prevent stress on operated site by decompressing.
5. To relieve vomiting and distention.
6. To collect gastric juice for diagnostic purposes.

Preliminary Assessment

Check

1. Doctor's order for any specific instruction.
2. Patients ability to follow instructions.
3. General condition of the patient.
4. Articles available in the unit.

CHAPTER 21: Nurse's Role in Diet Therapy

Preparation of the Patient and the Environment

1. Explain the sequence of procedure.
2. Arrange the articles at the bedside.
3. Provide privacy.
4. Provide comfortable position.
5. Place the Mackintosh and towel across the chest.
6. Remove the dentures, if any and place it in a bowel of clean water.
7. Give mouthwash and help them to clean the teeth.
8. Clean the nostrils, if there are secretions or crust formation, using swab stick dipped in saline.

Equipments

A tray containing:
1. Nasogastric tube of appropriate size.
2. k-basin.
3. Stethoscope.
4. Bowl with water.
5. Adhesive scissor.
6. Syringe 20 cc/10 cc.

Procedure

1. Wash hands thoroughly.
2. Measure distance of tube from tip of patient's earlobe to nose to the tip of xiphoid process (Fig. 21.2).
3. Mark the distance of the tube.
4. Lubricate the tube for about 6–8 inches with the lubricant, using a rag pieces or a paper square.

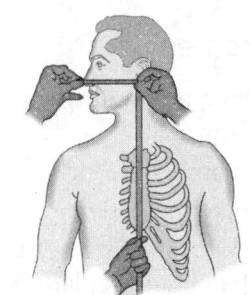

Fig. 21.2: Nasogastric tube measurement before insertion

5. Hold the coiled tube in the right hand and introduce the tip into the left nostril.
6. Pass the tube gently, but quickly, backwards momentary resistance may occur as the tube is passed into the nasopharynx.
7. When the tube reaches the pharynx, the patient may gag. Allow them to rest for a movement.
8. Have the patient take sips of water on command; advance the tube 3–4 inches each time patient swallows.
9. Make sure tube is in stomach.
10. Once location of NG tube insured, close other end of tube with spigot, secure tube on nose using adhesive in 'T' or butterfly.

Methods to Confirm Nasogastric Tube in the Stomach

1. Aspirate: Attach the syringe to the end of nasogastric (NG) tube and aspirate small amount of gastric contents.
2. Immerse distal end of tube into bowel of water and check for air bubbles. If the tube is in the trachea, air bubbles will coincide with the expiration of each breath.
3. Auscultate: Attach syringe to free end of NG tube, place diaphragm of stethoscope over left hypochondrium. Inject 10 mL of air and auscultate abdomen for gushing sound.

Aftercare

1. Offer a mouthwash, clean the face and hands and dry them.
2. Remove the Mackintosh and towel.
3. Make the patient comfortable in bed.
4. Take all the articles to the utility room; discard the waste, clean it and replace it in a proper place.
5. Wash hands.
6. Record the procedure in the nurse's record sheet (Fig. 21.3).

▶ GASTRIC GAVAGE

Gastric gavage or nasogastric tube feeding is given through the tube, which is inserted through patient's nose into stomach, when patient is unable to take food orally.

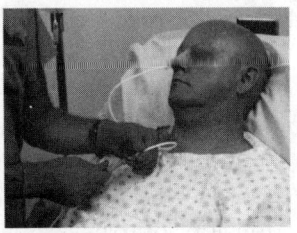

Fig. 21.3: Care of nasogastric tube

It is the administration of fluid food by means of tube passed into the stomach. It is also called gastric gavage.

Purposes

1. To provide adequate nutrition.
2. To give large amount of fluid for therapeutic purpose.
3. To assess tolerance of foods in postoperative patients.
4. To introduce food into stomach, when the patient is not able to take food in the usual manner.
5. When the condition of mouth or esophagus makes swallowing difficult.

Indications for Tube Feeding

1. Unconscious patient or semiconscious.
2. After certain surgeries of the mouth and throat.
3. Patients unable to swallow.
4. Premature babies.
5. When the patient is unable to retain the food, e.g. anorexia nervosa and vomiting.

General Instructions

1. Give mouthwash frequently to avoid complications of a neglected mouth.
2. Maintain intake and output chart accurately.
3. Measure and drain the feed (fluid) to avoid blockage in the tube.

4. Avoid introducing air into the stomach during each feed. Pinch the tube before the fluid run into the stomach completely from the tube.
5. Feeding may be given at intervals of 2, 3 or 4 hours and the amount is not exceeding 150–300 mL per feed.
6. Observe for complications such as nausea, vomiting, distension, diarrhea, aspiration pneumonia, asphyxia, fever and water and electrolyte imbalance.

Advantages of Tube Feeding

1. An adequate amount of all types of nutrients including distasteful foods and medication can be supplied.
2. Large amount of fluids can be given safely.
3. The danger of parenteral feeding is avoided, e.g. venous thrombosis.
4. Tube feeding may be continued for weeks without any danger to the patient.
5. The stomach may be aspirated at any time if desired.
6. Overloading of the stomach can be prevented by a drip method.

Principles Involved in Gastric Gavage

1. A thorough knowledge of the anatomy and physiology of the digestive tract and respiratory tract, ensures safe induction of the tube (avoid misplacement of the tube).
2. Tube feed is a process of giving liquid nutrients or medications through a tube into the stomach when the oral intake is inadequate or impossible.
3. Microorganism enters the body through food and drink.
4. Introduction of the tube into the mouth or nostrils is a frightening situation and the preparation of the patient facilitates introduction of the tube.
5. Systematic ways of working adds to the comfort and safety of the patient and help in the economy of material, time and energy.

CHAPTER 21: Nurse's Role in Diet Therapy

Preliminary Assessment

Chock

1. Identify the correct patient.
2. Check the doctor's order for any specific precautions.
3. Check the level of consciousness of the patient.
4. Check whether the feed is ready at hand.
5. Articles available in the unit.

Preparation of the Patient and the Environment

1. Explain the sequence of the procedure.
2. Provide adequate privacy.
3. Position the patient in sitting or semi-Fowler's position.
4. Place the Mackintosh and towel around the neck.
5. Arrange the articles at the bedside locker.
6. Clean the mouth by providing mouthwash.

Equipments

A tray containing:
1. Mackintosh and towel.
2. 20 cc syringe.
3. Stethoscope.
4. Bowl with water.
5. Adhesive with scissors.
6. Feeds and water.
7. Ounce glass.

Procedure

Syringe Method

1. Wash hands thoroughly.
2. Place towel around the neck in such a way that patients clothing and bed linen are protected.
3. Make sure the tube is in stomach before giving feeds.

4. Remove spigot; pinch tube to prevent air entry. Remove plunger from syringe and connect to tube.
5. Keep syringe about 12 inches above patient's head. Start feed with small measured amount of water and allow feed to follow slowly and steadily through the tube in such a way that air does not enter tube.
6. Do not force fluid, allow the flow by gravity.
7. At the end of feed the flush, tube by pouring small, measured amount of water. Remove syringe and replace spigot.

Syphon Method

1. Place towel around neck in such a way that patients clothing and bed linen are protected.
2. Make sure that tube is in stomach before giving feeds.
3. Immerse tip of tube in prepared feed immediately by avoiding air entry into tube.
4. Raise fluid container about 12 inches above patient's head and observe flow of fluid.
5. When feed is over flush the tube with small quantity of water.
6. Pinch tube and close with spigot.

Aftercare

1. Remove the Mackintosh and towel.
2. Place the patient in comfortable position.
3. Replace the articles to utility room, clean it and replace it.
4. Record the procedure in nurse's record sheet and intake output chart.

▶ GASTROJEJUNOSTOMY FEEDING

Gastrojejunostomy feeding is defined as enteral nutrition of a liquid food preparation directly into the stomach or small intestine via a tube.

CHAPTER 21: Nurse's Role in Diet Therapy

It is an ideal method of providing nutrition for the person who unable to swallow food and drink normally, but has intact gastrointestinal function.

It is the introduction of liquid food through a tube or catheter, which the surgeon has already introduced into the stomach through the abdominal wall.

Indications

1. Tumors or operations on the upper gastrointestinal tract.
2. Cancer of the esophagus.
3. Stricture of the esophagus caused by poisoning in case of fistula.

General Instructions

1. It is essential that the area of the skin around the tube be kept clean and dry.
2. A waterproof ointment such as zinc oxide may be applied around the tube to protect the skin from the irritation of the hydrochloric acid.
3. Foods given through the gastrostomy tube are same as those given by nasogastric tube and the same amounts are given at the same intervals.

Methods of Administration

1. Intermittent feeding given 4–6 times a day rather than continuously is delivered as a bolus through a longer lumen tube. Volume for formula usually 250–450 mL is placed in a large syringe and inserted into the proximal end of the tube.
2. Intermittent gravity drip administration delivers a similar volume 250–450 mL of feeding over 20–30 mL a minute, 4–6 times a day.
3. Continuous administration delivers fluid through a small lumen tube at a constant rate via orogastric and nasogastric

routes. The rate of flow is carefully regulated. The nurse should calculate the amount of fluid to be infused during an hour and regulates the infusion pump accordingly.

Preliminary Assessment

Check

1. The doctor's order for any specific instruction.
2. Level of consciousness of the patient.
3. Self-care ability of the patient.
4. Mental status to follow instructions.
5. Articles available in the unit.

Preparation of the Patient and the Environment

1. Explain the sequence of the procedure.
2. Provide privacy.
3. Arrange the articles at the bedside.
4. Place the patient in a comfortable position.
5. Keep the environment clean and tidy.
6. Keep ready with feed to be given.

Equipments

A clean tray containing:
1. A funnel, rubber tubing, glass connection screw and a clamp.
2. A glass of drinking water.
3. Required amount of feed, temperature 100°F.
4. Sterile lubricant to protect surrounding area.
5. Sterile dressing and forceps in a dressing tray.
6. Medicine as per order.
7. Kidney tray.
8. Many-tailed binder, if required.
9. Mackintosh and towel.
10. Stethoscope.
11. Syringe.

Procedure

1. Wash hands thoroughly.
2. Place the Mackintosh or towel; clean the surrounding area of the opening. Cover the wound with sterile piece of gauze.
3. Unscrew the clamp from the gastrostomy tube and attach the funnel and rubber tubing; keep the tube pinched to prevent air from setting in.
4. Aspirate the gastric contents by attaching a syringe.
5. Pour some clean water into the funnel and lower a little to let out air.
6. Then pour the feed before the funnel is empty.
7. If any medicines are ordered, these are given after feed.
8. Give water after giving medicines.
9. Disconnect the tabbing and funnel.
10. Clean and apply sterile instrument around the wound, dress it with sterile dressing and apply the binder.

Aftercare

1. Remove the Mackintosh and towel.
2. Position the patient comfortably.
3. Secure the tube with plaster.
4. Replace the articles to utility room.
5. Wash the hands.
6. Record the procedure in nurse record sheet.

▶ CONCLUSION

Food is an integral part of patient care and is a major contributor in his/her recovery. Therefore careful selection of foods, their preparation and ensuring that these are consumed by the patient is an important part of the therapy. The nurse is responsible for diagnosis and indicating the kind of modifications to be made in the normal diet in the view of condition of the patient.

Chapter 22

Fluid and Electrolytes

▶ INTRODUCTION

Water is vital for human existence. We can live without food for extended periods of time, but without water will result in death. Water is colorless calorie less compound of hydrogen and oxygen that virtually every cell in the body needs to survive. Water is closer, being a universal solvent than any other compound. Water is the largest single compound of the body and it is distributed as follows. Total body water content is mainly determined by total amount of salt in the body. Salt and water concentration in the body is controlled by the kidneys.

▶ IMPORTANCE OF WATER

The body's need for water is only at next to that of oxygen. One can live for weeks without food, but death is likely to follow deprivation of water for more than a few days. A 10% loss of body water is a serious hazard and death usually follows at a 20% loss. The water contents of an infant's body is as much as 70%, about 65% of body weight of lean adults is accounted by water and 55% or less of weight in obese adults is water. All body tissues contain water, but variations in tissue contents are wide. In our body, water is present in two forms—intracellular fluids (ICF), which are present within the cells, which accounts for about 45% of our body weight and extracellular fluids (ECF), which are present outside the cells, e.g. plasma, interstitial fluids, lymph's and the secretions of pancreas, the liver and gastrointestinal mucosa.

CHAPTER 22: Fluid and Electrolytes

▶ FUNCTIONS OF WATER

1. Water is an essential constituent of all the cells of the body and the internal environment.
2. Serves as a transport medium by which most of the nutrients pass into the cells and removes excretory products.
3. Water is a medium for most biochemical reactions within the body and sometimes a reactant.
4. It is a valuable solvent in which various substances such as electrolytes, non-electrolytes, hormones, enzymes, vitamins are carried from one place to another.
5. Plays a vital role in the maintenance of body temperature. Heat is produced when food is burnt for energy. Body temperature must be kept at 80°F–108°F, but for higher or lower body temperature than this can cause death. Body heat is lost through the skin, lungs, urine and feces.
6. It forms a part of fluids in body tissues. For example, the amniotic fluid that surrounds and protects the fetus during pregnancy.
7. Saliva is about 99.5% water. In healthy individuals it makes swallowing easier by moistening the food.
8. Water helps in maintaining the form and texture of the tissues.
9. Water is essential for the maintenance of acid-base and electrolyte balance. It should be noted that pure water consists of hydrogen ion (H^+) and hydroxyl ion (OH^-).

Substances dissolve in water as ions with positive and negative charge. They are called electrolytes. The common electrolytes in our body are sodium, potassium and chloride. Changes in electrolyte balance causes accumulation or depletion of water in ICF and ECF. The balance between the positively and negatively charged ions is essential for water flow and maintains osmolarity between the cells. This is called electrolyte balance. Acid-base balance is the dynamic state of equilibrium of hydrogen ion concentration. When pH falls below 7, it is termed acidity and when it increases above 7, it is termed alkalinity. Extremes of both cases results in death. The pH of the body should be maintained near neutrality. Enzymatic action depends on the pH. The digestion, absorption and utilization of nutrients are dependent on pH. Most body fluids are near neutral with the exception of gastric juice.

pH Value of Solutions

The pH value of some solutions is given below.

Acid

0 – Hydrochloric acid (HCL).
1 – HCL (0.1 mol dm^{-3}).
2 – Gastric juice.
3 – Vinegar, orange juice.
4 – Grapes.
5 – Bread, coffee.
6 – Urine (nearly neutral).
7 – Pure water, eggs, blood.
8 – Seawater.
14 – Sodium hydroxide.

Alkali

Water forms good source of macrominerals like calcium, magnesium, fluoride, iron and iodine.

▶ REQUIREMENTS

Requirements of water vary with climate, dietary constituents, activities and surface area of the body. As a rule, a person should take enough water to excrete about 1,200–1,500 mL of urine per day. In tropics because of greater water loss through perspiration, increased water intake is required to maintain urine volume. Normal intake of water ranges between 8 and 10 glasses per day.

Daily Water Input

In tropical countries like India, the daily water input, amounts to 2,400–3,000 mL of water through food, as fluid, drinks and as metabolic water:
1. As fluid drinks: Water, tea, coffee, milk, soups 1,500–1,750 mL.
2. Water intake through solid food 600–900 mL.
3. Oxidation of carbohydrate, fat, proteins (metabolic water) 300–350 mL.

Daily Output of Water

The total amount of output of water is 2,400–3,000 mL:
1. Urine: 1,200–1,500 mL (kidney).
2. Perspiration: 700–900 mL (skin).
3. Respiration: 400 mL (lungs).
4. Feces: 100–200 mL (intestine).

Therefore, the water intake and output is fairly kept constant. This is called water balance. The average adult metabolizes 2.5–3 L of water and a constant balance is maintained between intake and output. Inadequate water intake disturbs water equilibrium resulting in decreased urinary output, thereby causing changes in ECF and ICF. The water equilibrium is maintained by kidneys, lungs, intestine and pituitary gland. The water balance coordinated with both electrolyte and acid-base balance.

▶ DEHYDRATION

Causes and Effects of Dehydration

Causes

When water is constantly lost from the body as in severe vomiting, diarrhea, excessive sweating or excessive urine formation due to treatment with diuretics, the total water content of the body is reduced. ECF and ICF decreases leading to dehydration.

Effects

1. Tongue gets dry.
2. Pinch test is done by raising and releasing the skin. Slow return of skin to original position indicates decreased ECF.
3. Decrease in plasma volume reduces cardiac output and may lead to cardiac failure.

Prevention of Dehydration

Dehydration can be prevented by taking sufficient amounts of water as fluids. The correction of dehydration is called rehydration.

Oral Rehydration Therapy

Oral rehydration is the administration of fluid to prevent or correct dehydration.

Oral Rehydration Salt

World Health Organization (WHO), United Nations Children's Fund (UNICEF) formula consist of the NaCl 3.5 g, $NaHCO_3$ 2.5 g, KCl 1.5 g and glucose 20 g to be dissolved in 1 L of potable drinking water. The glucose present aids in the absorption of sodium chloride and potassium chloride apart from giving energy. This mixture is administered through the oral route at frequent intervals until the normal state is attained. Potable water is that water, which is safe and wholesome. It should be:

- Free from pathogenic agents
- Free from harmful chemical substance
- Pleasant to taste; free from color and odor
- Usable for domestic purpose.

▶ ELECTROLYTE

Electrolytes are substances whose molecules dissociate or split into ions when placed in water. These substances are found in ECF and ICF that dissociate into electrically charged particles known as 'ions'. 'Cations' are positively charged ions. For example, sodium (Na^+), potassium (K^+), calcium (Ca^{2+}) magnesium (Mg^+) and hydrogen (H^+) ions. 'Anions' are negatively charged ions. For example, bicarbonate (HCO_3^-), chloride (Cl^-) and phosphate (PO_4^{3-}) ions and proteins. The ionic charge is termed 'valence'. Cations and anions combine according to their valency. The concentration of electrolytes can be expressed in moles per deciliter (mol/dL), millimoles per liter (mmol/L) or milliequivalent per liter (mEq/L) (refer the normal level of electrolytes).

The role of electrolytes in cellular functions includes the following:

1. Regulation of water distribution and osmolality.
2. Regulation of acid-base balance.
3. Transmission of nerve impulses, i.e. neuromuscular activity.
4. Contraction of muscles.
5. Clotting of blood.
6. Enzyme reaction.

Regulation of Electrolytes

Electrolytes regulate water distribution, regulate acid-base balance and maintain a balanced degree of neuromuscular excitability. There are many different kinds of electrolytes in the body. These include sodium (Na), potassium (K), calcium (Ca), magnesium (Mg), chloride (Cl), bicarbonate (HCO_3), phosphate (PO_4), etc.

Electrolyte Imbalance

Human body contains quite large volume of water as ICF and ECF, and the fluid contains several inorganic ions such as sodium, potassium, chloride, bicarbonate, sulfate, phosphate, calcium and magnesium. The complex mechanism of human life maintains the concentration and volume of the body fluids at a constant level and in general, it is not influenced by dietary intake and metabolism, while kidneys play a vital role in maintaining the balance. When clients present with deficit or excess of sodium, potassium, calcium, magnesium and phosphate, special nursing care is required. A brief description of the common electrolyte imbalances are as follows.

▶ HYPONATREMIA

Hyponatremia refers to a sodium deficit in ECF caused by loss of sodium or a gain of water. It is a condition on lowered level of plasma volume. In this condition, osmotic pressure changes result in ECF, moving into the cells. When this occurs, an examiner's fingerprints tend to remain on the client's skin over the sternum where pressure is applied with the fingers. The related factors leading to hyponatremia are as follows:

1. Loss of sodium as in loss of Cl fluids, use of diuretics and adrenal insufficiency.
2. Gain of water as in excessive administration of dextrose 5% in water (D5W), diseases associated with syndrome of inappropriate antidiuretic hormone secretion (SIADH) pharmacological agents that impair renal water excretion.
3. Hyponatremia or sodium depletion occurs from loss of body fluids through sweating, vomiting, diarrhea, intestinal fistula and dialysis, and from aspiration of gastric contents.
4. Chronic pyelonephritis, chronic uremia, diuretic phase of acute renal failure, diabetic ketoacidosis, cystic diseases of the kidney and excessive or prolonged use of diuretics result in excessive loss of sodium through urine.
5. Endocrine diseases show as myxedema, Addison's disease, hyperaldosteronism and uncontrolled diabetes mellitus also leads to sodium depletion.
6. Excessive loss of sodium can also occur through the skins as in extensive burns, generalized dermatitis, etc. in children with cystic fibrosis.

Sodium is mainly an extracellular ion and its depletion causes migration of water in the intracellular compartments, making the ECF hypotonic. Consequently, plasma becomes hypo-osmolar and plasma volume falls.

Main Characteristics

- Anorexia
- Fingerprint over sternum
- Nausea and vomiting
- Muscular twitching
- Lethargy
- Seizures
- Confusion
- Coma
- Muscle cramps
- Serum sodium below 135 mEq/L.

This condition presents with tiredness, lethargy, muscular weakness, mental confusion and in severe cases convulsions and coma. The skin appears cold, pale and inelastic. Tongue gets dry. Reduction in plasma volume causes reduction in cardiac output and results tachycardia, fall of blood pressure and raising pulse rate. The eyeballs become soft due to reduced intraocular pressure, urine output is reduced and soon oliguria supervenes and finally leads to uremia. When the plasma serum concentration falls exaggeratedly to 120 mmol/L of blood or less, muscle cramps occur. It can produce acidosis and circulatory failure as complication.

Treatment

Mild cases are treated with frequent drinking of water with added sodium chloride or with isotonic (0.9%) saline solution by intravenous (IV) injection. In other cases, 2–4 L of isotonic saline solution is given IV infusion over 6–12 hours. More severe cases are treated with 2–3 L of IV isotonic solution in first 2–3 hours, followed by further 2–5 L within 24–48 hours. If there is associated water intoxication, water intake is restricted to 500–1,000 mL in 24 hours. In addition, the client is given treatment for the underlying condition.

Nursing Interventions

1. Identify clients at risk for hyponatremia.
2. Monitor fluid losses and gains. Look for loss of sodium-containing fluids, particularly in conjunction with low-sodium intake.
3. Monitor presence of gastrointestinal symptoms, such as anorexia, nausea, vomiting and abdominal cramping.
4. Monitor laboratory date for serum-sodium levels less than normal.
5. Check specific gravity of urine.
6. With clients able to consume a general diet, encourage foods and fluids with high-sodium content.
7. Be familiar with the sodium content of commonly used parenteral fluids.
8. Monitor client with cardiovascular disease receiving sodium-containing fluids closely for sign of circulatory overload, such as moist rales in the lungs.
9. Use extreme caution when administering hypertonic saline solution (3%–5% NaCl). Beware that these fluids can be lethal, if infused carelessly.
10. Avoid giving large water supplements to clients receiving isotonic tube feedings, particularly, if routes of abnormal sodium loss are present or water is being retained abnormally.

▶ HYPERNATREMIA

Hypernatremia or sodium excess refers to surplus of sodium in ECF that can result from excess water loss or overall excess of sodium in the body. Because of the increased extracellular osmotic pressure, fluids move from the cells, leaving them without sufficient fluid. It is a condition, where excess of sodium occurs in the ECF, giving rise to cellular dehydration. The related factors, which lead to hypernatremia are as follows:

1. Deprivation of water is most common in those unable to perceive or respond to thirst.
2. Hypertonic tube feeding with inadequate water supplements.
3. Increased insensible water loss (as in hyperventilation).
4. Ingestion of salt in unusual amounts.
5. Excessive parenteral administration of sodium-containing solution.
6. Hypertonic saline (3% or 5% NaCl).
7. 7.5% sodium bicarbonate.
8. Isotonic saline.
9. Profuse sweating.
10. Diabetes insipidus.
11. Heat stroke.
12. Drowning in seawater.

Hypernatremia also occurs when water losses the body exceeds from sodium loss; as that is seen in diabetes insipidus, marked glycosuria, hypercalcemia, hypokalemia, chronic renal failure and recovery phase of acute renal failure.

Sodium excess may occur along with water excess, when due to inadequate clearance of the kidneys both sodium and water accumulate in the extracellular space leading to edema, e.g. nephrotic syndrome, cardiac failure, nutritional or thiamine deficiency, cirrhosis of liver and in case of usage of drugs such as corticosteroids, androgens, phenylbutazone, oral contraceptive and carbenoxolone.

It causes retention of sodium, increased volume of ECF and edema in the interstitial compartment.

Main Characteristics

1. Thirst.
2. Elevated body temperature.
3. Tongue dry and swollen, sticky mucous membranes.
4. Disorientations.

SECTION 2: Dietetics

5. Hallucinations.
6. Lethargy, when disturbed.
7. Irritable and hyperactive when stimulated.
8. Focal or grand mal seizures, coma, low blood pressure, tachycardia, serum sodium above 145 mEq/L.
9. Urinary specific gravity 0.015 provided water loss from non-renal route.

It may produce hypernatremia, hyperglycemia and shock as complication.

Treatment

Management of the condition calls for an immediate attention and treatment instituted within 24–48 hours can avoid occurrence of cerebral edema. In mild cases, IV infusions D5W are given. Other cases need restriction of water and salt by mouth. Management of the condition depends upon the underlying condition. Diuretics and other measures are taken on the advice of the physician according to the condition of the patient.

Nursing Interventions

1. Identify clients at risk of hypernatremia.
2. Monitor fluid losses and gains. Look for abnormal losses of water or low water intake; and for large gains of sodium as might occur with ingestion of proprietary drugs with high sodium content. Also consider that prescription drugs may have high sodium content. Of course, one should look for excessive intake of high sodium foods.
3. Monitor changes in behavior such as restlessness, disorientation and lethargy.
4. Look for excessive thirst and elevated body temperature. If present, evaluate in relation to other signs.
5. Monitor serum sodium level.
6. Prevent hypernatremia in debilitated clients who are unable to perceive or respond to thirst by offering them fluids at regular intervals. If fluid intake remains inadequate, consult

the physician in order to plan and alternate route for intake, either by tube feedings or by the parenteral route.

7. If tube feedings are used, give sufficient water to keep the serum sodium and the blood urea nitrogen (BUN) level within normal limits. Beware, that the higher the osmolality of the feeding, the greater the need for water supplements.

▶ HYPOKALEMIA

Hypokalemia refers to a potassium deficit in ECF. When the extracellular potassium level falls, potassium moves from the cell, creating an intracellular potassium deficiency. Sodium and hydrogen ions are then retained by the cells to maintain isotonic fluids. These electrolyte shifts influence normal cellular functioning, the pH of ECF and function of most of the body systems. Skeletal muscles are generally the first to demonstrate a potassium deficiency. It is a condition associated with depletion of potassium characterized by muscular weakness, leg cramps, apathy, mental confusion and paralysis.

The related factors leading to hypokalemia are as follows:

1. It develops from excessive loss of potassium in the urine and stool, and from severe water depletion.
2. Potassium-losing diuretics, i.e. furosemide, thiazide, etc.
3. Steroid administration.
4. Use of carbenicillin, sodium penicillin, amphotericin B.
5. Hyperaldosteronism.
6. Hyperalimentations.
7. Poor intake as in anorexia nervosa, alcoholism, potassium-free parenteral fluids.
8. Osmotic diuresis (as occurs in uncontrolled diabetes mellitus or mannitol administration).

Main Characteristics

1. Fatigue.
2. Anorexia, nausea and vomiting.

3. Muscle weakness.
4. Decreased bowel motility (intestinal ileus) paralytic ileus.
5. Cardiac arrhythmia.
6. Increased, i.e. sensitivity to digitalis.
7. Polyuria, nocturia, dilute urine (if hypokalemia prolonged).
8. Mild hyperglycemia; serum K below 3.5 mEq/L.
9. Paresthesia or tender muscles.
10. Electrocardiogram (ECG) changes: Flattened T waves, ST segment depressions.
11. Respiratory hyperventilation.

Treatment

Management of the condition requires adequate management of the underlying conditions.

Nursing Interventions

1. Beware of clients at risk for hypokalemia and monitor for its occurrence.
2. Assess digitalized clients at risk for hypokalemia especially closely for symptoms of digitalis toxicity.
3. Take measures to prevent hypokalemia, if possible.
4. Prevention may take the form of encouraging extra potassium intake for at risk patient (when the diet allows).
5. When hypokalemia occurs due to abuse of laxatives or diuretics, education of the client may help alleviate the problems.
6. Administer oral potassium supplement when prescribed.
7. Beware that clients may not need potassium supplements, if they are using salt substitutes, because these substances usually contain sizable amounts of potassium.
8. Be thoroughly familiar with the critical facts related to administering potassium intravenously.

CHAPTER 22: Fluid and Electrolytes

▶ HYPERKALEMIA

Hyperkalemia refers to a condition with excess of potassium in ECF, characterized by conduction defect in the heart and myoneural junction of the muscle.

The related factors, which lead to hyperkalemia, includes the following:

1. Decreased potassium excretions.
2. Oliguric renal failure.
3. Potassium-conserving diuretic usage.
4. Hypoaldosteronism.
5. High potassium intake, especially in presence of renal insufficiency.
6. Improper use of oral potassium supplements.
7. Rapid excessive administration of IV potassium.
8. High-dose potassium penicillin.
9. Foods high in potassium (such as dried apricots).
10. Shift of potassium out of cells due to acidosis, tissue trauma and malignant cell lysis.
11. Excess potassium also occurs in acute renal failure, severe crush injuries and burns, severe hemorrhages and adrenal insufficiency.
12. It is also seen in diabetic ketoacidosis.

Main Characteristics

1. Vague muscular weakness is usually first sign.
2. Cardiac arrhythmias, bradycardia and heart block can occur.
3. Paresthesias of face, tongue, feet and hands.
4. Flaccid muscle paralysis (spreads from legs to trunk and arms, respiratory muscle may be affected).
5. Gastrointestinal symptoms such as nausea, intermittent intestinal colic or diarrhea may occur.

6. The ECG changes falls, peaked T waves, P waves absent widened QRS complex.
7. Serum K, above 5.0 mEq/L (mmol/L).
8. It can produce cardiac arrest, metabolic acidosis and respiratory acidosis as complications.

Treatment

Management of the condition is done by replacement of water loss and correction of electrolyte imbalance. The client is given diet with restricted protein, but with as much as fat and carbohydrate, and also managing the underlying condition.

Nursing Interventions

1. Beware of clients at risk for hyperkalemia and monitor for its occurrence. Hyperkalemia is life-threatening; it is imperative to detect it easily.
2. Take measures to prevent hyperkalemia, when possible by following guidelines for administering potassium safely, both intravenously and orally.
3. Follow rules for safe administration of potassium.
4. Avoid administration of potassium, conserving diuretics, potassium supplements or salt substitutes to client with renal insufficiency.
5. Caution client to use salt substitute sparingly, if they are taking other supplementary form of potassium or taking potassium-conserving diuretics (e.g. spironolactone, triamterene and amiloride).
6. Caution hyperkalemic clients to avoid foods high in potassium content. Some of these are coffee, cocoa, tea, dried fruits, dried beans, whole-grain breads.

▶ HYPOCALCEMIA

Hypocalcemia refers to a calcium deficit in ECF. If the condition is prolonged, calcium gets lessen from bones. This results in osteomalacia, which is characterized by soft and pliable bones. Common signs and symptoms for hypocalcemia include numbness and tingling of fingers, muscle cramps and tetany.

The related factors leading to hypocalcemia are as follows:
1. Surgical hypoparathyroidism (may follow thyroid surgery or radical neck surgery for cancer).
2. Malabsorption.
3. Vitamin D deficiency.
4. Acute pancreatitis.
5. Excessive administration of citrated blood.
6. Primary hypothyroidism.
7. Alkalytic states (decreased ionized calcium).
8. Hyperphosphatemia.
9. Medullary carcinoma of thyroid.
10. Hypoalbuminemia (as in cirrhosis, nephrotic syndrome and starvation).
11. Hypomagnesemia.
12. Increased/decreased ultraviolet exposure.

Main Characteristics

1. Numbness, tingling in fingers, circumoral region and toes.
2. Cramps in the muscle of extremities.
3. Hyperactive deep tendon reflexes (such as patellar and triceps).
4. Trousseau's sign.
5. Chvostek's sign.
6. Mental changes such as confusion and alteration in mood and memory.
7. Convulsions, usually generalized, but may be focal.
8. Spasm of laryngeal muscles.
9. The ECG shows prolonged QT interval.
10. Spasms of muscles in abdomen (can simulate acute abdominal emergency).

11. Total calcium level below 8.5 mg/dL or ionized level below normal (below 50%).
12. Hypocalcemic state occurs when calcium loss occurs causing a fall in serum calcium level. This may eventually cause tetany and teeth.
13. It is usually asymptomatic and the neurological manifestations develop slowly.
14. It then gives rise to diffuse encephalopathy, depression and psychosis.
15. In severe cases, there may be laryngospasm and general convulsion.
16. It may also give rise to papilledema and cataract.

Treatment

Most cases respond well to adequate or supplement calcium and phosphorus. The patient may be given calcium carbonate 2.52–3.78 g daily orally or calcium gluconate 0.5–1.5 g along with calciferol 15.45 mg daily orally. Otherwise, 10 mL of 10% calcium gluconate is given by slow IV. Adequate management and control of predisposing causes can prevent the occurrence of the condition.

Nursing Interventions

1. Beware of clients at risk for hypocalcemia and monitor its occurrence.
2. Be prepared to take seizures precautions.
3. Monitor condition of airway closely because laryngeal stridor can occur.
4. Take safety precautions, if confusion is present.
5. Beware of factors related to the safe administration of calcium replacement salts.
6. Educate people in high-risk groups for osteoporosis (especially postmenopausal women not on estrogen therapy).

If adequate amounts are not consumed in the diet (as is often the case), calcium supplements should be considered.
7. Educate people at risk for osteoporosis about the value of regular physical exercise in decreasing bone loss.
8. To prevent osteoporosis in later years, educate young women about the need for a normal diet to ensure adequate calcium intake. Also discuss the calcium-losing aspects of alcohol and nicotine use.

▶ HYPERCALCEMIA

Hypercalcemia refers to an excess of calcium in ECF. It presents as an emergency situation because this condition often leads to cardiac arrest. It is a condition of excess of calcium and is characterized by polyuria, polydipsia, skeletal muscle weakness and hypertension. The related factors that lead to hypercalcemia are as follows:

1. Hyperparathyroidism.
2. Malignant neoplastic disease.
3. Prolonged immobilization.
4. Large doses of vitamin D.
5. Overuse of calcium-containing antacids or calcium supplements thiazide diuretics.
6. Milk-alkali syndrome.
7. Sarcoidosis.
8. It is also seen in person with Paget's disease, myxedema, Addison's disease and osteoporosis in aged persons.

Main Characteristics

1. Muscle weakness.
2. Tiredness, restlessness, lethargy.
3. Constipation.
4. Anorexia, nausea and vomiting.
5. Decreased memory span, decreased attention span and confusion.

6. Polyuria and polydipsia.
7. Renal stones.
8. Neurotic behavior progressing to frank psychosis may occur (reversible with correction of hypercalcemia).
9. Cardiac arrest may occur in hypercalcemic crisis.
10. The ECG shows shortened QT interval.
11. Serum calcium over 10.5 mg/dL.
12. It may produce renal failure, shock and death in complication.

Treatment

In mild cases, adequate rehydration is often effective. Management of the condition also includes management of the underlying conditions. In other cases, intravenous infusion of isotonic saline is given to promote calciuria. Calcium is also eliminated or maintained in the lower level by giving sodium phosphate 1–2 g orally daily and client is encouraged to take more fluids.

Nursing Interventions

1. Beware of clients at risk for hypercalcemia and monitor its occurrence.
2. Increase client mobilization when feasible.
3. Encourage the oral intake of sufficient fluids to keep the client well-hydrated.
4. Discourage excessive consumption of milk products and other high-calcium foods.
5. Encourage adequate bulk in the diet to offset the tendency for constipation.
6. Take safety precautions if confusion or other mental symptoms by hypercalcemia are present.
7. Beware that cardiac arrest can occur in clients with severe hypercalcemia; be prepared to deal with this emergency.
8. Beware that bones may fracture more easily in clients with chronic hypercalcemia because bone resorption has been

excessive, weakening the bony structure. Transfer clients cautiously.
9. Educate home-bound oncology clients with a predisposition for hypercalcemia and their families, to be alert for symptoms that occur with this condition and to report them to the healthcare providers before they become severe.
10. Be alert for signs of digitalis toxicity when hypercalcemia occurs in digitalized clients.
11. Help prevent formation of calcium renal stones in clients with longstanding hypercalcemia or immobilization by:
    a. Forcing fluids to maintain dilute urine, thus avoiding super saturation of precipitates.
    b. Encouraging fluids that yield an acid ash (prune or cranberry milk) because a urinary pH less than 6.5 favors calcium deposits.
    c. Preventing urinary stasis by turning the immobilized client, elevating head of the bed and having the client sit up, if this can be tolerated.

▶ HYPOMAGNESEMIA

Magnesium is an important and plentiful cation, and is essential for many enzymatic system associated with protein, carbohydrate and lipid metabolism.

Hypomagnesemia refers to magnesium deficit. It is a condition of low plasma concentration of magnesium, characterized by neuromuscular and central nervous system (CNS) hyperirritability.

The related factors, which lead to hypomagnesemia, are as follows:
1. Chronic alcoholism.
2. Intestinal malabsorption syndrome.
3. Diarrhea.
4. Nasogastric suction: Prolonged.

5. Aggressive refeeding after starvation [as in total parenteral nutrition (TPN)].
6. Prolonged administration of magnesium-free IV fluids.
7. Uncontrolled diabetes mellitus (diabetic ketoacidosis).
8. Hyperaldosteronism.
9. Drugs: Prolonged use of diuretics, aminoglycoside, antibiotics (e.g. gentamicin), cisplatin excessive dose of vitamin D or calcium supplements.
10. Citrate preservative in blood products pancreatitis, thyrotoxicosis, hyperparathyroidism, severe osteitis fibrosa, protein-energy malnutrition (PEM).

Main Characteristics

1. It presents with multiple metabolic and nutritional deficiency.
2. It gives rise to anorexia, lethargy, vomiting, weakness and tetany neuromuscular irritability.
3. Increased reflex.
4. Course tremors.
5. Positive Chvostek's and Trousseau's signs.
6. Convulsions.

Cardiac manifestations include:
1. Tachyarrhythmia's.
2. Increased susceptibility to digitalis toxicity.
3. The ECG changes in severe cases, PR and QT interval prolongation, widened QRS complex, ST segment depression and T-wave inversion.
4. Mental changes.
5. Disorientation in memory.
6. Mood changes.
7. Intense confusion.
8. Hallucination.
9. Serum magnesium level below 1.3 mEq/L.

Treatment

Repletion of the cases is done through magnesium sulfate and chloride. It is customary to give double the amount required, because half of magnesium given is excreted by the kidneys. The repletion is done gradually and is given orally or intravenously; in severe cases, IV only.

Nursing Interventions

1. Beware, client at risk for hypomagnesemia, especially closely for symptoms of digitalis toxicity, because a deficit of magnesium predisposes to toxicity.
2. Be prepared to take seizure precautions.
3. Monitor condition of airway, because laryngeal stridor can occur. Take safety precautions if confusion presents, be familiar with magnesium replacement salts and factors related to these safe administrations.
4. Beware that magnesium-depleted clients may experience difficulty in swallowing.
5. When magnesium deficit is due to abuse of diuretics in laxatives, educating the client may help alleviate problem.
6. Beware that most commonly used IV fluids have either no magnesium or relatively small amount. When indicated, discuss the need for magnesium replacement with physicians.
7. For clients experiencing abnormal losses, but able to consume a general diet, encourage intake of magnesium-rich foods (such as green leafy vegetables, nuts, legumes and fruits such as bananas, oranges and grape fruits).

▶ HYPERMAGNESEMIA

Hypermagnesemia refers to excess of magnesium in ECF. It can occur especially in end-stage renal failure. When kidneys fail to excrete magnesium and excessive amounts are administered therapeutically. It is a condition associated with excess of magnesium and is characterized by muscular weakness and ECG changes.

SECTION 2: Dietetics

The related factors, which lead to hypermagnesemia, are as follows:
1. Renal failure (particularly when magnesium-containing medications are administered).
2. Adrenal insufficiency.
3. Administration of excessive magnesium during the treatment of eclampsia.
4. Hemodialysis with excessively hard water or with dialysate inadvertently high in magnesium content.

Magnesium has a direct action on the myoneural junction. Its excess produces blockage causing impairment of neuromuscular transmission and that results diminished excitability of the muscle cells.

Main Characteristics

1. Early signs (serum level of g of 3–5 mEq/L).
2. Flushing and a sense of skin warmth (due to peripheral vasodilation).
3. Hypotension (due to blockage of sympathetic ganglia).
4. Depressed respiration.
5. Drowsiness, hypoactive reflexes and muscular weakness.
6. Cardiac abnormalities—cardiac arrest may develop.
7. Weak or absent cry in newborn.
8. The ECG shows prolonged PR interval, widened QRS complex and elevated T-wave amplitude.
9. Elevated serum magnesium level.

Treatment

In severe cases and also in other cases, cardiac and respiratory support is given by IV injection of 10–20 mL of 10% calcium gluconate. Maintenance of adequate hydration is essential. The client is also given furosemide by IV injection to promote excretion of magnesium. In more severe cases, hemodialysis is done.

Nursing Interventions

1. Beware of client at risk for hypomagnesemia and assess for its presence. When it is suspected, assess the following parameters:
   a. Vital signs: Look for low blood pressure and shallow respirations with periods of apnea.
   b. Level of consciousness: Look for drowsiness, lethargy and coma.
2. Do not give magnesium-containing medication to clients with renal failure or compromised renal function.
3. Be particularly careful in following 'standing order' for bowel preparation for X-ray, because some of these include the use of magnesium citrate.
4. Caution clients with renal disease to check with their healthcare providers before taking over the counter medication.
5. Beware of factors related to safe parenteral administration of magnesium salts.

▶ HYPOPHOSPHATEMIA

Hypophosphatemia refers to a below normal serum concentration of inorganic phosphorus. It is a clinical manifestation of phosphate depletion, characterized by progressive encephalopathy and osteomalacia. The related factors, which lead to hypophosphatemia, are as follows:

1. Inadequate intake or absorption of phosphorus: Malabsorption.
2. It is associated with vomiting and diarrhea.
3. Prolonged injection of aluminum hydroxide or bicarbonate.
4. It is also seen in prolonged use of glucose insulin, fructose and administrations.
5. Refeeding after starvation.

SECTION 2: Dietetics

6. Hyperalimentation.
7. Alcohol withdrawal.
8. Diabetic ketoacidosis.
9. Respiratory alkalosis.
10. Use of phosphate-binding antacids.
11. Recovery phase after severe burns.
12. Use of anabolic steroids.
13. Chronic hemodialysis.

Main Characteristics

1. Progressive encephalopathy.
2. Paresthesias.
3. Muscle weakness.
4. Muscle pain and tenderness.
5. Mental changes, such as apprehension, confusion, delirium coma.
6. Cardiomyopathy.
7. Acute respiratory failure.
8. Seizures.
9. Decreased tissue oxygenation.
10. Joint stiffness.
11. Serum phosphate below 2.5 mg/dL.
12. Phosphate compounds are present in all normal foods and are essential for metabolism of carbohydrate, protein and fat. They are also responsible for changes, transfer or depletion occurs from prolonged negative phosphate balance and from chronic malnutrition.

Treatment

Management of the condition includes treatment of the underlying cause, repletion of phosphate and maintenance of body fluids.

Nursing Interventions

1. Identify clients at risk for hypophosphatemia.
2. Severely malnourished clients.
3. Alcoholic clients.
4. Clients with diabetic ketoacidosis.
5. Monitor clients at risk for the presence of hypophosphatemia.
6. Beware that severely hypophosphatemic clients are thought to be at greater risk of infection, because of changes in white blood cells (WBCs).
7. Administer IV phosphate products cautiously.
8. Beware that in adults the usual maintenance dose of phosphorus is 10–15 mmol/L of TPN solution.
9. Beware of the need to introduce hyperalimentation gradually in clients who are malnourished.
10. Because it is possible to give too much phosphorus when administering phosphate solutions, monitor for signs of hyperphosphatemia and of the salt in which it is administered.
11. Monitor for diarrhea in clients taking oral phosphorus supplements; consult physician if it persists or is severe.
12. Powdered oral phosphorus supplements with chilled or ice water to make them more palatable.

▶ HYPERPHOSPHATEMIA

Hyperphosphatemia refers to above normal serum concentrations of inorganic phosphorus. It is a condition associated with increased level of phosphate and is characterized by hypocalcemia. The related factors, which lead to hyperphosphatemia, are as follows:

1. Excessive intake of phosphate.
2. Hypervitaminosis D: Large vitamin D intake, acute renal failure.
3. Chronic renal insufficiency.
4. Chemotherapy, particularly for acute lymphoblastic leukemia and lymphoma.

5. Large intake of milk.
6. Use of cow's milk in infants.
7. Excessive intake of phosphate-containing laxatives.
8. Overzealous administration of phosphorus supplements (oral or IV).
9. Excessive use of Fleet's phospho-soda as enema solution, particularly in children and people with slow bowel elimination.
10. Hypoparathyroidism.
11. Hyperthyroidism.

Main Characteristics

Hyperphosphatemia condition by itself does not give rise to any symptoms, but manifested with that of hypocalcemia. This includes:

1. Short-term consequences: Symptoms of tetany, such as tingling of fingertips and around mouth, numbness and muscle spasms.
2. Long-term consequences: Precipitation of calcium phosphate in non-osseous sites; such as kidney, joints, arteries, skin or cornea.
3. Serum phosphate above 4.5 mg/dL.

Treatment

Management of the condition requires correction of underlying condition.

Nursing Interventions

1. Identify clients at risk for hyperphosphatemia.
2. Monitor signs of tetanus and other features of hypocalcemia.
3. Beware that soft-tissue calcification can be long-term complication of a chemically elevated serum-phosphate level. Calcification may occur in site such as kidney, arteries, joints, etc.

4. Administer prescribed oral or IV phosphate supplements cautiously and monitor serum phosphorus levels periodically during their use.
5. When appropriate, instruct clients that use of phosphate- containing laxatives may result in acute phosphate poisoning.
6. Beware that phosphate-containing enema can result in hyperphosphatemia if used injudiciously, particularly in children and those with slow bowel emptying, instruct clients accordingly.
7. When low-phosphorus diet is prescribed, instruct clients to avoid foods high in phosphorus content. Such foods include hard cheese or cream, nuts and nut products, whole grain cereals, dried fruits, dried vegetables, special meats such as kidneys, sardines, sweet breads and desserts made with milk.

▶ CONCLUSION

Water is the commonest liquid with the most uncommon properties. Water content of the body changes with age. Water content is more in brain tissues and less in adipose tissue. Water intake and output must be balanced. Water requirements of a person vary with climate, age, activity, dietary habits and body build. Water depletion occurs when water loss is not met by water intake. Acid-base balance refers to the regulation of the hydrogen ion concentration of body fluids. Electrolytes are substances that become ions in solution and acquire the capacity to conduct electricity. Human body contains quite a large volume of water as ICF and ECF and the fluid contains several inorganic ions such as sodium, potassium, chloride, bicarbonate, sulfate, phosphate, calcium and magnesium. Electrolytes are present in the human body and the balance of the electrolytes in bodies is essential for normal function of the cells and organs. Electrolytes regulate water distribution, regulate acid-base balance and maintain a balanced degree of neuromuscular excitability.

SECTION 3

Infant and Child Nutrition

Chapter 23

Nutritional Needs of Infants

▶ INTRODUCTION

Nutrients, which are needed by the body for good nutritional status, are provided by food. An individual nutritional status is dependent on the provision of sufficient nutrients and the good utilization of these nutrients. Power status of nutrition may be caused by eating that is inadequate in amount and kind or it may be caused by failure in digestion and utilization of these nutrients. Adequate nutrition during infancy is essential for lifelong health and well-being. Infants should be exclusively breastfed for the first 6 months of life to achieve optimal growth, development and health. Thereafter, to meet their evolving nutritional requirements, infants should receive nutritionally adequate and safe complementary foods, while continuing to breastfeed for up to 2 years or more.

▶ NEED OF INFANT NUTRITION

Malnutrition is responsible directly or indirectly for about one third of deaths among children under age 5. Well-above two thirds of these deaths often associated with inappropriate feeding practices occur during the 1st year of life. Nutrition and nurturing during the 1st year of life are both crucial for lifelong health and well-being. In infancy, no gift is more precious than breastfeeding, yet rarely one in three infants is exclusively breastfed during the first 6 months of life.

The World Health Organization (WHO) recommends that infants start breastfeeding within 1 hour of life, are exclusively breastfed for 6 months, with timely introduction of adequate, safe and properly fed complementary foods while continuing breastfeeding for up to 2 years of age or beyond. Promoting sound feeding practices is one of the main program areas that the Department of Nutrition for Health and Development focuses on. Activities include the production of sound, evidence-based technical information, development of guidelines and counseling courses, provision of guidance for the protection, promotion and support of infant and young child feeding at policy, health service and community levels, production of appropriate indicators and maintenance of a Global Data Bank on infant and young child feeding.

▶ DIETARY REQUIREMENTS

It is important to recognize that people's dietary needs change during their life span. A suitable balanced diet for a small child will not be suitable for an adult or older person, so needs must be taken into account when caring for different individuals.

Energy

Three basic nutrients—carbohydrates, proteins and fats supply the body's caloric needs. Protein promotes cellular growth and maintenance, aid metabolism and contributes to many protective substances. Fats provide concentrated energy storage, transport essential nutrients (such as fatty acids needed for neurological growth and development) and insulate vital organs. Carbohydrate, which contains 4 cal/g, should provide 35%–55% of the neonate's total calories; fats that contain 9 cal/g provide 30%–55% and proteins, which contain 4 cal/g, the remaining calories.

Vitamins and Minerals

Vitamins regulate metabolic processes and promote growth and maintenance of body tissues. Fat-soluble vitamins (A, D, E and K) in excess of amount can be stored in the body to some extent and normally are not excreted; therefore reserve may accumulate. Water-soluble vitamins (C, B_1, B_2, B_6, B_{12}, niacin, folic acid, pantothenic acid and biotin) are stored only in small amounts. Consequently, if these vitamins are not ingested regularly, deficiencies may develop relatively quickly.

All major minerals and trace minerals are essential for a wide range of body functions, including regulation of enzyme metabolism, acid-base balance and nerve and muscle integrity. Calcium and iron are particularly important for growth—calcium for the rapid bone mineralization of the 1st year and for hemoglobin synthesis.

Fluid

Neonate's difficulty in concentrating urine plus a high extracellular water content result in a much greater need for fluid (150 mL/kg/day) compared to the adult (20–30 mL/kg/day). The neonate has limited gastric capacity. Also, fat absorption does not reach adult level until ages 6–9 months. For the 1st month, limited splitting of the starch salivary enzyme called ptyalin and absence of pancreatic amylase restrict digestion of complex starches found in solid foods.

Although the basic components of the neurological system are present at birth, myelination is incomplete. Only breast milk, infant formula and whole milk contain enough linoleic acid to facilitate myelination. Therefore, the milk that contains less than 2% milk fat is not recommended before age of 1 year.

▶ INFANCY

At birth, babies rely only on milk to meet their nutritional requirements. Breast milk is the ideal food for newborns because it contains nutrients for all the baby's needs in the right amounts. Although it is low in iron and copper, the baby has enough of these stored until it starts eating solid foods. In addition, breast milk provides immunity, and is clean, readily available and does not have to be prepared. Some mothers are either unable or choose not to breastfeed and use formula milk, which is modified cow's milk. This must be made up to the right concentration to prevent damage to the immature kidneys. The equipment used must be sterilized to prevent infection.

SECTION 3: Infant and Child Nutrition

Weaning should not be done before about 4 months of age as doing it early may cause later obesity or allergies. Different foods can be introduced gradually such as cereals, then fruit and vegetables, egg yolk and finely minced meat. By about 12–18 months, the children should be eating the same food as the rest of the family, with no extra salt or sugar added. It is usually advised that up until the age of 2 years, children should be given whole milk, but after this they can be given semi-skimmed milk. Skimmed milk should not be given until the age of 5. The amount of milk drunk will decrease as the child eats more and more solid food.

▶ CHILDHOOD

Children aged between 4 and 10 years of age tend to be very active and are growing fast. Although, their energy requirements are not high as adults, they need almost the same amount of some vitamins and minerals. Some children seem to have big appetites—this is not due to greed, but to the fact that they have high nutritional needs. During childhood, children should be encouraged to eat healthy meals consisting of meat, fish or eggs and potatoes, pasta or rice with plenty of vegetables and fruits. They should not eat too many sweets, crisps, biscuits and fizzy drinks, as these can lead to obesity and tooth decay. Signs that babies are hungry include:

1. Moving their heads from side to side.
2. Opening their mouths.
3. Sticking out their tongues.
4. Placing their hands, fingers and fists to their mouths.
5. Puckering their lips as if to suckle.
6. Nuzzling against their mother's breasts.
7. Showing the rooting reflex (when a baby moves its mouth in the direction of something that's stroking or touching its cheek).

▶ EXCLUSIVE BREASTFEEDING

Breastfeeding is an unequalled way of providing ideal food for the healthy growth and development of infants; it is also

CHAPTER 23: Nutritional Needs of Infants

an integral part of the reproductive process with important implications for the health of mothers. Review of evidence has shown that on a population basis, exclusive breastfeeding for 6 months is the optimal way of feeding infants. Thereafter, infants should receive complementary foods with continued breastfeeding up to 2 years of age or beyond.

To enable mothers to establish and sustain exclusive breastfeeding for 6 months, WHO and United Nations Children's Fund (UNICEF) recommend:

1. Initiation of breastfeeding within the first hour of life.
2. Exclusive breastfeeding—that is the infant receives only breast milk without any additional food or drink, not even water.
3. Breastfeeding on demand—that is as often as the child wants, day and night.
4. No use of bottles, teats or pacifiers.

Breast milk is the natural first food for babies, it provides all the energy and nutrients that the infant needs for the 1st months of life and it continues to provide up to half or more of a child's nutritional needs during the second half of the 1st year and up to one third during the 2nd year of life.

Breast milk promotes sensory and cognitive development, and protects the infant against infectious and chronic diseases. Exclusive breastfeeding reduces infant mortality due to common childhood illnesses such as diarrhea or pneumonia and helps for a quicker recovery during illness. These effects can be measured in resource poor and affluent societies. Breastfeeding contributes to the health and well-being of mothers; it helps to space children, reduces the risk of ovarian cancer and breast cancer, increases family and national resources is a secure way of feeding and is safe for the environment.

While breastfeeding is a natural act, it is also a learned behavior. An extensive body of research has demonstrated that mothers and other caregivers require active support for establishing and sustaining appropriate breastfeeding practices. WHO and UNICEF launched the Baby-friendly Hospital Initiative (BFHI) in 1992, to strengthen maternity practices to support breastfeeding. The foundation for the BFHI is the 10 steps to successful breastfeeding described in protecting, promoting and supporting breastfeeding—a joint WHO/UNICEF Statement. The evidence for the effectiveness of the 10 steps has been summarized in a scientific review document.

Breastfeeding

Most infants start feeding by first few hours of birth. Early feeding helps to maintain normal metabolism and growth, promotes maternal infant bonding, and decreases risk of hypoglycemia, hyperkalemia, dehydration, fever and hyperbilirubinemia. Breast milk is wholesome food for the baby. Breastfeeding is the most effective way to provide baby with a caring environment and complete nutrition. It meets the nutritional as well as emotional needs of the baby. UNICEF and WHO recommends exclusive breastfeeding to babies until 6 months of age.

Physiology of Lactation

Human milk is produced due to interaction between hormones and reflexes. During pregnancy, the glandular tissue of breast is stimulated to produce milk due to hormones—oxytocin and prolactin. Also two reflexes mediated by these hormones come into play:

1. **Milk secretion reflex (prolactin reflex):** Prolactin produced by anterior pituitary gland is responsible for milk secretion by alveolar cells of breast. When the baby suckles, the nerve endings in the nipple carry message to anterior pituitary, which in turn releases prolactin. This cycle from stimulation to secretion is called 'milk secretion reflex or prolactin reflex'.

2. **Milk ejection reflex (oxytocin reflex):** Oxytocin produced by posterior pituitary is responsible for contraction of breast tissue leading to ejection of milk from the gland into the lactiferous and ducts. This hormone is produced in response to stimulation of nerve endings in the nipple by suckling as well as by the thought, sight or sound of the

baby. Since, this reflex is affected by mother's emotions, a relaxed and confident attitude helps in 'milk ejection'.

Initiation: After delivery when the mother is still in the delivery room, she should have an opportunity to hold her baby for 10–15 minutes. As soon as the mother is ready to feed, she should be encouraged to give breastfeeding.

First milk: Toward the end of the pregnancy, the alveolar cells secrete yellow fluid called colostrum. It contains fluid secretion partly of whole and fragmental alveolar cells and some white blood cells. These cells produce antibodies, which can protect both the breast itself and the intestines of the baby against infections.

During pregnancy, the hormones produced by the ovary and placenta inhibit milk production. Immediately after delivery, there is a rapid decrease in the inhibitory hormones. With the stimulus of suckling by the newborn, the production of milk starts. The mature and full milk production may occur within about 10 days. The milk secretion depends on reflexes as follows.

Milk producing reflex: The breast of the mother produces milk for the baby according to baby's need and demand in response to its suckling. When the baby suckles, the sensory nerves ending in the breast are stimulated and impulses are carried by the vagus nerve to the hypothalamus. This causes the anterior pituitary to release prolactin into the blood. Prolactin acts on the milk producing cells of the breasts. The more the baby suckles, the more the milk is secreted.

The sensory nerve impulses that start when the baby suckles on the nipple cause the posterior pituitary to release oxytocin, make the myoepithelial cells around the alveoli and ducts contract. This squeezes milk from the alveoli, ducts and sinuses toward the nipple. Therefore, when the baby suckles at the nipple, it stimulates the nipple that produces milk flow. The ejection reflex is called 'let-down' reflex (Figs 23.1A and B).

Factors affecting let-down reflex:
1. When the mother thinks happily or affectionately about her baby, milk may start to flow.

SECTION 3: Infant and Child Nutrition

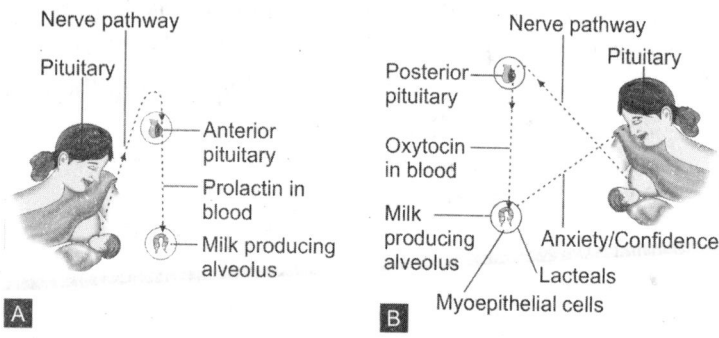

Figs 23.1A and B: The milk-ejection reflex ('let-down' reflex). **A.** Affects of anterior pituitary and prolactin in milk ejection; **B.** Affects of posterior pituitary and oxytocin in milk ejection.

2. A hungry baby suckles more often, more vigorously and longer than the satisfied baby. The baby's hunger is therefore the regulatory mechanism of the milk production.
3. Fear, excitement, anger and embarrassment may inhibit let-down reflex, and prevent milk present deep in the gland from coming down to the nipple.

Types of Breast Milk

The composition of breast milk (Table 23.1) varies at different stages of postnatal period, to suit the needs of the baby:

1. **Colostrum:** It is the milk secreted during the first 3 days after delivery. It is thick and yellow in color and rich in antibodies and vitamin A, D, E and K.
2. **Transitional milk:** It is the milk secreted during the next 2 weeks. The immunoglobulin and protein content decreases, white fat and sugar increases.
3. **Mature milk:** It follows transitional milk. It is thinner and watery, but has all nutrients for optimum growth of baby.
4. **Foremilk:** It is the milk secreted at the start of a feed. It is rich in proteins, sugar, vitamins and water.
5. **Hindmilk:** It comes later, toward the end of a feed, and is rich in fat and energy and satisfies the baby's hunger.

CHAPTER 23: Nutritional Needs of Infants

Table 23.1: Nutrition in human and cow's milk

Nutrients	Human milk	Cow's milk
Protein	1.2 g	3.5 g
• Casein	0.4 g	2.8 g
• Lactalbumin	0.8 g	0.7 g
Lactose	6.5 g	4.5 g
Fat	3.5 g	3.5 g
Calcium	34 mg	22 mg
Phosphate	15 mg	90 mg
Calories	67 kJ	67 kJ
Vitamin A	64 µg	53 µg
Vitamin B	0.03 µg	0.03 µg
Vitamin E	0.3 µg	0.7 µg
Vitamin C	5 µg	1 µg
Water	87.5%	88%

Initiation of Breastfeeding

Breastfeeding should be started within first ½–1 hour of birth or as soon as possible after normal delivery, whereas in case of cesarean section delivery, within 4 hours. Rooming-in and bedding-in should be done with mother and baby to prevent separation and promote breastfeeding.

Techniques of Breastfeeding

Initially the mothers need help in breastfeeding:
1. Position of mother and baby:
    a. Help the mother to get into a comfortable and relaxed position—sitting or lying down.
    b. Explain the mother to hold the baby, keeping in mind the four key points:
        i. Head and body of baby should be straight.
        ii. The baby's nose should be opposite to the nipple.
        iii. Baby's body should be close to her body.
        iv. Whole body of the baby must be supported.

c. Mother should than support her breast with her fingers flat against her chest wall under her breast.
2. Latching or attachment of baby to the breast: After proper positioning, the baby's cheek is touched with the nipple. Due to rooting reflex, baby quickly turns face toward the breast and starts suckling and the baby suckles, pauses and suckles again.

Signs of good attachment:
a. Baby's mouth is wide open.
b. Baby's chin touches the breast.
c. Much of the areola is not visible as it is in the baby's mouth.
d. Baby's cheeks are full and not hollow.

Signs of poor attachment:
a. Only the nipple is in the baby's mouth not the areola.
b. The baby's tongue is back inside mouth and cannot reach the ducts to press on them.
c. Suckling with poor attachment may be uncomfortable or painful for the mother.

Breastfeeding Methods

Breastfeeding methods are of four types showing in Figure 23.2:

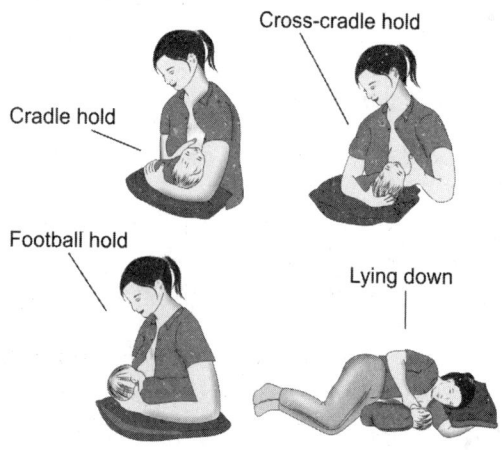

Fig. 23.2: Methods of breastfeeding

1. Cradle hold.
2. Cross-cradle hold.
3. Football hold.
4. Laying down.

Important Precautions for Breastfeeding

1. The mother's desire to feed is the first requirement for successful lactation. She should be psychologically prepared to feed. She should drink milk, juice or water before feeding.
2. She must wash her hands before feeding.
3. She should be physically and emotionally relaxed and comfortable.
4. She can sit comfortably with a support at the back. It is advisable to hold the baby in her lap.
5. If she is unable to sit, she may feed by lying on her side with a pillow under the shoulder.
6. She must check whether the baby has soiled the linen. If required the baby should be cleaned and dried to make the baby comfortable, before feeding.
7. The baby's head should be supported and slightly raised. The baby may be held in a semi-sitting position with his/her head close to the breast and supported with one arm.
8. The cheek of the baby should touch the nipple so that by rooting reflex the baby can get to the nipple and let-down reflex is encouraged.
9. If the breast is firm and full, it should be pressed with the first finger to prevent pressing of the baby's nose. Both breasts should be fed at each time, alternately, using each breast first. If possible one breast (which is given first) should be completely emptied at the alternate feeding.
10. During the first few days most of the babies fall asleep after taking a few suckle. They should be aroused by gentle tickle behind the ear or on the sole of the foot.

11. Before removal of the baby from the breast, it is necessary to break suckling by putting a little finger into the corner of the baby's mouth.
12. Every baby swallows some air during the feeding and should be held upright and patted on the back until the air is belched. If too much air is swallowed and not removed, the baby may have vomiting, colic or fretfulness. After feeding, if required, the diaper should be changed.
13. After feeding, the baby must be positioned on a right side or on the abdomen.

Factors Inhibiting Breast Milk

1. **Psychological factor:** A shock, strong pain, anger, anxiety or worry can affect the 'let-down' reflex. The mother should be encouraged, and given support by a calm and positive attitude to develop a confidence that any difficulties may be overcome. She should be explained the proper technique of relaxation and feeding.

   She should make sure that the neonate is suckling and should be encouraged to feed more often to increase suckling stimuli. In a case of severe anxiety, sedative may be ordered by the doctor for a short time.

2. **Early breast engorgement:** During the early period after delivery, breasts may be felt full and uncomfortable. Some mothers get hard engorged breasts with the pain. This problem can be solved by application of warm compresses to the breast and then expressing the excess milk. Later, the milk production gets adjusted according to demand of the baby.

3. **Flat and inverted nipple:** If nipples are flat and it is difficult for the baby to get hold of the nipple and pull it into the mouth, stimulation of the suckling reflex may be interrupted. A flat or inverted nipple may be pulled outward with the fingers to stimulate erection. After making the nipple erect, the baby can be gently put to the breast. If it is not successful, the nipple shield may be used.

CHAPTER 23: Nutritional Needs of Infants

Some babies who get accustomed to the nipple shield may be reluctant to return to the mother's nipple. Therefore, wearing a specially prepared plastic cup between the feeding may be helpful.

4. **Sore nipple:** Nipples may be sore because of faulty suckling technique, such as the baby takes an insufficient amount of areola surrounding the nipple into the mouth, while nursing. Also, it may be sore due to the long period of vigorous suckling, suckling in a bad position, engorged breast, fissures and oral thrush of the baby. Sore nipples are very painful.

Sore nipples can be prevented by proper antenatal care. Decreasing the length of the feeding time and increasing the frequency of feeding may also help. The use of soap on the breast should be avoided as it causes drying. The cream may be used by the doctor's advice or any edible oil can be applied on the nipples between feed.

Factors Influencing Breastfeeding

1. Milk producing reflex is influenced by the psychology of the mother.
2. Confidence of the mother about her ability for lactation stimulates the milk production.
3. Love and affection of the mother for her baby, through the close contact develop a psychological bond between the mother and the baby.
4. Frequent feeding stimulates the production and ejection reflex.
5. Feeding habits and technique are important to improve the close contact, positioning, comfort and regulate the demand for feeding.
6. Social factors such as not feeding the colostrum, delays the first suckling of the baby, thus affects the milk production.
7. The diet of the mother containing extra proteins and calcium is necessary. Pregnancy during the early lactation period affects the lactation.

8. Faulty suckling and the weak baby may cause inadequate stimulation. If the baby does not have suckling reflex; the express milk can be fed by tube feeding method. In case where, mother's milk is not available for some reason, the milk may be obtained from the substitute mother or a milk bank.

The value of the human milk is very high and cannot be substituted. If in any situation, it is not possible to obtain breast milk, cow milk may be used. Sometime because of saturated fats in the cow milk, neonates cannot digest and absorb it.

Contraindication for Breastfeeding

Mother
1. Breast diseases, e.g. mastitis, breast abscess.
2. Cardiac diseases and active tuberculosis.
3. Infectious diseases.
4. Mental illness of mother.
5. Unconscious mother.

Baby
1. Babies with cleft lip and cleft palate.
2. Premature and sick babies, who have poor suckling reflex.
3. Oral thrush.

General Instructions

1. Mother should keep her body clean and wear clean clothes.
2. Before each feed, clean the breasts and hands of the mother.
3. Mother should be in comfortable position during feeding.
4. Hold the nipple between index and middle finger.
5. Feed the baby on demand; it helps the baby to gain weight.
6. Feed the baby for minimum 10 minutes on each breast.
7. Instruct the mother to feed even when the baby is ill.
8. Burping should be done after each feed to expel the air from the baby's stomach.
9. When the baby is 4–6 months old start weaning, because mother's milk is not sufficient to sustain growth after 6 months of age.

CHAPTER 23: Nutritional Needs of Infants

10. If the baby's napkin is wet, dirty, change the napkins and clothes before each feeding.
11. Weigh the child every month and record it.
12. Teach the mother to have adequate rest to avoid tension, fatigue and stress.

Advantages of Breastfeeding

Breastfeeding is ideal for the neonates. It has several advantages both for the baby and mother.

Advantages for baby

It is a wholesome food for the baby as it contains all the nutrients that a baby needs in first 6 months of life for optimum growth and development.

Proteins: Human milk has low protein (1.2 g/dL) than cow's milk (3.5 g/dL), which lowers the solute load on kidneys of baby (Table 23.2). Also, human milk protein mainly lactalbumin is more easily digested than cow's milk protein (casein).

Table 23.2: Difference between human milk and cow's milk

Ingredients	Human	Cow
Carbohydrate	7%	4%
Protein	1.5%	4%
Fat	3.5%	4%

Fat: Higher content of monounsaturated fatty acids especially, linoleic acid in human milk promotes brain growth and protects individuals from atherosclerosis in later life.

Minerals: Human milk contains a smaller, but more balanced proportion of calcium and phosphorus as compared to cow's milk.

Lowers risk of infection: Human milk contains high level of lysozyme and IgA, which offers protection to the baby against several viral and bacterial diseases. Breast milk especially colostrums contains numerous host defense factors like macrophages, granulocytes, T and B lymphocytes. Lactoferrin present in breast milk protects the baby from enteric infections. Para-aminobenzoic acid (PABA) present in breast milk protects the baby from malaria.

Advantages of breastfeeding for baby and mother

1. Infant derives the sense of security and belongingness by the comfort of being held in the arms during the process of breastfeeding. There is an unbreakable bond created between the two.
2. It is economical to breastfeed the infant as it is naturally available food, which is clean and hygienic.
3. Breastfeeding helps in birth control. The hormone prolactin that stimulates milk production will also decrease the synthesis of various hormones. It is a cost-effective method of contraception. By breastfeeding the uterus comes back to normal size and would stop bleeding by the secretion of oxytocin. It also helps to reduce weight in mothers.
4. Risk of breast cancer is higher in women who have not breastfed their babies.
5. There is proper development of jaws and teeth, and they are not crowded as the infant must suckle hard to extract milk.
6. Reduced likelihood of child being allergic to milk, as human milk proteins do not cause allergies.
7. There is less danger of the feed being contaminated, which could lead to gastrointestinal problems. Mortality rates are lower among breastfed infants.
8. Human milk contains bacterial and viral antibodies including high concentration of secretary IgA, which provide local gastrointestinal immunity.
9. It is available at correct temperature and needs no time for preparation.
10. It is convenient to feed the baby when it is in the mother's arms.
11. It protects the babies from obesity.
12. There is rapid maturation of the gastrointestinal tract due to the presence of growth factors and certain hormones.

13. The fats and proteins present are more easily digestible and there is less chance of child developing gastric and intestinal distress.
14. Milk has other anti-infective proteins due to the presence of macrophages, complement, lysozyme and lactoferrin. All these provide protection against diarrhea and respiratory infections.
15. The breast milk also provides many biochemical advantages like prevention of neonatal hypoglycemia.

Conditions when mothers are advised not to breastfeed: Septicemia, nephritis, active tuberculosis, typhoid fever, malaria, renal failure, grade IV cardiac failure and severe neurosis.

Breastfeeding Policy

Ten steps to successful breastfeeding. Every facility providing maternity services and care for newborn infants should:

1. Have a written breastfeeding policy that is routinely communicated to all healthcare staff.
2. Train all healthcare staff in skills necessary to implement this policy.
3. Inform all pregnant women about the benefits and management of breastfeeding.
4. Help mothers initiate breastfeeding within half an hour of birth.
5. Show mothers how to breastfeed and how to maintain lactation even if they should be separate from their infants.
6. Do not give food or drink to newborn infants other than breast milk, unless medically indicated.
7. Practice rooming-in—allow mothers and infants to remain together—24 hours.
8. Encourage breastfeeding on demand.
9. Do not give artificial teats or pacifiers (also called dummies or soothers) to breastfeeding infants.
10. Foster the establishment of breastfeeding support groups and refer mothers to them on discharge from the hospital or clinic.

SECTION 3: Infant and Child Nutrition

▶ ARTIFICIAL FEEDING

Artificial feeding (Table 23.3) is given to infants instead of breast milk; breast milk is often substituted by cow's milk. The cow's milk is substituted by dried milk, evaporated milk, etc.

Table 23.3: Artificial feeding and its frequency

Age of infant	Artificial feeding	Frequency
0–2 week	Cow's milk dilution 1:1	3 hourly
2–4 week	2:1 (2 parts of milk to 1 part of water)	3 hourly
1–3 month	3:1	4 hourly (if the baby demands 3 hourly needs to be adjusted)
3–6 month	Undiluted cow's milk	4 hourly

Preparation Formula

The milk formula should be planned to meet the nutritional requirement of the infant, which is based on infant age and weight:

1. Caloric requirement: 110 cal/kg of body weight.
2. Fluid requirement: 165 mL/kg of body weight.
3. Milk requirement: 100–130 mL/kg of body weight.
4. Number of feeds in 24 hours: 7 feeds.
5. Time interval between each feed: 2–3 hours.

Preparation of Milk Formula for a Day

Take 460 mL of milk, 140 mL of water and add 9 teaspoonful of sugar and boil it and keep it in the refrigerator, for each feed, take 85 mL of milk, warm it and feed the baby.

Different Ways of Artificial Feeding an Infant

1. By using the feeding bottle and teat.
2. By nasal tubes.
3. By belcroy feeder.

CHAPTER 23: Nutritional Needs of Infants

4. By dropper.
5. By using spoon.

Disadvantages of Artificial Feeding

1. Contamination: Artificial needs are often contaminated with bacteria, especially if the mother uses a feeding bottle, which she does not clean and boil properly.
2. Animal milk does not contain living white blood cells and antibodies to protect the baby against infections. Artificially fed babies fall ill more often with diarrhea and respiratory infections.
3. Animal milk may not contain enough vitamins for a baby.
4. The iron from animal milk is not absorbed as completely as the iron from human milk.
5. An artificially fed baby may develop anemia.
6. Animal milk contains too much salt, which may result in fits. Animal milk also contains excessive calcium and phosphates, which may cause tetany, i.e. twitching.
7. Animal milk contains more saturated fatty acids and does not contain enough essential fatty acids, which are vital for proper growth and development.
8. Animal milk contains too much casein, which is difficult for a baby's immature kidneys to excrete.
9. Animal milk is more difficult to digest, as it does not contain the enzyme lipase, which helps digest the fat.
10. Babies fed on animal milk may develop allergies.
11. Animal milk is expensive and the family might not be able to afford it.

Any supplement started before the baby is 4 months of age, increases the risk of infection and even death.

Methods of Artificial Feeding

Babies can be fed artificially by following ways:

1. Bottle feeding.
2. Katori and spoon feeding.

3. Cup feeding.
4. Gavage or nasogastric feeding.

Bottle Feeding

Bottle feeding is a common practice in India, to which babies become addicted. A prolonged bottle feeding may lead to 'baby bottle tooth decay'. Also it is difficult to wean bottle fed babies. At times bottle is contaminated or inadequately cleaned resulting in gastrointestinal infection causing diarrhea. Despite of these negative factors, if bottle feeding is practiced, it must be done cautiously.

Principles of bottle feeding

The following principles must be kept in mind while bottle feeding the baby:

1. After washing the bottle with brush and clean water, it should be boiled for about 10 minutes. The milk or cream sticking to nipple can be easily removed by rubbing with common salt.
2. Hand should be washed thoroughly before touching the bottle and preparing the feed.
3. The hole of teat should be such that drip rate is one drop/second. A hole smaller than this makes feeding difficult, exhausts the child and results in swallowing of air leading to vomiting and abdominal distension. A big hole, on other hand will result in choking, vomiting and abdominal distension.

Techniques of bottle feeding

1. After cleaning the teat and bottle, it should be sterilized and kept covered.
2. Prepare the formula as per requirement, when the baby is hungry (Table 23.4).
3. Change the soiled diaper and make the baby comfortable.
4. Wash hands and test flow of milk and its temperature, by sprinkling a few drops on inner aspect of wrist.
5. Sit in a comfortable position with baby on lap. Head of the baby should be higher than rest of the body.

CHAPTER 23: Nutritional Needs of Infants

Table 23.4: Quantity of reconstituted or cow's milk and its frequency of feeds

Quantity of reconstituted or cow's milk	Frequency of feeds
120–150 mL/kg/day	7 time/day × 1st 2 month 6 time/day × next 2 month 5 time/day × next 3 month

6. If any medication is to be administered, it should be given before feeding.
7. The teat should be touched to the corner of baby's mouth and when baby opens mouth, teat should be inserted in mouth.
8. The bottle should be held at an angle that teat is completely filled and there is no air in the teat.
9. The baby should be burped during and after the feeds.
10. After burping, make the baby lie in right lateral position.

Instructions to the mother

1. The mother should be explained about the type of formula, its preparation and sterilization of the feeding bottle and teats.
2. She should also be told about the selection of the proper bottle, technique of feeding, position of the baby during and after the feeding and how to burp the baby.
3. The mother should be explained about the need for additional fluids during periods of hot weather and when the baby has a fever, diarrhea or vomiting.
4. Mother should be told about the common potential problems related to feeding such as overfeeding, underfeeding, difficulty in digestion, improper feeding techniques and colic. In such a case, she should seek the doctor's help.

Development of healthy food habits

1. The healthy food habits should be started from the birth. The breastfeeding should be given regularly at least for 4–6 months.

2. Children should feel secured, satisfied and loved during the feeding.
3. Weaning should be started gradually. It is recommended that breast/bottle feeding should be discontinued by the age of 1 year.
4. Feeding from the cup can be started by the age of 8–10 months.
5. By the age of 1 year, children may eat with the family.

Health instructions on nutrition

In general, people may have very little knowledge about the nutritive value. It is the responsibility of health workers to provide appropriate information to the people, in the community, hospitals and clinics, at various levels of child development. Parents should be made aware of their role in practicing healthy food habits.

Demonstrations on the preparations of simple multipurpose food can create interest in the mothers. Discussion on variety of preparations with balanced diet with the reasonable cost can help people in daily feeding of children.

Katori and Spoon Feeding

When the neonate cannot suckle on the breast due to prematurity or any congenital malformation or when breast milk is obtained from sources others than mother, feeding with katori and spoon is the best method.

Technique of katori and spoon feeding:
1. The katori and spoon should be washed thoroughly and boiled for 10 minutes.
2. Take required amount of feed in the cup and keep it covered.
3. Change soiled diaper.
4. Wash hands and hold the baby semi-upright in lap and wrap a bib or soft cloth around the neck.
5. Touch the spoon to the corner of the mouth and when the baby opens mouth, feed is given. The first bolus is allowed to swallow, before the next is given. Feed from the corner

of the mouth and constantly observe the baby to prevent aspiration and control feeding.
6. After feeding, burp the baby, wipe the mouth and make him/her lie in right lateral position.

Cup Feeding

Another good method of feeding the baby is directly by cup. A baby, who feeds by cup, should be given 5 mL extra at each feed to allow for spillage from cup.

Techniques of cup feeding:
1. Wash the cup thoroughly and boil it for 10 minutes.
2. Take the required amount of feed with 5 mL extra to allow for spillage from the cup.
3. Hold the baby in lap after changing of soiled diaper, supporting baby head and shoulders.
4. Hold the cup of milk resting on the lower lip so that the rim of cup touches the baby's upper lip.
5. Tilt the cup so that the milk just reaches baby's lips.
6. A term baby will suck the milk, spitting some of it.
7. Do not pour the milk into baby's mouth; let the baby suck it.
8. When the baby has had enough, he/she doses the mouth and stops taking feed.
9. Wipe off the face and burp the baby.
10. Make the baby lie in right lateral position.

Gavage Feeding

For gavage feeding, size 5 Fr feeding catheter is required for nasogastric or orgiastic placement. For nasogastric insertion, the catheter is measured from external nares to the tragus of the ear and from there to the xiphisternum. This length of tube should be inserted from nose. For orogastric insertion, distance is measured from angle of mouth to the tragus and from there to the xiphisternum. During nasogastric or orogastric tube insertion, the head is slightly raised and a wet (not lubricated) catheter is passed gently though the nose or mouth into the esophagus and then to stomach. Position of the nasogastric tube is verified by aspirating the gastric contents.

The tube is then fixed through an adhesive tape. At the time of feeding, a 5 or 10 mL syringe without plunger is attached to the tube and milk is given through it. After feeding, place the baby in right lateral position. There is no need to burp the baby after gavage feed. A nasogastric or orogastric tube can be left in situ for up to 7 days.

Problems Associated with Artificial Feeding

The problems associated with artificial feeding are:
1. Constipation due to undigested protein. This can be relieved by adding sugar to the milk.
2. Underfeeding.
3. Overfeeding.
4. Aerophagy (swallowing of air) leading to distension of abdomen, colic and aspiration.
5. Low pH formulas may lead to acidosis.
6. Malnutrition, if feeds are overdiluted.
7. It is expensive and its preparation is tedious.
8. High incidence of infection, if hygiene is not maintained.
9. Cow's milk contains higher sodium and phosphorus leading to increased solute load on kidneys, which predispose babies to hypertonic dehydration.
10. Artificially fed infants are at higher risk of gastroenteritis, anemia, hyperphosphatemia, hypocalcemia and latent or clinical scurvy.

General Instructions

1. Plan the formula according to the nutritional requirement of the baby.
2. The feeding bottle, teat and other articles used for the feeding should be sterile.
3. The milk feed should be warm.

CHAPTER 23: Nutritional Needs of Infants

4. The mother and the child should be in a comfortable position.
5. Ensure a slow and steady flow of milk by making a hole in the teat neither too big nor too small.
6. Change the napkin before the feed, it if is wet or soiled.
7. The feeds should be given at regular intervals.
8. The mother should wash her hands thoroughly before preparing the feed and feeding the child.
9. Offer a small quantity of water at the end of each feed.
10. Never pinch the nose to make baby to open the mouth instead press cheeks.

Preliminary Assessment

Consider the following:
1. Check the doctor's order for any specific instructions.
2. Plan the formula according to the nutritional needs of the infant.
3. Time at which the last feed was given.
4. General condition of the baby.
5. Baby's ability for sucking.
6. Articles available in the unit.

Preparation of the Infant and the Environment

1. Arrange the articles at the bedside.
2. Provide privacy.
3. Change the napkin if it is wet.
4. Bath the baby if necessary.
5. Keep the feeding bottle ready.

Equipments

A tray containing:
1. Mackintosh and towel.
2. Baby dress and napkin.

3. Feeding bottle and teat in a sterile container.
4. Required amount of feed (sterile).
5. Sterile water in a bottle.
6. A piece of clean towel or flannel.
7. Gown and mask for the nurse.

Procedure

1. Wash hands thoroughly.
2. Hold the baby in a position similar to one used for breast-feeding.
3. Check the temperature of the feed by dropping few drops on the inner aspect of the wrist joint.
4. Hold the bottle in an angle of 45° and bring the teat to the lips and then into the mouth of the baby.
5. Take care to keep the teat filled with milk throughout the feeding.
6. Break the wind (burping) in between the feeds.
7. When the feed is finished, give sterile water to the baby.

Aftercare

1. Keep the baby on the shoulders and pat over baby's back.
2. Wipe the face.
3. Remove the towel and lay the baby in the cradle.
4. Replace the articles in the proper place after cleaning.
5. Wash hands.
6. Record the procedures in the nurse's record sheet.

▶ COMPLEMENTARY FEEDING

When breast milk is no longer enough to meet the nutritional needs of the infant, complementary foods should be added to the diet of the child. The transition from exclusive breastfeeding to family foods, referred to as complementary feeding, typically covers the period from 6 to 18 or 24 months of age and is a very vulnerable period. It is the time, when malnutrition starts in many infants, contributing significantly to the high prevalence of malnutrition in children under 5 years of age worldwide. WHO estimates that two out of five children are stunted in low-income countries.

Complementary feeding should be timely, meaning that all infants should start receiving foods in addition to breast milk from 6 months onwards. It should be adequate meaning that the complementary foods should be given in amounts, frequency and consistency, and using a variety of foods to cover the nutritional needs of the growing child while maintaining breastfeeding. Foods should be prepared and given in a safe manner, meaning that measures are taken to minimize the risk of contamination with pathogens. And they should be given in a way that is appropriate, meaning that foods are of appropriate texture for the age of the child and applying responsive feeding following the principles of psychosocial care.

The adequacy of complementary feeding (adequacy in short for timely, adequate, safe and appropriate) not only depends on the availability of a variety of foods in the household, but also on the feeding practices of caregivers. Feeding young infants requires active care and stimulation, where the caregiver is responsive to the child clues for hunger and also encourages the child to eat. This is also referred to as active or responsive feeding.

The WHO recommends that infants start receiving complementary foods at 6 months of age in addition to breast milk, initially 2–3 times a day between 6 and 8 months, increasing to 3–4 times daily between 9–11 months and 12–24 months with additional nutritious snacks offered 2–3 times per day, as desired.

Inappropriate feeding practices are often a greater determinant of inadequate intakes than the availability of foods in the households. WHO has developed a protocol for adapting feeding recommendations that enables program managers to identify local feeding practices, common problems associated with feeding and adequate complementary foods. The protocol builds upon available information and proposes household trials to test improved feeding recommendations. WHO recommends that the protocol be used to design interventions for improved complementary feeding and is included as part of adaptation process of the Integrated Management of Childhood Illness (IMCI) strategy.

Guiding Principles

Breast milk alone is not sufficient to meet the nutritional requirements of the baby after 6 months. Also infants are developmentally ready to take other foods at about 6 months. By 6–8 months teeth eruption begins, and the baby learns to bite and chew (Fig. 23.3). The digestive system becomes mature enough to digest starch, protein and fat in non-milk diet. Very young infants push food out with their tongue, but by the age of 6–9 months they are able to hold food in their mouths. Hence, 6 months is the recommended age for weaning.

The energy needed in addition to breast milk is about 200 kcal/day in infants of 6–8 months, 300 kcal/day during 9–11 months and 550 kcal/day during 12–23 months of age. So, baby needs extra food in addition to breast milk.

Principle 1

Practice exclusive breastfeeding from birth up to 6 months of age and introduce complementary foods after 6 months of age along with breastfeeding.

Principle 2

Continue frequent on demand breastfeeding until 2 years of age or beyond.

Principle 3

Practice responsive (active) feeding applying the principles of psychosocial care.

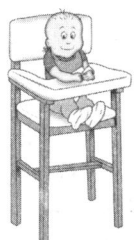

Fig. 23.3: Infant feeding technique

CHAPTER 23: Nutritional Needs of Infants

Feed child slowly and patiently, and encourage them to eat, but do not force them. If the child refuses to eat food, experiment with different food combinations, tastes and textures. Minimize distractions during meals if the child loses interest easily.

Principle 4

Practice good hygiene and proper food handling to reduce the risk of diarrhea.

Principle 5

Start at 6 months of age with small amounts of food and increase the quantity as the child gets older, while maintaining frequent breastfeeding.

Principle 6

Gradually increase food consistency and variety as the infant grows older, adapting to the infant's requirements and abilities. Begin liquids at 6 months. By 8 months child can eat semisolids and by 12 months he/she can eat solid foods as consumed by rest of the family members.

Principle 7

Increase the number of times the child is fed complementary food, as the child gets older. A breastfed infant, who is 6–8 months old, needs 2–3 meals a day and at 9–23 months he/she needs 3–4 meals a day.

Principle 8

Need a variety of nutrient rich foods to ensure that all nutrient needs are met. Complementary foods should provide sufficient energy, protein, vitamins, iron and micronutrients. Complementary food should include animal products, dairy products, pulses, fruits, vegetables and oil.

Principle 9

Give micronutrient rich complementary foods or vitamin and mineral supplements to the infant as needed.

Principle 10

It is advisable to start one or two teaspoons of new food at first, which should be given when baby is hungry, just before regular feeding, during day time. It may be continued for a few days until the child gets used to the same. Then the new food item may be started, one at a time.

▶ CONCLUSION

Nutrition during infancy lays the foundation for health. Infancy is a period of rapid growth. During the first few days of birth the infant loses weight, but slowly regains weight. Tissues and organ synthesis rate is high in infants. Therefore meeting the nutritional needs require careful planning. A healthy newborn baby doubles in birth weight by the 5th month and triples by 1 year. Infant in the age group of 0–3 months are mostly breast-fed. Scientific studies have shown that watery human milk is what the human infant needs. Malnutrition impairs the growth and development of the baby, such babies show reduction in working efficiency in adult life.

Chapter 24

Premature Infant Feeding

▶ INTRODUCTION

The premature infant's nutritional requirements are substantially different from those of the term infant and meeting their unique needs can be challenging. Early care in the neonatal intensive care unit (NICU) is focused on vital organ development; nutrition may be introduced only gradually in the 1st week of life in recognition of the risk of intolerance due to immaturities of the infant's digestive system and feeding abilities. On the other hand, optimizing nutrition early in life is essential to improve survival and promote growth and development. Avoiding early malnutrition can have both short-and long-term benefits for the infant.

▶ IMPORTANCE OF PRETERM NUTRITION

Proper nutrition in infancy is essential for normal growth, resistance to infection, long-term health and optimal neurologic and cognitive development. Providing adequate nutrition to preterm infants is challenging because of several problems, some of them are unique to these small infants. These problems include immaturity of bowel function, inability to suck and swallow, high risk of necrotizing enterocolitis (NEC), illnesses that may interfere with adequate enteral feeding [e.g. respiratory distress syndrome (RDS), patent ductus arteriosus (PDA)] and medical interventions that preclude feeding (e.g. umbilical vessel catheters, exchange transfusion, indomethacin therapy).

Physiology and Pathophysiology

The gut has formed and has completed its rotation back into the abdominal cavity by 10 weeks of gestation. By 16 weeks, the fetus can swallow amniotic fluid. Gastrointestinal (GI) motor activity is present before 24 weeks, but organized peristalsis is not established until 29–30 weeks and is facilitated by antenatal corticosteroid treatment. Coordinated sucking and swallowing develops at 32–34 weeks.

By term, the fetus swallows about 150 cc/kg/day of amniotic fluid, which has 275 mOsm/L, contains carbohydrates, protein, fat, electrolytes, immunoglobulin and growth factors, and plays an important role in the development of GI function. Preterm birth interrupts this development. Even if nutrients are provided parenterally, lack of enteric intake leads to decreased circulating gut peptides, slower enterocyte turnover and nutrient transport, decreased bile acid secretion and increased susceptibility to infection due to impaired barrier function by intestinal epithelium, lack of colonization by normal commensal flora and colonization by pathogenic organisms. For fat digestion, the newborn depends on lingual lipase, which is stimulated by sucking and swallowing, and by nutrients in the stomach, but not the small bowel.

Physical Challenges to Optimal Nutrition

Providing adequate nutrition to the preterm infant is complicated by immature organ systems, particularly the GI system and metabolic processes. GI immaturities in the preterm infant include inability to coordinate breathing, sucking and swallowing:
- Low esophageal sphincter (LES) pressure
- Delayed gastric emptying
- Slower upper and lower intestinal motility
- Immature digestion and absorption of carbohydrates, proteins and lipids.

In addition, prior to birth the GI tract is sterile and therefore, immunologically immature. Normal gut colonization acquired through contact with the mother and feeding, may be delayed or absent following birth due to isolation of the infant and residence in the NICU setting. Preterm infants may therefore be at risk of acquiring abnormal bacterial flora and developing nosocomial infections.

Premature Infants

A premature infant is a baby born before 37 completed weeks of gestation (more than 3 weeks before the 'due date'). Health conditions in the mother, such as diabetes, heart disease and kidney disease, may contribute to preterm labor. Often, the cause of preterm labor is unknown. About 15% of all premature births are multiple pregnancies (twins, triplets, etc).

Risk of Preterm Labor or Early Delivery

1. A weakened cervix that begins to open (dilate) early, also called cervical incompetence.
2. Birth defects of the uterus.
3. History of preterm delivery.
4. Infection (such as a urinary tract infection or infection of the amniotic membrane).
5. Poor nutrition right before or during pregnancy.
6. Preeclampsia: High blood pressure and protein in the urine that develop after the 20th week of pregnancy.
7. Premature rupture of the membranes (placenta previa).

Other Factors Affecting Premature Delivery

1. Age of the mother (mothers who are younger than 16 or older than 35).
2. Being African/American.
3. Lack of prenatal care.
4. Low socioeconomic status.
5. Use of tobacco, cocaine or amphetamines.

Clinical Manifestations

A premature infant may have signs of the following problems:

1. Anemia.
2. Bleeding into the brain or damage to the brains white matter.
3. Infection or neonatal sepsis.
4. Low blood sugar (hypoglycemia).
5. Neonatal respiratory distress syndrome, extra air in the tissue of the lungs (pulmonary interstitial emphysema) or bleeding in the lungs (pulmonary hemorrhage).
6. Newborn jaundice.
7. Problems breathing due to immature lungs, pneumonia or PDA.
8. Severe intestinal inflammation (NEC).

A premature infant will have a lower birth weight than a full-term infant. Common signs of prematurity include:

1. Abnormal breathing patterns (shallow, irregular pauses in breathing called apnea).
2. Body hair (lanugo).
3. Enlarged clitoris (in female infants).
4. Less body fat.
5. Lower muscle tone and less activity than full-term infants.
6. Problems feeding due to trouble sucking or coordinating swallowing and breathing.
7. Small scrotum that is smooth and has no ridges, and undescended testicles (in male infants).
8. Soft, flexible ear cartilage.
9. Thin, smooth, shiny skin that is often transparent (can see veins under skin).

Management

When premature labor develops and cannot be stopped, the healthcare team will prepare for a high-risk birth. The mother may be moved to a center that is set up to care for premature infants in a NICU.

After birth, the baby is admitted to a high-risk nursery. The infant is placed under a warmer or in a clear, heated box called

CHAPTER 24: Premature Infant Feeding

incubator, which controls the air temperature. Monitoring machines track the baby's breathing, heart rate and level of oxygen in the blood.

Premature infant's organs are not fully developed. The infant needs special care in a nursery until the organs have developed enough to keep the baby alive without medical support. This may take weeks to months.

Infants usually cannot coordinate sucking and swallowing before 34 weeks gestation. A premature baby may have a small, soft feeding tube placed through the nose or mouth into the stomach. In very premature or sick infants, nutrition may be given through a vein until the baby is stable enough to receive all nutrition through the stomach.

▶ NUTRITIONAL REQUIREMENTS

1. Preterm infants have higher nutrient requirements than term infants (Table 24.1).
2. Energy requirements for preterm infants are estimated to be around 110–150 kcal/kg.
3. These recommendations for requirements are for infants lesser than 1,500 g birth weight, although most infants born lesser than 2,000 g will benefit from these nutrient recommendations. Use the patient's actual weight when calculating nutrient requirements, unless the actual weight is lower than the birth weight in which case birth weight should be used.
4. Most preterm infants weighing less than 1,500 g will need parenteral nutrition (PN) to meet energy and nutrient requirements, while enteral feeds are introduced and progressing.
5. Careful and early consideration should be given to the need for PN in preterm infants, and once the decision to commence PN is made it should be started without undue delay and should meet the infant's requirements.

Energy intake above the infant's requirement will lead to higher weight gain as a result of fat deposition and is not recommended.

SECTION 3: Infant and Child Nutrition

Table 24.1: Daily requirements of preterm baby

Nutrients	Amount/day	Condition
Proteins	3–4 g/kg	
Calories	1 week 60 cal/kg/day after 2 week 120–150 cal/kg/day	
Fluids	90–100 cc/day	
Vitamin A	1,000 IU	Orally after 2 week
Vitamin C	35 mg	Orally after 2 week
Vitamin D	400 IU	Orally after 2 week
Folic acid	50 μg	Orally after 2 week
Vitamin K	0.5 mg	At birth biweekly, if infant is receiving total parenteral nutrition (TPN) antibiotics
Vitamin E	15 IU	If the infant weight is less than 1,500 g, this should be given for 36 week
Zinc	800–1,200 mg/kg	If breast milk is not given, this supplementation is needed
Iodine	4–5 mg/kcal	If breast milk is not given, this supplementation is needed
Copper	100–200 μg/kg/day	If breast milk is not given, this supplementation is needed
Sodium	4–8 μg/kg	If breast milk is not given, this supplementation is needed

6. Higher energy requirements may be necessary in circumstances such as:
    a. Increased respiratory rate [as seen in chronic lung disease (CLD)].
    b. Low body temperatures.
    c. Cardiac conditions.

For infants with intrauterine growth restriction (IUGR) or faltering growth the upper ranges of suggested nutrient requirements should be used, i.e. 150 kcal/kg/day of actual weight.

Protein accretion rate is achieved in preterm infants at around 2 g/kg/day with a protein intake of 3–4 g/kg/day as long as energy intake is at least 110 kcal/kg/day (i.e. minimum protein energy ratio 11% 15%). There is incomplete utilization of protein if more than 4.5 g/kg/day.

Long-chain polyunsaturated fats (LCPs) are conditionally essential in preterm infants and are less efficiently absorbed from formula than breast milk, while breast milk contains probiotics, there is currently insufficient evidence for the addition of these to preterm infant formulas.

▶ GOALS OF NUTRITION

Feeding tolerance, digestibility and progression to full feeds are key goals in nutrition of the preterm infant. The nutritional guideline for postnatal nutrition in preterm infants, established by the American Academy Pediatrics (AAP) in 1985, aimed to duplicate normal in utero growth rates. But, while weight gain has been seen as a primary goal for optimal nutrition of the preterm infant, the emphasis has expanded to include enhancement of neurodevelopment, organ maturity and functioning, prevention of infection and development of immune function.

Contraindications to Feeding

Do not start feeds, if the infant:
1. Is receiving indomethacin or received it within the previous 48 hours.
2. Has a hemodynamically significant PDA.
3. Has either an umbilical arterial or venous catheter. Do not start feedings until the catheters have been removed for ≥ 8 hours is polycythemic.
4. Has significant metabolic acidosis.
5. Has severe respiratory instability or there is impending endotracheal intubation.
6. Has hemodynamic instability as evidenced by clinical signs of sepsis, hypotension.
7. Is receiving dopamine (at a dose > 3 μg/kg/min) or other vasopressor drugs.

8. Received an exchange transfusion within the past 48 hours.
9. Has abdominal distension or other signs of GI dysfunction.
10. Had an episode of severe asphyxia (perinatal or postnatal) in the previous 72 hours.

▶ FEEDING PROTOCOL

The following are the guidelines for initiation and advance of enteral feedings in preterm infants.

Methods of Feeding

Because these infants usually have not yet developed coordinated sucking and swallowing, they must be fed by gavage:

1. Orogastric tubes are usually used. Because infants are obligate nose breathers, it is best not to occlude the nares with a tube. In addition, repeated insertion of a nasal gastric tube can cause inflammation of the nose with subsequent obstruction.
2. Estimate length of tube that must be inserted to reach the stomach.
3. Insert the tube and aspirate to see if gastric contents are returned. While listening over stomach with stethoscope, inject ~5 cc of air. If tube is in stomach, bubbling is heard as air is infected. If bubbling is not heard, tube may be in the trachea. Therefore, do not feed infant until certain that tube is in stomach.
4. Do not use duodenal or jejunal tubes for gavage feedings as feedings are less well-tolerated and do not stimulate secretion of lingual lipase. In addition, residuals are no longer useful in assessing tolerance of feedings.
5. Nipple feedings can be considered as the infant matures. The best judge of when to start nipple feedings is an experienced nurse.

Content of Feeding

Begin with either breast milk (preterm breast milk is 290 mOsm/L) or formula for preterm infants (e.g. Premature Enfamil® or Similac Special Care®, 260 mOsm/L):

1. Some physicians use half-strength feedings, but there is no evidence that this is beneficial. In fact, hypo-osmolar solutions may slow gastric emptying leading to increased incidence of residuals and feeding intolerance.
2. Remember that fetuses swallow amniotic fluid, which is 275 mOsm/L and this swallowing begins at 16 weeks gestation.

Guidelines for Feeding

Initiation of feedings, their volume and the rate of advance of feedings are related to birth weight, gestational age and how the infant has tolerated feeds to date. General guidelines include:

1. Initial volume is 2 cc/kg per feeding with a minimal absolute volume of 2 cc.
2. Do not advance feedings, if there are any signs that the baby is not tolerating feeds. Aggressive advances of feedings increase the risk of NEC.
3. A small volume, even if not advanced, is much better than nothing at all. Even very small volumes stimulate maturation of gut motility and production of enteric peptides.
4. Bolus feedings are preferable to continuous feedings.
5. The goals for 'full feedings' are:
   a. Volume: 150–160 cc/kg/day.
   b. Calories: 110–120 kcal/kg/day.
   c. Some small for gestational age (SGA) infants will require a higher caloric intake to achieve consistent weight gain.

Fortifying Feedings

Fortifying feeding not only provides more calories but also improved intake of calcium, phosphorus and protein. Fortify feedings (breast milk and formula) as follows:

1. When infant is tolerating ≥ 100 cc/kg/day, feedings may be fortified to 22 cal/oz.
2. When infant has been tolerating ≥ 150 cc/kg/day for at least 2nd feedings may be fortified to 24 cal/oz.

▶ INTOLERANCE TO FEEDINGS

Intolerance to feeding is common among very small preterm infants and most such infants will have episodes that require either temporary discontinuation of feedings or a delay in advancing feedings. Although, most episodes resolve spontaneously and without sequelae, any signs of feeding intolerance should be regarded as potentially serious because of the increased risk of NEC among these infants. Signs that indicate possible intolerance of feeding include:

1. Gastric residuals or emesis: Abdominal distension.
2. Blood in the stool (gross or occult): 'Loose stools' or diarrhea.
3. Metabolic acidosis: Temperature instability.
4. Onset of apneic episodes: Hyperglycemia.

Management of Feeding Intolerance

Management of feeding intolerance should be related to the type and severity of the presenting signs as described below:

1. Gastric residuals:
   a. Non-bilious residuals:
      i. If these are smaller than the volume of a feeding and are not increasing in volume, and if the infant otherwise appears well, feeding can continue, but the infant should be observed carefully for other signs of feeding intolerance. If the infant has any other worrisome findings, hold the feedings, consider obtaining an abdominal radiograph and observe the infant.
      ii. If the residuals are greater than the volume of a feeding or are progressively increasing in volume, hold the feedings and observe closely.

b. Bilious residuals:
   i. These are a serious sign. Hold feedings, evaluate infant closely and consider further work up including abdominal radiograph, complete blood count (CBC) and platelets.
2. Abdominal distension is a serious sign. Discontinue feedings, obtain abdominal radiograph and consider further evaluation and treatment.
3. Blood in stools: Discontinue feedings; consider obtaining clotting studies and abdominal radiograph.
4. If metabolic acidosis occurs, hold feedings, evaluate closely for NEC, sepsis, hypotension and a PDA. Metabolic acidosis in the presence of NEC is a grave prognostic sign.
5. Loose stools, temperature instability, apnea and hyperglycemia: Hold feedings and evaluate infant carefully.

If feedings have to be stopped for any of these reasons, notify the neonatology fellow and/or the attending physician, so that they can follow the infant's condition with you.

If there is any doubt about how well an infant is tolerating feedings, it is best to hold feedings, evaluate the infant and discuss the case with the other members of the team.

Parenteral Nutrition

Preterm infants have low energy reserves and require support soon after birth to meet their needs for energy, as well as protein and lipids. The goal of parenteral nutrition is to meet the infant's energy needs to prevent catabolism, while providing sufficient protein and lipids to avoid early deficiencies. However, while early parenteral nutrition provides crucial nutritional elements, while avoiding putting stress on an immature GI system with prolonged parenteral nutrition these digestive processes are not receiving the very stimulation that will help to mature and initiate normal GI functioning.

Minimal Enteral Nutrition

Growing recognition of the importance of enteral feedings in stimulating growth and development of the GI tract has prompted a number of studies that have shown the benefits and safety of early minimal enteral nutrition as a supplement to parenteral nutrition.

Minimal enteral nutrition refers to enteral feeding of breast milk, formula or a combination of the two. Even at very low volumes, enteral nutrition is considered beneficial to the preterm infant in large part, because of its role in stimulating GI function including maintaining mucosal mass and function, supporting fluid and electrolyte balance, nutrient absorption and immune defenses. A strategy of early parenteral nutrition, followed by combined parenteral and enteral nutrition, then phasing to complete enteral nutrition is currently a common practice.

Enteral Nutrition

Studies suggest that minimal enteral nutrition can be started within the 1st day of life in many preterm infants, particularly those who are clinically stable. Extremely small volumes may be initiated to 'prim' the digestive system, increasing the volume as the infant becomes more stable and tolerance is confirmed. Breast milk provides the same advantages to the preterm infant as to the full-term infant. Early immune system development is particularly important for the preterm infant to help protect against infection, including NEC and the contributions of breast milk to immune development are well -confirmed. The nutrient content of breast milk may not be sufficient to meet the needs of the preterm infant, particularly for calcium, phosphorus and protein and energy in the form of fat content, and nutrient fortifiers are often recommended. Monitoring of the infant's nutritional status is important to ensure that breast milk is meeting the infant's needs.

If breast milk is not available or not in sufficient quantity then recommend a preterm formula containing 24 calories/oz.

Concerns about feeding tolerance with cow's milk formula—characterized by vomiting, larger gastric residuals, gas and constipation—have prompted studies on the implications of protein source and type. In term formulas, improved digestibility has been observed with hydrolyzed formulas as compared to formulas with intact protein and protein-based formula has been shown to promote a faster gastric emptying rate than casein.

It is difficult to develop optimal recommendations for minimal effective volumes and quantity of volume increases considering that preterm infants differ widely with respect to developmental stage, particularly GI maturity. One study comparing minimal feeding volumes with advancing volumes found that 10% of infants receiving advancing feeding volumes developed NEC versus 1.4% receiving minimal volumes. Compared with later introduction of enteral feedings, early minimal enteral nutrition does not increase the incidence of NEC, shortens the time to full enteral feedings, improves weight gain and produces lower rates of feeding intolerance, while promoting maturation of GI functioning.

▶ CONCLUSION

The preterm babies are those who are born before 37 weeks of gestation. Low-birth-weight babies are born with a birth weight of less than 2,500 g. The incidence of low-birth-weight babies in India is 30%. The feeding is one of the major challenges in the care of premature infants. Goal of feeding is to achieve a growth rate that approaches the normal growth rate. The problem facing by premature are poor sucking and swallowing reflexes, relatively high calorie requirement with small stomach capacity, poor gag reflexes and incompetent cardioesophageal sphincter leading to aspiration, decreased absorption of essential nutrients.

Chapter 25

Weaning and Supplementary Feeding

▶ INTRODUCTION

Good nutrition is essential for the growth and development that occurs during an infant's 1st year of life. When developing infants are fed the appropriate types and amounts of foods, their health is promoted. Positive and supportive feeding attitudes and techniques demonstrated by the caregiver help infants develop healthy attitudes toward foods, themselves and others.

▶ WEANING

Weaning is a process in which infant's diet pattern is gradually changed from liquid food like breast milk and substitute milk preparations to cooked solid foods. This process can be started from the age of 3–4 months. The time of introduction of weaning is greatly influenced by the maturity of the infants, its appetite, digestion and the absence of tendency toward food allergies. After 6 months, breast milk does not provide all the nutrients that the growing baby needs, in particular iron and calories that solid foods provide. For other sources of nourishment, the mother should try to gradually introduce semisolid or solid foods for the baby. Hence weaning provides the child a nutritional balance for proper growth and development.

Definition

Weaning is the process by which the baby moves or shifts from having breast milk to consuming semisolid or solid foods. There is a gradual reduction in the intake of breast milk and/or baby formula and more often starts taking more solid food.

CHAPTER 25: Weaning and Supplementary Feeding

Weaning is one of the many milestones in the process of development. It is very important for the health and development.

Importance of Weaning

1. Though breast milk is the best and safest food for an infant this can sustain the growth only for first 3 months, and so breast milk alone cannot satisfy the growing infants on nutritional basis.
2. Storage of iron and vitamin A in liver gets used by 3 months and thus supplements are needed.
3. Taste buds, which at first are immature, become more sensitive to different taste.
4. In the second half of the 1st year, primary dentition begins as more solid diet provides a stimulus for chewing, which helps new teeth to erupt.
5. Supplementary foods promote physical and cognitive growth and development.
6. Proper infant nutrition prevents malnutrition by which infant mortality rate is reduced.

Weaning Problems

1. If breastfeeding is stopped, suddenly, it can have psychological and nutritional effect on the young children.
2. Solid foods can cause diarrhea, if prepared unhygienically or not digested properly.
3. If weaning foods are too poor to provide adequate nutrients, the children can develop malnutrition.

For some babies the breastfeeding may be sufficient for 4 months, while others may feel hungry even after the breastfeeding and may not gain weight.

Introduction to Solid Foods

To start weaning foods, the consistency of food should be gradually increased from liquid to semisolid and then from semisolid to solid foods. It is advisable to start one or two spoons of the new food at first. It should be given when a child is hungry, just before the regular feeding during the day time. It may be continued for a few days until the child gets used to the same. Then the new food item may be started, one at a time. Always, the fresh food should be given. The amount should be increased gradually. The child should never be forced to eat.

Children may spit out initially. As children like to participate in feeding, their hands should be washed. Those who feed the child must wash their hands. Clean utensils must be used to prepare the food. The food should be always covered. The solids should be fed gradually, regularly and according to children's likes. It should be observed for an indigestion, abdominal pain, diarrhea or rash because some children may be allergic to certain food. Such problems related to feeding, should be reported to the doctor.

Points to be Kept in Mind

During weaning the following points should be kept in mind and the foods should be included in infant's diet daily:

1. One can start weaning with cereal foods provided the food is cooked soft and smooth and solid foods, such as mashed vegetables, fruits like papaya, oranges and banana may be gradually introduced during weaning.
2. The child can be given mashed potato with little addition of lime juice and salt. The introduction of fruits and vegetables will correct the deficiency of vitamin C and iron.
3. Only a small quantity of food must be given to the baby in the beginning. Do not force the baby to take more; otherwise baby will reject it in course of time.
4. There should be proper variety in supplementation.
5. The quantity of vitamin D in the diet helps in the digestion of calcium and phosphorus.

Choosing of Weaning Foods

A food chosen for the weaning should be suitable to the family. It should be easily available, low in cost and used frequently in

CHAPTER 25: Weaning and Supplementary Feeding

most households. The local methods of food preparation may be advised. Cooking methods that use minimum fuel and less time should be recommended. Rules of food hygiene should be followed to prevent infection, by the age of 1 year; the infant can eat solid foods. The toddler can eat with the family. For the infants and toddlers, the volume of the meal should not be large. The toddler can eat 200 mL of foods at a time. If children are eating only three small meals a day, one of those must have high-concentrated calories and proteins to meet their needs for 24 hours.

Weaning Foods

Following are the examples of weaning foods that may be started according to child's ability to feed:

1. **Liquids:** Soup of vegetables, tomato, pulses (dals) and fruit juices.
2. **Semisolids food:** Potato, pulses and root vegetables can be well-cooked and mashed before feeding. A banana can be mashed and fed. Soft-cooked rice and soft-cooked fish can be mashed before feeding.

    To increase the nutritive value, preparations can be used, such as:
    - Ragi
    - Jaggery
    - Bengal gram (chana) powder, jaggery and ghee
    - Sugar will supply proteins, calories and iron.
3. **Solid foods:** Cooked rice, chapati, idli, bread, biscuits, groundnuts, roasted chana and banana. Solid food can be started when the children learn to chew properly.

Types of Weaning

Baby-led Weaning

An approach to introducing solid foods that allows baby to control intake of solid foods by self-feeding from the very beginning of the process. Parents do not make purees or mash up food.

They introduce self-feeding finger foods, which helps babies explore texture and taste, and allows for a natural transition to solids. Baby may pick up or lick food before moving onto putting into mouth or eating. There is no spoon feeding unless baby holds spoon for self. 'Until they are one, it is just for fun' – nutrition comes from breastfeeding, so it is okay to allow time for baby to feed self and explore food.

Gradual Weaning

"Gradual weaning allows to gradually substituting other kinds of nutrition, affection and attention to compensate for the loss of nursing" – Kellymom. In gradual weaning, mother encourages weaning by providing distractions and other nourishment in place of breastfeeding. This type of weaning is recommended when mother is ready to wean (or knows she will want/need to wean), but child is not ready or not expressing readiness signs. Gradual weaning is best, if it is gentle, patient, flexible and respectful of child's needs.

Partial Weaning

A compromise between frequent nursing and weaning entirely in which you keep one (or more) feeding a day and eliminate the rest. One method of partial weaning is night weaning – eliminating nighttime nursing from time child goes to sleep for a period of at least 7 hours.

Natural Weaning

"Baby-led weaning occurs when a child no longer has a need to nurse nutritionally or emotionally" – Kellymom. Though no two weanlings are alike, generally children that are allowed to wean themselves gradually cut down nursing over a matter of months, slowly dropping feedings and then going longer and longer between feedings. "Natural weaning means allowing the child to outgrow nursing on their own timetable." How weaning happens before completely weaning, a child may go

CHAPTER 25: Weaning and Supplementary Feeding

months (or years) nursing one to three times a day, typically at bedtime, waking and nap.

Benefits of natural weaning: The transition is easy because it happens over time, the breastfeeding relationship is allowed to come to a satisfying conclusion because the child is able to fulfill and outgrow their needs, mother learns to trust child's timetable and development, and the child feels a sense of control over her life.

Sudden or Abrupt Weaning

Stop breastfeeding suddenly rather than gradually. This is usually mother led unless there is an emergency involved. Possible challenges include engorgement, plugged ducts or mastitis, drastic hormonal changes, feelings of regret and sadness, exhaustion and power struggles with child. Child may be aggressive, angry or have tantrums, unwilling or unable to accept substitutions for nursing, regress adopt a security object, have increased night waking, clingy and demand attention and begin sucking on other things (fingers, toys, pacifier). The child may also exhibit anxious attachment and be afraid of separations from mother. Methods of abrupt weaning that can be particularly damaging to the child include weaning by desertion leaving child with another caregiver including dad, so that child not only loses milk, but mom also; the 'spicy burrito' method of putting something spicy or bitter tasting on nipple; the fear method of painting (with lipstick or the like) a frightening image on the breast, so that child will be too scared to want to nurse again; and crying it out.

Child's Readiness Signs for Weaning

1. Child is at least 1 year old.
2. Child gradually showing less interest in nursing.
3. Child is eating a variety of foods.
4. Child is secure in relationship with mother.
5. Child accepts other ways of being comforted besides nursing.

6. Child can be reasoned with (at least part of the time) to not nurse at certain times or places.
7. Sometimes the child falls asleep or goes to sleep without nursing.
8. Child shows little anxiety when gently encouraged not to nurse.
9. When offered a choice, child prefers to read, play or do something else with mom other than nurse.

Problems During Weaning

Several problems may be encountered during weaning, which are as follows:

1. If on starting weaning, breastfeeding is stopped suddenly, it can have adverse psychological effect on the child.
2. Weaning food, if prepared unhygienically or not digested properly can cause diarrhea.
3. If weaning foods are not nutrient rich, the child can develop malnutrition.
4. Children may develop indigestion, abdominal pain, diarrhea or rashes if they are allergic to certain foods.

Weaning Foods for Various Age Groups

4–6 Months

The stomach capacity is 86–130 mL approximately. The supplementary feeding should be started at 4 months in the form of liquids like fresh juices and soups from green leafy vegetables. At around 4–5 months of life, frequency of breastfeeding is reduced to 3–4 times per day and substituted with animal milk.

The semisolid food should preferably be given after breastfeeding at day time in the form of mashed fruit like banana or cereals like kanji, if not available 'porridge' can be made with wheat flour (atta), ragi, millet, etc.

Fruits like banana, papaya and mango can be given in a mashed or juices. The apple and pear can be given after cooking them few minutes.

- **Liquid foods:** Tomato juice, vegetable soup
- **Semisolid foods:** Rice porridge, wheat porridge
- **Solid foods:** 1/2 cup of cereal, 2–4 fruit slices and 2–4 spoon vegetables.

6–8 Months

The stomach capacity is approximately 130–180 mL. Introduce solids and after usual breast milk or formula.

Iron is much important for babies brain rice mixed with formula or breast milk to make a runny solution on a rubber-tipped soft spoon once a day and then finish with milk feed. When baby is eating 2–3 spoons cereals/day, then try adding another food.

Avoid 'gluten' containing foods, such as oats, wheat, rye and barley-based foods, in order to reduce risk of developing 'celiac diseases. As the baby's eating skills grow, increase the thickness of foods offered to include soft lumps and mashed foods.

Common foods for 6–8 months: Ragi porridge, mashed potato, egg yolk, biscuits, wheat porridge, sago kanji, suji kheer, bread, idli, milk (dilute), dal rice.

8–10 Months

At about 8 months, baby is ready for finger foods (cut into bite-sized bits), it will great the baby to hold things and allow baby a degree of control.

Introduce a wider range of starchy foods like bread, pasta, oats, potatoes, rice, breakfast cereals and baby breadsticks. Give two to three servings a day of starchy foods and begin to introduce dairy products like cheese. It is serving of protein rich food/day.

Avoid peanuts. Include the citrus fruits like oranges and satsumas. Dilute it one part of juice to nine part of boiled and cooled water, and use a beaker with soft spout.

Give mashed or minced foods include some lumps. So baby can get used to chewing or gumming. Well-cooked eggs and fish, shellfish can also be in the baby's diet. Add other protein rich foods.

Common foods for 8–10 months: Cereals, eggs, egg yolk, fruits, vegetables and biscuits, well-cooked fish and shellfish and cheese.

10–12 Months

Stomach capacity is approximately 190–260 mL; at least three meals and two snacks per day. Progression of foods from munched to finely chopped. Breast milk intake is at least 600 mL/day. Include energy dense foods like nuts, butter regularly. Give iron rich foods daily and a fruit serving for better absorption. Avoid tea, wheat with iron sources. Cow's milk is not recommended before 1 year as main milk diet for the infant. Give proteins, iron, vitamin A and C content diets to prevent deficiency problems.

Major Weaning Foods and Nutritive Values

1. **Cereals:** It containing 7%–12% of proteins and about 75% of carbohydrates. These are cheaper than most of other foods and usually consumed by family. While preparing some oil or fat, or sugar should be added to make it richer in calories and easier to swallow and digest, and commonly made as 'porridge'.
2. **Tubers and starchy roots:** These are rich in carbohydrates, e.g. potato, sweet potato and tapioca, etc. These contain approximately more than 70% of carbohydrates.
3. **Pulses:** Their protein content is 20%–25%. Dry legumes are much richer source than immature legumes, and also good source of vitamins and minerals. The legumes like Bengal gram, black gram, red gram, horse gram, etc.
4. **Vegetables:** These are poor in calories and protein, but good sources of vitamins especially vitamin A, B and C and minerals like iron, calcium, etc.
5. **Fruits:** The fruits like mango, papaya are contains vitamin A, guava is one of the fruit, which contains rich calcium and commonly banana supplies about 800 cal/100 g. The citrus fruits like orange contain vitamin C in more amounts.

CHAPTER 25: Weaning and Supplementary Feeding

6. **Juices:** The juices like oranges, sweet lime, grapes are supplementing the protective nutrients such as vitamins and minerals in high quantity to the baby.
7. **Fish:** The fish liver oil is good source of vitamin A and D.

Foods of animal origin are nutritious and high quantity and quality of protein, vitamin B_{12}, iron and easily digestible.

▶ BABY-FRIENDLY HOSPITAL INITIATIVE

Baby-Friendly Hospital Initiative (BFHI) was launched jointly by World Health Organizations (WHO) and UNICEF in March 1992 in order to encourage and promote exclusive breastfeeding. BFHI was launched to resurrect the dwindling practice of breastfeeding. BFHI aims at improving the knowledge, attitude and practices of healthcare workers by providing them with knowledge and skills to promote exclusive breastfeeding among infants up to the age of 6 months.

Minimum Global Criteria

The following ten steps are recognized as minimum global criteria for attaining the status of a baby friendly hospital.

Step 1

Have a written breastfeeding policy that is routinely communicated to all health staff. A written policy consisting of ten steps for successful breastfeeding should be displayed in the maternal and child health (MCH) area of the hospital. The policy statement should be available both in English and local language.

Step 2

Train healthcare staff in skills necessary to implement this policy. The healthcare staff should get practical training to implement ten steps of breastfeeding. They should be taught the skills needed to assist the nursing mothers for expression of breast milk, correct positioning and attachment of baby during breastfeeding.

Step 3

Inform all pregnant women about the benefits and management of breastfeeding. During antenatal period mothers should be informed and educated about the advantages of breastfeeding for both mother and baby. The problems like retracted, small or cracked nipples should be managed during antenatal period.

Step 4

Help mothers to initiate breastfeeding within half hour of birth. Establish mother-baby bonding soon after delivery and encourage all mothers to initiate breastfeeding their half an hour of birth. Mothers should be advised not to administer prelacteal feeds.

Step 5

Show mothers how to breastfeed and how to maintain lactation, if they are separated from their infants. Mothers should be taught the art of breastfeeding including position and technique of feeding. They are taught the correct technique of expression of breast milk manually or with the help of breast pump in order to maintain adequate lactation.

Step 6

Give newborn infants no food or drink other than breast milk, unless medically indicated. Prelacteal feeds should be given to the newborn. Only breastfeeding should be given. In case breast milk; not available supplementary feeding is given.

Step 7

Practice rooming-in and allow mothers and infants to remain together round the clock. Keeping mother and newborn together promotes bonding between mother and baby and also helps in timely 'initiation of breastfeeding'.

Step 8

Encourage breastfeeding on demand. Mothers should breastfeed the babies whenever they are hungry and not according to the clock.

Step 9

Give no artificial feeds or pacifiers to the baby. Pacifiers should not be given to babies due to the risk of infection and non-nutritive sucking. Expressed breast milk (EBM) or any other medically indicated fluid should be administered through katori/spoon or paladai, but not feeding bottle.

Step 10

Foster the establishment of breastfeeding support groups and refer mothers to them on discharge from hospital. Women breastfeeding support group should be established in the community for promotion of breastfeeding. Follow-up support for all breastfeeding mothers is necessary after they are discharged from the hospital.

The BFHI movement is active in India under a National Task Force comprising of Government of India, UNICEF, WHO, voluntary organizations and many professional bodies.

Recognition as Baby-friendly Hospital

For recognition of a hospital as baby friendly, it has to follow three steps:
1. A hospital that conducts a minimum of 250 deliveries per year can seek the recognition. After implementation of the ten steps for promotion of breastfeeding, a duly completed self-assessment form and registration form should be sent to BFHI secretariat.
2. The hospital/nursing home meeting all the ten criteria is visited by an 'assessor' for on the spot checks and to interview

the mothers and healthcare staff. The assessor sends their report and observations to BFHI secretariat, which is reviewed by the review committee for final recommendation.
3. The hospital fulfilling the national BFHI requirements are recognized as 'Baby Friendly'. The National Task Force organizes a public ceremony for presentation of BFHI certificate and a logo. The hospitals that is unable to fulfill the criteria for certification can reapply for it later on, after eliminating all shortcomings.

▶ SUPPLEMENTARY FEEDING

The first solid foods are introduced at 5– 6 months of age (Table 25.1). The foods given are cereals, cereal milk or cereal dahi preparations such as suji halwa, rice milk, upma, rice dahi, khichdi, pongal, bread, rice flakes/poha, etc. Fruits such as ripe banana, mango, papaya, which are soft and pulpy are also given. Well-cooked non-fibrous vegetables such as ash gourd, potato, pumpkin are fed along with rice.

Most of the problems of food acceptance begin in the toddler stage. The child will show a remarkable decrease in appetite in the 2nd year as compared to the 1st year. So, it is important to give small portions of food and let the child enjoy the food. Allow the child home freedom to decide when he/she is satisfied. Allow some flexibility in choices and help the child form good food habits.

Definitions

1. **Supplementary feed:** Where a breastfed infant has been given one or more fluid feeds, including infant formula. EBM is considered a supplementary feed.
2. **Hypoallergenic/hydrolyzed formula:** Cow's milk based formula that has been processed to breakdown most of the proteins, which cause symptoms in cow's milk allergic children.

CHAPTER 25: Weaning and Supplementary Feeding

Table 25.1: Supplementary feeding for various age groups

Age	Energy needed in addition to breast milk	Consistency	Frequency	Amount at each meal
6–8 month	200 kcal/day	Start with liquids and pureed food	2–3 time/day	Start with 2–3 tablespoons per feed and increase to about 125 mL
9–11 month	300 kcal/day	Finely chopped or mashed foods, finger foods	3–4 time/day	Half cup of 250 mL
12–23 month	550 kcal/day	Solid family food, chopped or mashed, if needed	3–4 meals/day	Quarter to full cup of 250 mL

Supplementary for Toddlers

Children can share family meals, by the time they are 2 years old. A few alterations may be needed when the family makes highly spiced food. Toddler should not be given foods, which are too fatty or too sweet. Such foods may fill his limited space, without providing the nutrients needs. The child may be encouraged to eat sweets towards the end of the meal, so that he may not eat these to the exclusion of other foods. It is good to give appetizing beverages, such as fruit juices and milk to the children. It is good to serve part of his milk needs in the form of soups, kheer, custard or ice cream. Fruits are ideal snacks. Crisp crackers or toast are liked and children can eat these without help, which help him feel independent.

Supplementary Feeding Program

Direct distribution of supplementary foods has been employed by UNICEF among children. The supplementary food should

be distributed to the vulnerable groups through the following channels:
- The MCH centers
- Outpatient departments of hospitals
- Schools
- Crèches
- Nutritional rehabilitation centers.

Maternal and Child Health Centers

These can serve as convenient centers for the distribution of infant foods to infant and protein foods to weaned infants preschool children, expectant and nursing mothers. Nutritional education should be imparted to the mothers through films and charts on the nutritional requirements of infants, children and mothers and the value of protein foods and supplements to poor diets and for curing deficiency diseases.

Outpatient Departments of Hospitals

These can serve as centers for the distribution of protein foods to malnourished children and mothers, who come there for treatment.

Schools

School lunch is a measure for improving the health and nutrition of children. School lunch is based on locally available foods.

Crèches

All industrial concerns employing women as workers should establish crèches where infants and preschool children of the workers will be fed with nutritious foods daily during the working hours.

CHAPTER 25: Weaning and Supplementary Feeding

Nutritional Rehabilitation Centers

Children suffering from moderate degrees of malnutrition are not usually considered ill enough for being treated in hospitals. Malnourished children attending these centers can be given processed protein foods, vitamin A capsules and iron tablets.

▶ CONCLUSION

Breastfeeding alone is not able to provide sufficient amounts of the nutrients needed to maintain growth after first 6 months. Weaning begins from the moment supplementary food is started and continuous till the child is taken off the breast completely. Solid food added to an infant's diet is called beikost. There is an increase in activities of enzymes at the time of weaning. Introduction of weaning food too late can lead to undernutrition and increased diarrheal morbidity.

Chapter 26

Nutritional Assessment

▶ INTRODUCTION

Assessment of the nutritional status of pediatric patients, while in the hospital setting is important for identifying the goals of nutritional intervention, increasing the quality of care and diagnosing malnutrition. Nutritional status can be determined by the assessment of body weight, growth, adipose tissue, skeletal muscle, visceral protein stores and cellular immune function.

▶ CONCEPT

1. Nutritional status is the balance between the intake of nutrients by an organism and the expenditure of these in the processes of growth, reproduction and health maintenance. Because this process is highly complex and quite individualized, nutritional status assessment can be directed at a wide variety of aspects of nutriture (Fig. 26.1).

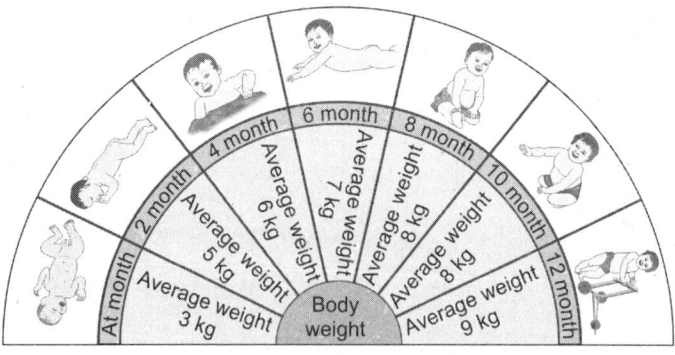

Fig. 26.1: Infant nutritional assessment

CHAPTER 26: Nutritional Assessment

2. These range from nutrient levels in the body to the products of their metabolism and to the functional processes they regulate.
   Nutritional status can be measured for individuals as well as for populations. Accurate measurement of individual nutritional status is required in clinical practice. Population measures are more important in research.
3. The assessment of nutritional status is commonly summarized by the mnemonic American born confused desi (ABCD), which stands for anthropometric measurement, biochemical or laboratory tests, clinical indicators and dietary assessment. This review will focus on anthropometric and dietary techniques.

▶ ASSESSMENT OF NUTRITIONAL STATUS

Definition

Assessment is an evaluation of information obtained from diet survey, clinical examination, anthropometry and laboratory investigations that help to find out the nutritional condition of the child or an individual.

Purposes

1. To assess the growth of children.
2. To monitor the impact of the nutritional programs.
3. To find out the magnitude of the problem.
4. To assess the extent of prevalence of clinical signs and symptoms due to dietary deficiencies.
5. To analyze the reasons for the nutritional disorders.
6. To suggest ways of overcoming overnutrition and undernutrition in the community.

Types of Surveys

1. Longitudinal-section of individuals/family and duration should be more than 1 year.

2. Cross-sectional sample of the population should be in a given point of time.

Methods of Nutritional Assessment

- Clinical examination of the nutritional disorders
- Nutritional anthropometry
- Dietetic survey
- 24-hour recall
- Socioeconomic condition
- Vital events
- Certain laboratory investigations.

Clinical examination of the child from head to foot and in the most essential part of all nutritional surveys, to minimize the errors in clinical examination, standard survey and forms should be used covering all areas of the body. The subject is examined from head to foot in good ventilation.

Anthropometric Measurements and Indices

Nutritional anthropometry is concerned with the measurements of the variations of physical dimensions and body composition at stages of life cycle, and different planes of nutrition. It is a field-oriented method, which can be easily adopted and interpreted (Fig. 26.2).

The basic measurements, which should be made on all age groups are weight in kilograms, length/height and arm circumference in centimeters. In young children, it should be supplemented by measurements of head and chest circumference.

Weight

Weight gain is an indicator of growth in children. It is measured with the help of the weighing scale. Body weight should be determined after the first void and before ingestion of food.

The weight for age can be compared with the standards of Indian Council of Medical Research (ICMR) and the nutritional status can be interpreted.

CHAPTER 26: Nutritional Assessment

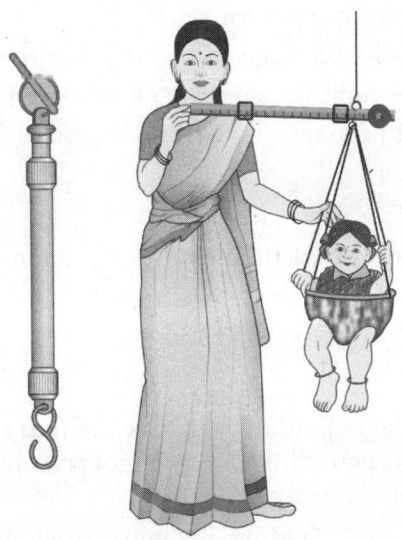

Fig. 26.2: Infant weight measurement technique

The standard reference body weight (kg) of Indians of different age groups is given in the Table 26.1.

Table 26.1: Reference body weight (kg) of Indians of different age

Sl No	Age group	Age (year)	Male	Female
1.	Infants	0–½	5.4	5.4
2.	Children	½–1	8.6	8.6
		1–3	12.61	11.81
		4–6	19.20	18.69
		7–9	27.00	26.75
		10–12	35.54	37.91
3.	Adolescents	13–15	47.88	46.66
		16–18	57.28	49.92
4.	Adults	20–50	60	50

Weight for Age

The nutritional status can be interpreted using Gomez classification as follows:

- > 90% weight-for-age normal
- 76%–90% weight-for-age grade I malnutrition
- 61% < 75% weight-for-age grade II malnutrition
- < 60% weight-for-age grade III malnutrition.

Linear Measurements

Two types of linear measurements are commonly used:
1. Height or length of the whole body.
2. Circumference of the head and the chest.

Height

The height of the individual is the sum of four components—leg, pelvis, spine and skull. The height of an individual is measured using a stadiometer.

For infants and children recumbent length (crown-heel length) is measured. The measurement is compared with the standards of the ICMR to assess nutritional status.

The desirable birth weight and length of an infant is 3 kg and 50 cm respectively. By the time the baby turns the first birthday, the birth weight is doubled and an increment of 25 cm in length is reached (Fig. 26.3).

Head circumference

The measurement of head circumference is a standard procedure to detect pathological condition in children. Head circumference is related mainly to brain size. At birth, the circumference of head is greater than that of the chest.

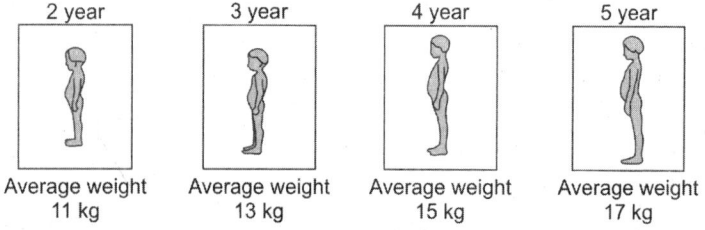

Fig. 26.3: Average weight of 2–5 years age

Chest circumference

The circumference of the head and the chest are about the same at 6 months of age. After this the skull grows slowly and the chest more rapidly.

Therefore between the ages of 6 months and 5 years the chest and head circumference ratio of less than one may be due to failure to develop or due to wasting of muscle and fat of chest.

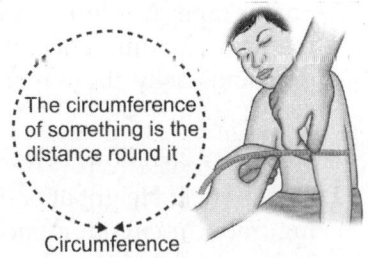

Fig. 26.4: Midarm circumference measurement technique

In nutritional anthropometry, the chest and head circumference ratio is of value in detecting undernutrition in early childhood.

Midupper arm circumference

Midupper arm circumference (MUAC) at birth in a healthy child is between 10 and 11 cm. Over the 1st year, the increment in MUAC is 3-4 cm as the muscles of the arms start to develop. In the preschool age the increase in MUAC is only 1 cm. Hence, there is not much difference between the MUAC of a 3 years old from that of a 5 years old. So, MUAC is an age independent index. The field workers in nutrition in our country have fixed the desirable value for MUAC as 12 cm for Indian preschool children (Fig. 26.4).

The WHO has recommended 14 cm as a desirable value for MUAC for preschool children. Hence, in screening malnourished children in a community this method is used with ease. When the value of MUAC is less than 12 cm among 1-5 years old children, they are designated as malnourished. In the field condition, a bangle with a diameter of 4 cm can be used as a tool to detect malnutrition. When the bangle moves smoothly over the midupper arm of the child, it indicates malnutrition. The bangle test can be conducted with ease in field condition to screen malnourished children.

SECTION 3: Infant and Child Nutrition

1. Shakir tape: A colored coated tape is used to measure the midarm circumference in children. The mothers can understand easily about their child's nutritional status:
   a. 3.5–16 cm: Green.
   b. 12.5–13.5: Yellow, below 12.5: Red.
2. Quack stick: Height at one side of the rod and corresponding midarm circumference on the other side are marked. This is available in pediatric wards.

▶ ANTHROPOMETRIC APPROACH

Anthropometric approaches to nutritional status assessment:

1. Anthropometric approaches are, for the most part, relatively non-invasive methods that assess the size or body composition of an individual. For adults, body weight and height are used to evaluate overall nutritional status and to classify whether individuals are at healthy or non-healthy weights.

   In children, growth charts have been developed to allow researchers and clinicians to assess weight and height-for-age, as well as weight-for-height. For children, low height-for-age is considered stunting, while low weight-for-height indicates wasting. In addition to weight and height, measures of midarm circumference and skinfold measured over the triceps muscle at the midarm are used to estimate fat and muscle mass.

2. Anthropometric measures of nutritional status can be compromised by other health conditions. For example, edema characteristic of some forms of malnutrition and other disease states can conceal wasting by increasing body weight. Head circumference can be measured in children 36 months and younger to monitor brain growth in the presence of malnutrition. Brain growth is better spared than either height or weight during malnutrition.

3. To interpret anthropometric data, they must be compared with reference data. The choice of the appropriate reference has been discussed by Johnston and Ouyang. Because

well-nourished children in all populations follow similar patterns of growth, reference data need not come from the same population as the children of interest. It is of greater importance that reference data be based on well-defined, large samples, collected in populations that are healthy and adequately nourished. These have been adopted as international standards by the World Health Organization (WHO).

▶ NUTRITIONAL ASSESSMENT GUIDELINES

The assessment is mainly made for the caloric and protein intake of the child and individual. The calculation for other nutrients, i.e. iron, calcium, vitamin A and vitamin B are only approximate. The nutritive values given in any standard Indian nutrition book of 'Nutritive Value of Indian foods' LC Gopalan may be referred for the values of any uncooked food. The values of cooked foods (common ones) are given in the hand is attached to this. It may be referred for those items only.

Dietary Approach to Nutritional Status Assessment

1. Several techniques exist for collecting dietary data with which to estimate nutritional status. Because these techniques vary in cost for data collection, burden on the respondent and which aspects of diet they are designed to measure. It is important to clearly articulate the goals of dietary assessment of nutritional status before choosing an assessment strategy.
2. The primary consideration in choosing a dietary assessment method is the specific type of data needed. "Is the research intended to document intake of foods" or of 'nutrients'? If the answer is foods, the method must take account of the population's footways. These include variability in food intake patterns (e.g. day-to-day, seasonal, ritual cycles); differences in food consumption by sex, age and ethnicity, and what items the population considers to be legitimate 'food'. If the objective is to measure

nutrient intake, the method must take into account several additional factors such as food, preparation techniques including the addition of condiments and the effects of the technique on nutrient composition of the food, sources of error in the determination of amounts of food consumed, differentiation distribution of nutrients among foods, and the contribution of 'non-food' consumption (such as betel nut, laundry starch, vitamin and mineral supplements) to total nutrient consumption.

3. Another important consideration is the time period the data are intended to represent. If the period is a relatively discrete one, it may be possible to document diet quite precisely. However, if the interest is in measuring 'usual' diet, the methods must allow this abstract concept to be estimated statistically.

4. Population measures of dietary status can be derived either from data describing the entire population or population subgroup, or from data describing samples of individuals. Population-wide data include food availability figures, which allow the assessment of food balance; the amount of food produced or imported by a population less than that exported or used as non-human food. Such measures are necessarily crude, as they do not measure consumption directly. Another approach to measure dietary status of groups has been to focus on the household. Indirect data on household food intake can be derived from records of foods brought into the household or from pantry inventories. Because of variations in intrahousehold distribution of foods, such techniques cannot be used to estimate individual intakes.

5. By far the most precise way of measuring dietary intake is to gather data on individuals. These methods depend on identifying a period of time for which data are needed, measuring food quantities consumed and then translating these into nutrient amounts, either through direct chemical analysis or (more commonly) using food composition tables.

CHAPTER 26: Nutritional Assessment

Dietary Data Collection

1. The most valid or accurate dietary methods are prospective methods. These involve keeping records of foods consumed over the period of time of interest. This can be done by individuals themselves or by others observing them.
2. Sometimes the foods are weighed before eating and then plate waste is weighed and subtracted.
3. A similar method is to prepare two duplicate meals, one is consumed by the subject and the other is analyzed for nutrient content.
4. Another method is the dietary record in which the subject records estimated amounts of foods consumed. In any case, these methods are highly reactive because individuals may alter usual behavior to make their diet more socially desirable or to simplify the process of record keeping.
5. Recall methods are the most widely used type of dietary data collection method. They are less reactive, but also less accurate than record methods. 24-hour recalls in which the previous day's intake is queried in detail (for instance, foods, amounts, preparation techniques, condiments) are easiest for individuals to complete.
6. The data reported are converted from foods to nutrients with the use of food composition tables. Because a single day is not representative of usual intake, multiple 24-hour recalls are frequently used.
7. These multiple recalls can be thought of as sampling from an individual's ongoing food behavior. The number necessary to reliably measure diet depends on the nutrient of interest. Nutrients widely distributed in food (such as carbohydrates) require fewer days than nutrients not widely distributed (such as cholesterol).
8. The number of recalls needed also depends on the nature of the diet. In societies where day-to-day and season-to-season food intake varies, more days are needed than where diets are more monotonous.
9. The semiquantitative food frequency is a recall method in which an individual summarizes the diet to produce a

measure of usual intake. For a list of foods commonly eaten, the individual estimates how frequently the food has been eaten in the time period in question (often, 1 year) and in what amount. Food composition tables are then used to estimate the usual daily intake.
10. This method combines low burden on the individual with low cost. It has been widely used and studied, as it is the foremost method used in nutritional epidemiology.

Socioeconomic Condition

It is necessary to collect certain background information such as family size, occupations, income, education, housing and prices of food. They are useful index of nutrition. Food consumption patterns are likely to vary among various socioeconomic groups.

Vital Statistics

The vital events provide an indirect means of nutritional assessment of human groups. The following parameters are necessary to assess the nutritional status of children in a community infant mortality, neonatal morbidity rate, stillbirth rate, perinatal mortality rate, preschool mortality rate, family size, fertility rate, incidence and prevalence of chronic illness like tuberculosis and malaria. In developing countries, it is well-known that these rates are low in well-nourished populations.

Malnutrition and undernutrition are not always due to shortage of foods too often, there is starvation in the midst of plenty. People choose poor diets when good ones are available because of cultural influences, poverty and ignorance. In order to find out the nutritional disorders of the individuals, the nurse have the responsibility to assess the nutritional status in the family and also in the community.

Laboratory Methods of Investigation

Deficiency of any nutrients leads to biochemical changes, which then manifests. Finally, tissue changes, serum protein levels are often investigated, but blood tests are time consuming and cannot be applied on a large scale in the community. Hemoglobin test, RBC count, stools and urine examinations are often carried out in nutritional surveys. Hemoglobin level is a useful index of the overall state of nutrition irrespective of its significance in anemia.

Stool tests are carried out to rule out worm infestation. Other blood tests are carried out in the clinical testing such as:

- Serum albumin content
- Serum transferrin
- Serum amino acid
- Blood urea
- Serum copper
- β-lipoprotein.

▶ ROAD-TO-HEALTH CHART

The weights of many children can be put on one chart. This is described as a 'Pass port' to child health care. The chart is made on the basis of weight records because weight is the most important single measurement, which reflects the growth and which itself is an index of the nutritional status of the child (Figs 26.5A and B).

The top line on the road-to-health card represents the 50th percentile of the Harvard standard, which is generally accepted as reference standard and the lower lines represent 80%, 70% and 60% of that weight. If the child is growing normally, the growth curve is parallel to the road-to-health. In addition, the card helps in the grading of malnutrition as follows:

- Up to 80%—satisfactory
- Between 80% and 71%—1st degree malnutrition
- Between 70% and 61%—2nd degree malnutrition
- Under 60%—3rd degree malnutrition.

The road-to-health chart helps to identify 'at a glance' any growth failure and the degree of malnutrition, if any. Space is also provided on the card to record important events such

SECTION 3: Infant and Child Nutrition

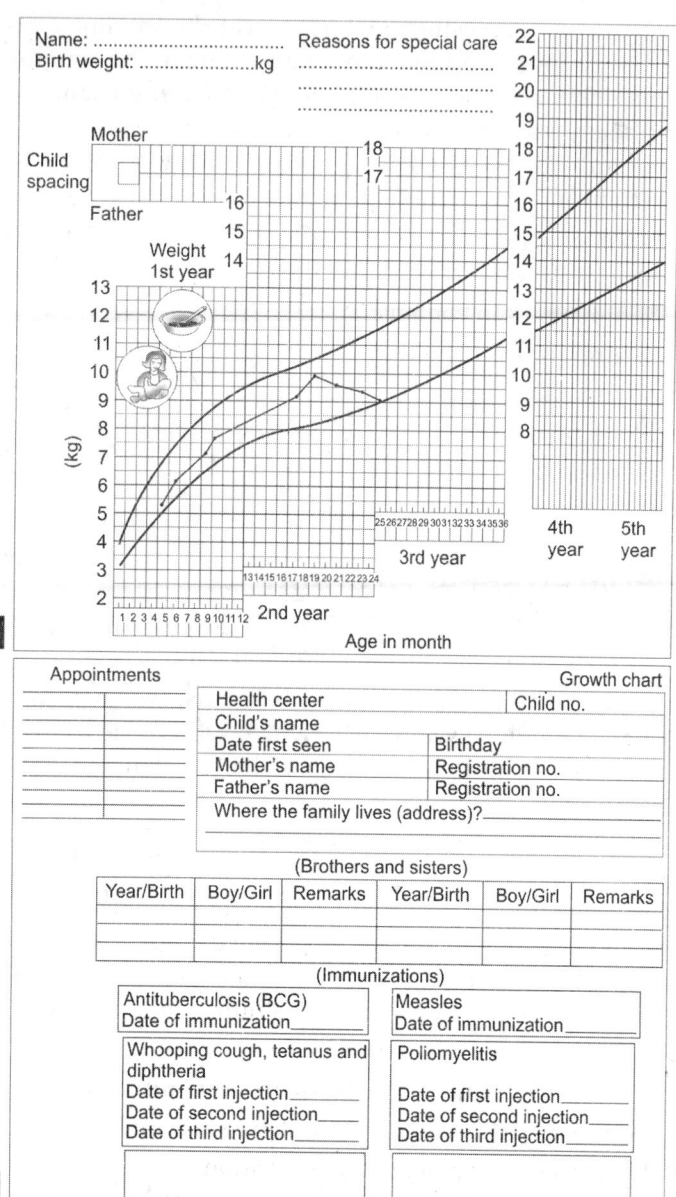

Figs 26.5A and B: Road-to-health chart

as immunization, birth history, illness, if any treatment given, IFA, deworming, vitamin 'A' solution and special immunization, if any. This chart is widely recognized and used in many developing countries. The card should be in thick paper and is contained in a plastic cover and it has to be kept by the mother for a period of 5 years.

Mothers should be addressed to bring the card every time they bring the child to the immunization clinic, so that appropriate entries can be made. The card has been found to be effective in motivating mothers to avail of the special services offered to the children through the less than 5 years clinics and in detecting early onset of malnutrition among children. It is envisaged as a tool for health education of parents.

▶ CONCLUSION

The aim of nutritional assessment is to know the magnitude of malnutrition, to analyze the factors responsible for it and to effectively plan to control and eradicate them to maintain good nutrition. Malnutrition and undernutrition affects adversely the growth and health of children. Anthropometric approaches are relatively non-invasive methods that assess the size or body composition of an individual.

Chapter 27

Nutrition for Sick Child

▶ INTRODUCTION

From the nutritional point of view, the Indian society is actual society, consisting of a small group of well-fed and a very large group of undernourished. The high-income groups are sharing diseases of affluence, which one finds in developed countries.

▶ EFFECTS OF ILLNESS ON FOOD

Food acceptance is affected by the following factors.

Stress of Illness

The sick person is stressed with many thoughts, such as the outcome of the illness, the cost of treatment, concern about depending on others, restrictions in physical movement and dietary restriction. Hospitalization exerts additional stress on a sick person. For some it is easy to get adjusted to the new environment, where as for others it is difficult.

Illness Modifies Food Acceptance

Hospitalization is a major factor, which affects the food acceptance. During sickness an individual needs family support, but when in the hospital he/she is forced to eat alone without family members around. The meal timings may be different than what he/she is accustomed to; the food served may not be familiar with respect to choice, flavor or portion, size, etc. may affect the food acceptance. Some patients may use food as a means of drawing attention of the hospital personnel and family members. Food acceptance may be affected by the disease process itself. Some foods may cause nausea, others may cause abdominal distention and some may irritate the gastrointestinal tract and so on.

Nutritional Stress

Emotional stress causes increased losses of nitrogen and calcium. Immobilization is also a stressful condition for many, which causes increased losses of nitrogen and calcium. Patients who are immobilized due to chronic or long-term illness may suffer from serious demineralization of bones. Excessive losses of nutrients also occur in trauma to the body such as burns, bone fractures, fever and wound injury. The hormonal secretions are increased, thus increasing the needs for vitamins for metabolic processes.

▶ SPECIAL FEEDING METHODS

The patients, who are terminally ill, are unable to consume fluids orally. Therefore, special feeding methods can be used to administer nutrients to them to prevent nutritional deficiencies. There are two methods commonly used to administer fluids namely:

1. Enteral feeding.
2. Parenteral feeding.

Enteral Feeding

Enteral feeding refers to provision of nutrients into the gastrointestinal tract through a tube when oral intake is insufficient. Enteral nutrition can be used in patients who have at least 2–3 feet of functional gastrointestinal tract, but the oral intake is inadequate to maintain optimal nutritional status. Figure 27.1 shows the enteral tube placement.

Enteral Access (Short Term)

- Nasogastric
- Nasoduodenal
- Nasojejunal.

SECTION 3: Infant and Child Nutrition

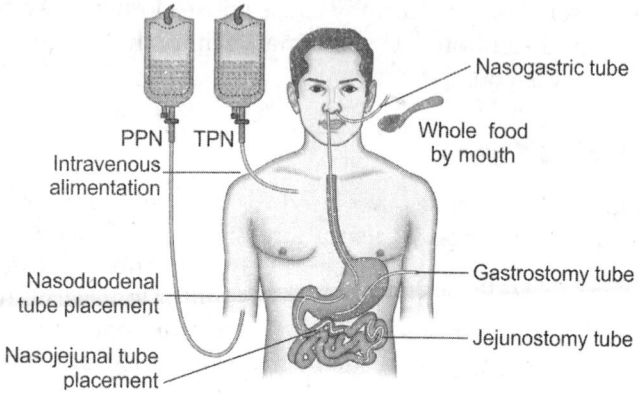

Fig. 27.1: Enteral tube placement

Nasogastric: This method is for short term, i.e. 3–4 weeks. A nasogastric tube is passed through the nose into the stomach. Patients who have normal gastrointestinal function and gag reflex tolerate this method. Feeds can be administered by bolus injection or intermittent or continuous infusion. Tube placement can be verified by aspirating gastric contents or it can be confirmed radiological for its tip location.

Nasoduodenal and nasojejunal: These methods can be used for short term, i.e. 3–4 weeks in patients with gastric motility disorders, esophageal reflux or persistent nausea and vomiting. The tube is passed through the nose and esophagus, and inserted into the stomach, and the tip of the tube reaches into the small intestine via peristaltic movements. Tube placement can be verified radiologically.

Enteral Access (Long Term)

- Gastrostomy
- Jejunostomy.

Gastrostomy and jejunostomy: In this method small opening (stoma) is made directly into the stomach or jejunum and enteral feeds are administered directly at the time of operation. The patient suffering from carcinoma of esophagus should be fed through gastrostomy (Fig. 27.2). The jejunostomy feeding

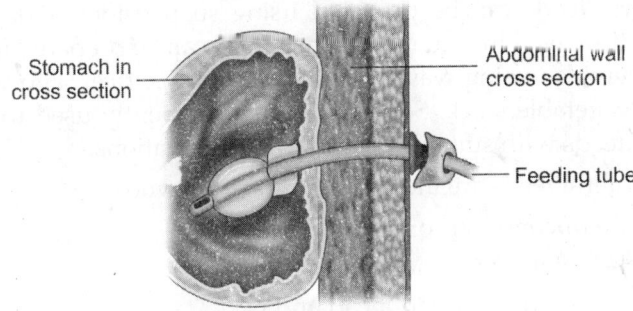

Fig. 27.2: Gastrostomy feeding tube placement

can be done to patients suffering from carcinoma of stomach along with the carcinoma of esophagus or after partial resection or total gastrectomy. Since the food bypasses the mouth and the stomach, salivary and gastric digestion is completely eliminated. Therefore, it becomes essential to give small frequent feeds, i.e. 100 mL every half an hour. The kinds of foods, which can be used are homogenized milk, glucose, pre or partially digested proteins, carbohydrates, vitamins and mineral supplements.

Enteral Access (Long-term Illness)

Percutaneous endoscopic gastrostomy or jejunostomy: Percutaneous endoscopic gastrostomy (PEG) is a non-surgical technique. The tube is directly placed into the stomach through the abdominal wall. This procedure is performed using an endoscope and the patient is given local anesthesia. The tube is endoscopically guided into the stomach or jejunum and then brought out through the abdominal wall to provide the access route for enteral feedings. This route of feeding is preferred for patients who require tube feeding for more than 3–4 weeks. This method takes less time to insert, limited need for anesthesia and it has minimal wound complications. Percutaneous endoscopic jejunostomy is also possible, but this procedure has higher degree of risk. PEG can be used in many clinical situations, such as carcinoma of esophagus due to which swallowing may be difficult, malabsorption syndrome, partial bowel obstruction, inflammatory bowel disease, hepatic failure, etc.

Enteral feeds can be prepared using suspensions and powders dissolved in water. These formulas can be prepared in the kitchen also using washed pulses, soybeans, rice, sago water and vegetable stock. Soy milk is also frequently used to prepare feeds with suitable commercial preparations.

Enteral feeds are indicated for patients who:
1. Are unconscious or semiconscious.
2. Have persistent anorexia, nausea and vomiting.
3. Have/had surgery of head and neck.
4. Have/had gastrointestinal surgeries.

Methods of Enteral Feeding

The kind of formula selected depends on the condition of the patient. Enteral feeding can be done by various methods.

Bolus method: This method is chosen when the patient is clinically stable and has a functional stomach. Syringe bolus feeding is always preferred overpump or gravity bolus as it is less expensive. This method should be encouraged if feed is being tolerated. Ordinarily a 60 mL syringe is used to infuse the formula. About 50 mL per minute and a volume of 350 mL per meal are given. The number of feeds depends on the nutritional needs of the patient. The patient who has normal gastric function usually tolerates up to 500 mL of feeds at each time. Normally, 3–4 bolus feeds per day can provide daily requirements for the patients.

Intermittent drip method: These feedings can be given by pump or gravity drip. Normally, 4–6 feedings per day are administered for 20–60 minutes. The formula is initially started at 100–150 mL per feeding and gradually increased as tolerated.

Continuous drip method: Continuous infusion requires a pump. This is an ideal method for patients who do not tolerate large volumes of feeds administered through either bolus or intermittent method. The total volume is administered over 8–20 hours. Initially it is started with 50 mL per hour and gradually increased to 125 mL per hour.

Parenteral Feeding

Parenteral nutrition can be defined as the provision of nutrients directly into the bloodstream intravenously. The patients who cannot be fed through enteral route are the appropriate candidates for parenteral nutrition. After this, it is necessary to choose between central and peripheral access. In the central access, the catheter tip is placed in a large high-blood flow, vein such as superior vena cava. This is known as total parenteral nutrition (TPN) (Fig. 27.3). And in the peripheral access the catheter tip is placed in a small vein of the arm. Peripheral veins do not tolerate concentrated solutions, thus it becomes necessary to infuse large volumes of diluted feeds to meet nutritional requirements. Patients with volume restrictions such as renal or hepatic failure and cardiopulmonary failure are not good candidates for partial parenteral nutrition (PPN).

Parenteral Access

Peripheral access: The feed can be infused through a peripheral intravenous catheter placed in a vein. PPN is a good nutrition support for mildly malnourished patients. It can be used as a supplement along with the enteral feeding. It is generally given through the small veins in the arm. Various types of solutions are used for short period of time, which provides fluids and electrolytes.

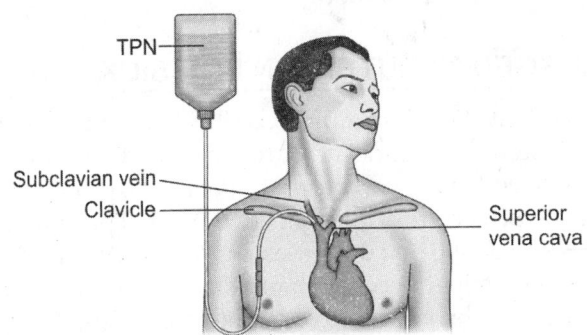

Fig. 27.3: Total parenteral nutrition infusion

Central access: By the use of aseptic technique, catheters are inserted into the subclavian vein and proceeded until the catheter tip reaches the superior vena cava. It is essential to verify the tip site radiologically before infusion of nutrients is initiated. After inserting the tube successfully at the right place, TPN can be started. TPN is indicated when the gut is totally non-functional or obstructed. Patients with severe malnutrition, with electrolyte imbalance, massive surgery, burns or sepsis and excessive vomiting are the candidates for TPN. Large amounts of nutrients such as glucose, amino acids, fatty acids and vitamins can be administered through this method. Various types of commercially prepared formulas are available in the market and can be selected based on the patients' need.

Advantages of TPN
1. It provides more adequate amounts of nutrients.
2. All the nutrients are precalculated for various conditions.
3. It is easy to administer.
4. Nutritional adequacy is easily monitored.

Disadvantages of TPN
1. It is very complicated as compared to enteral method.
2. Regular biochemical testing is needed.
3. It is difficult to operate. More skilled professionals are required.
4. It demands regular medical and nursing attention.
5. It is not a natural method.

▶ EMERGENCY NUTRITION FOR SICK

The goal of nutritional therapy in a critically ill infant or child is to provide sufficient calories and protein (Table 27.1) to spare mobilization of body reserves, prevent catabolism, promote wound healing and protect from infection. In the initial phase of trauma or illness, metabolic rate decreases and the body becomes catabolic. As the patient becomes more stable, exogenous calories and protein can be utilized to promote anabolism. It is important to avoid both underfeeding, which can compromise healing and overfeeding, which can lead to refeeding syndrome.

CHAPTER 27: Nutrition for Sick Child

Table 27.1: Calorie and protein requirements of infant and children

Calorie and protein needs of infants and children age	Calories/ kg	Grams of protein/kg	
		Tube feeds or by mouth (PO)	Parenteral nutrition
Infants 0–1 year	80–120	2.5–3.5	2.0–2.5
1–10 year	60–90	2.0–2.5	1.7–2.0
11–18 year	30–75	1.5–2.0	1.0–1.5

Tube Feedings

Use an age-appropriate product, if available. Standard adult formulas are acceptable in children older than 1 year. Protein content will be 1.5–2 times that of pediatric products. Avoid exceeding 4 g of protein per kg. Higher protein concentrations will stress the kidneys, so be sure that fluid intake is adequate. Minimum calories can usually meet even, while giving this maximum amount of protein. Additional calories can be given using vegetable oil (100 kcal/15 mL) and sugar (48 calories per 15 mL).

Goal rate for enteral feedings depends on caloric and fluid needs. If patient is on intravenous fluids, adjust volume as enteral feeds are advanced, so do not exceed calculated fluid requirements (Table 27.2).

Nutrient Needs in Specific Conditions

1. **Burns and open wounds:** High protein, supplement with vitamin C and zinc, if available; otherwise, use a standard multivitamin mineral supplement.

Table 27.2: Continous tube feeding guidelines

Guidelines for initiating and advancing continuous feedings age	Initial infusion	Incremental advances
Infant to 1 year	1–2 mL/kg/h	10–20 mL/kg/day
1–6 year	1 mL/kg/h	1 mL/kg 2–8 h
> 7 year	10–25 mL/h	25 mL 2–8 h

2. **Ventilated and sedated:** Lower end of caloric needs goal protein.
3. **Sepsis:** Mid range of calories, goal protein. Sepsis with fever, use upper range of calories and goal protein.

▶ NUTRITIONAL PROBLEMS OF THE CHILD

The specific nutritional problems in the country are:
- Protein-energy malnutrition
- Nutritional anemia
- Low birth weight
- Xerophthalmia
- Iodine deficiency disorder and others.

Undernutrition or malnutrition is a worldwide problem of today. It is not only an important cause of child mortality and morbidity but it also leads to permanent impairment of physical and mental growth of those who survive. The main target of undernutrition is the preschooler, pregnant and nursing mothers.

Malnutrition, a major problem, has been receiving progressive attention through all the 5 year plans with further extension and intensification in the seventh 5 years plan. More emphasis has been laid for uplifting the weaker and the vulnerable section of population with a focus on the tribal and the scheduled castes. Malnutrition being a multifaceted problem, a combination of approaches like nutritional education, fortification and enrichment of foods extending the existing food supplies and health measures are being emphasized in policy making and program implementation.

Malnutrition among children and women is seriously danger today. Nutrition is the science of nourishment and is therefore, the sum total of those processes by which the living organism received and utilizes the materials necessary for the maintenance of life. Nutrition is the function of food, the nutrients and other substances therein. Their action, interaction and balancing are in relation to health and diseases. Nutrition is a positive physiological state of well-being.

CHAPTER 27: Nutrition for Sick Child

In addition, it is concerned with social, economic, cultural and psychological implications of food and eating. In the absence of proper nutrition, a state of malnutrition occurs leading to one or more of the following states (Table 27.3):

1. An increased risk of mortality and morbidity.
2. A reduced life expectancy.
3. A generalized functional impairments.
4. Disabilities.
5. Adverse influences on mental and physical development.

Table 27.3: Signs of a well-nourished child as against of an ill child

Sl No	Signs of well-nourished child	Signs of ill child
1.	Skin is smooth, pliable and elastic and of a healthy color	Lack of color of skin —paleness
2.	Bright and clear eyes, and pink eye membranes	Pale, dark red, or purple mucous membrane lining the eyes. Failing eyesight
3.	Firm pink nails	Rigid brittle nails
4.	The hair is lustrous and firmly attached to the scalp	Dull hair lacking sheen, dry and can be easily plucked
5.	Healthy gums and membranes of the mouth	Pale, dark red or purple color of gums
6.	Reddish pink tongue, not coated, pink lips	Sores on skin, lip or tongue, pale lips
7.	Desirable height for age and desirable weight for height.	Stunted growth and weight deficit
8.	Good appetite and sound nutrition	Loss of appetite, digestive disturbances, undernutrition
9.	Normal body temperature, pulse rate and breathing rate	Above normal body temperature, shortness of breath while performing normal activity
10.	Healthy children are alert	Listless, irritable and depressed

SECTION 3: Infant and Child Nutrition

▶ MALNUTRITION

Malnutrition has been defined as a pathological state resulting from an absolute or relative deficiency or excess of one or more essential nutrients. Malnutrition may be an outcome of undernutrition, overnutrition or imbalance:

1. **Undernutrition:** It is a state of absolute deficiency of one or more nutrients. An undernutrition of a less severe kind results in nutritional adaptation in children, which may manifest as wasting, stunting or a combination of both.
2. **Overnutrition:** It is a state of one or more nutrients, over nutrients, resulting from absolute excess of nutrients over a period of time, leads to obesity and its associated complications. It can also occur in case of certain vitamins and minerals. Examples of selective overnutrition are hypervitaminosis A, hypervitaminosis D and fluorosis.
3. **Imbalance:** It is an outcome of relative deficiency, or excess of one or more nutrients in a diet. The proportion of nutrients resulting in excess in one and deficiency in the other can cause malnutrition through imbalance. If the carbohydrate intake is not adequate, the proteins in the diet shall be sacrificed by the body in yielding energy resulting in protein wastage and malnutrition due to imbalance.

Causes of Malnutrition

1. Person suffered by diseases and infections.
2. Individual habits, dietary idiosyncrasies, cooking methods, religion, personal likes and dislikes, customs, traditions, etc.
3. Low standard of living among women, low female literacy.
4. Poverty, lack of education, unemployment, population explosion and lack of information.
5. Lower production of food or its unavailability.
6. Unhealthy behavior.
7. Lack of nutrition education, etc.

Effects of Malnutrition

1. Malnutrition borne diseases like kwashiorkor, marasmus, xerophthalmia, nutritional anemia, goiter, etc. these are five main malnutrition borne diseases.
2. Diseases due to deficiency of vitamins and minerals, e.g. scurvy, rickets, etc.
3. Higher maternal and infant mortality.
4. Stunted growth and improper development of children.
5. Reduction of expectancy of life.
6. Reduced working capacity of a person.
7. Fall in health status of the country or a blow to the 'healthy citizen, healthy nation' belief.

Assessment of Malnutrition

A comprehensive assessment of malnutrition problem demands:

1. The execution of a three-dimensional survey, comprising of an appraisal of the nutritional status.
2. Appraisal of the dietary intake.
3. Appraisal of the ecological background of malnutrition:
   a. Appraisal of the nutritional status: As the population is based on the finding of its anthropometric assessment, clinical assessment and biochemical assessment.
   b. Appraisal of dietary intake: The diet survey is carried out on a sample of population treating family as the unit of survey. Given that the diet of a family is usually repeated every week, the survey is carried out for 7 consecutive days. A dietary survey may be conducted by recall method or weighment method. Assessment of dietary intake also is done by chemical analysis method.
   c. Appraisal of ecological background: The information is collected on diverse areas of the population under survey such as health and disease profile, morbidity and mortality patterns, primary healthcare services, public

healthcare program activities, fertility profile and fertility regulation, health and nutritional awareness, socioeconomic and sociocultural milieu, water supply and sanitation, agricultural produce and farming practices and nutrition intervention programs.

Prevention and Control of Malnutrition

Malnutrition and undernutrition are serious problems affecting the health of weaned infants and preschool children in India. The contributory causes are:

1. Inadequate production of different categories of foodstuffs.
2. Large increase in population.
3. Poverty.
4. Illiteracy.

All the factors are responsible for the inadequate and ill—balanced diets consumed by the preschool children of low-income groups. Studies carried out in India have shown that when preschool children consume adequate amounts of the customary diets, they grow well and supplementation of the diets with processed food on cereals, oil seeds and legumes bring about marked improvement in the growth and nutritional status of children. The solution to the problem of malnutrition lies in the production of adequate amounts of cereals and makes them available to low-income groups at subsidized rates as part of their wages.

Supplementary feeding programs using conventional food should be instituted through MCH centers and balwadis. Other measures, which will help in overcoming malnutrition include:

1. Increased production of processed foods based on oil seed meals and their distribution through hospitals and health centers.
2. Nutrition education of mothers: In addition to the above, improvements should be effected on the economic, social educational and cultural aspects of the low-income groups

of the population as these factors influence profoundly the food habits of the people.

▶ CONCLUSION

Optimal health of patients relies on good nutrition from all ends of the spectrum. Nutrition plays key role in the care of the critically ill, those with inadequate gut function, eating disorder, patients with food intolerance, the obese and a vast range of other clinical problems. It is often necessary to cater to a patient's appetite, since many individuals become especially hard to please when sick. A tactful and observant nurse can be of great benefit to the physician and dietetian in carrying out the dietary regimen. This is important to meet the changing needs of the sick individual's ability to make use of foods.

Chapter 28

Child Nutrition Programs

▶ SPECIAL NUTRITION PROGRAM

Special Nutrition Program is primarily a food distribution program, initiated 1970 in India as a crash program. Diet surveys conducted among preschool children in several regions had clearly indicated that the primary factor in the home diets of a majority of Indian children suffering from various grades of protein calorie malnutrition.

The government of India in 1970 initiated, on a priority basis, the Special Nutrition Program for tribal and urban slum children in different parts of the country.

Objectives

1. The program is operated through the Ministry of Social Welfare and Community.
2. It was suggested that the supplement should provide approximately a minimum of 300 calories and 9 g of protein per day per child.
3. The supplement actually consisted of cereal, pulse, oil seed and jaggery (wheat 60 g, Bengal gram 10 g, groundnut 10 g and jaggery 30 g, provides 400 calories and 12 g protein).

Types of Special Nutrition Program

The Government of India has launched several nutritional programs for the prevention of nutritional diseases:
1. Supplementary Feeding Program.
2. Balwadi Nutrition Program.
3. Mid-day Meal Program.

4. Integrated Child Development Services (ICDS) Scheme.
5. Anemia Control Program.
6. Vitamin A Prophylaxis Program.
7. National Goiter Control Program.
8. Tamil Nadu Integrated Nutrition Project.

Supplementary Feeding Program

Supplementary Feeding Program was started in 1970 for nutritional benefit of preschool children (6 months to 6 years), pregnant women and nursing mothers. The supplementary food supplies 300 calories of energy and 10–12 g of protein per child per day. The beneficiary mother receives daily 500 calories and 25 g of protein. This supplement is provided to them for about 300 days in a year.

Balwadi Nutrition Program

Balwadi Nutrition Program is being organized by the Central Social Welfare Board from the year 1970–71. National level organizations give active support in Balwadi Nutrition Program and provide help to the voluntary agencies for implementation of the same. These organizations are Indian Tribal Caste Association, Indian Council for Child Welfare, Kasturba Gandhi National Memorial Trust and Harijan Sevak Sangh.

Balwadi were established in rural areas for providing preparatory education to children in the age group of 3–6 years. The supplement provided to the beneficiaries supplies 300 cal and 10 g of protein per child per day.

Mid-day Meal Program

Mid-day Meal Program has an important role in providing balanced diet to school children. Since 1960s this is an effort taken by Government of India, to provide at least one nutritious meal and diet supplements to children in primary and middle schools. It was first organized in 1957 in Tamil Nadu successfully.

In this program one third of the child's daily requirement can be fulfilled. Child and Adolescent Resources and Education (CARE), UNICEF and many international, governmental voluntary agencies give their contribution in this. The primary objective of Mid-day Meal Program is to improve the nutritional status of children and imparting nutritional education and to ensure universal primary education.

Concept of Mid-day Meal program:
1. In India, the Mid-day Meal Program was first started at Madras city in 1961.
2. The Mid-day Meal Program was launched in the country as a whole in 1962–1963.
3. Nearly 12 million children benefited by this program in 1947 and 16 million children in 1979.
4. Food material consisting of corn, soymilk and salad oil supplied by CARE has been the sheet anchor of the school lunch program in a majority of places.

Integrated Child Development Service Scheme

Integrated Child Development Service (ICDS) Scheme. This project was started in the year 1975 in pursuance of the national policy for children. The beneficiaries are preschool children below 6 years, pregnant and lactating mothers.

Vitamin A Prophylaxis Program

Vitamin A Prophylaxis Program was launched by Ministry of Health and Family Welfare in 1970. For the success of the National Program for Control of Blindness, it is necessary to prevent disease due to deficiency of vitamin A. For these children less than 5 years of age are given vitamin A containing 200,000 IU orally, every 6 months, through this program in India every year. The primary responsibility of implementation of this program rests on the maternal and child health using of the Health and Family Welfare Department. ICDS have an important role in the implementation of this program.

Anemia Control Program

Anemia Control Program consists of distribution of iron and folic acid tablets to pregnant women and young children (1–12 years). Mother and child health (MCH) centers in urban areas, primary health centers in rural areas and ICDS projects are engaged in the implementation of this program.

National Goiter Control Program

The National Goiter Control Program was launched by the Government of India in 1962 in the conventional goiter belt in the Himalayan region with objectives of identification of goiter endemic areas to supply iodized salt.

Tamil Nadu Integrated Nutrition Project

Tamil Nadu Integrated Nutrition Projects Program was started in 1980. This provides a package of health and nutrition services to the rural pregnant and lactating mothers and their children in the rural blocks of Tamil Nadu. The second phase the targets were revised and expanded with the implementation of ICDS everywhere, the blocks will be converted into ICDS blocks.

▶ APPLIED NUTRITION PROGRAM

The concept and philosophy of the Applied Nutrition Program (ANP) arose early in the 1950s, out of the realization that the problem of improving nutritional condition and preventing malnutrition could not be solved by scattered, uncoordinated activities mainly of a relief nature, such as the free distribution of food to the vulnerable segments of the population.

Applied Nutrition Program has been defined as coordinated educational activities among health, agricultural and educational departments, and other interested agencies with the active participation of the people to help them. Emphasis is placed on community action and the production of low cost productive foods.

SECTION 3: Infant and Child Nutrition

Their utilization for vulnerable groups in the family, especially infants and small children is emphasized, sometimes through community supplementary feeding programs, with or without externally provided foods. The implementation should be continuously adapted to changing conditions.

Objectives

1. To increase the production of protective foods, e.g. milk, fruits, vegetables eggs and fish, etc.
2. To ensure effective utilization of these protective foods by pregnant and nursing women, preschool and school children.
3. Nutritional education of ANP in community development blocks.
4. To assist in the extension of ANP in community development blocks.
5. To promote sound and hygienic practices for production, preservation, and use of protective foods through demonstration and education among village communities.

Activities

1. **Training of personnel:** As a first phase facilities for conducting practical courses in poultry management, dairying, fisheries (inland and marine) horticulture and home science, and in the teaching of applied human nutrition are being strengthened in selected training institutions such as rural extension training centers.
2. **Program at the state level:** As soon as the subsidiary plan of operation is signed for a state government a coordination committee is established at the state, district and block levels. The state nutrition officer, in consultation with the officer in charge of the ANP in the state, formulates a training program for different categories of persons employed in the implementation of this program.

CHAPTER 28: Child Nutrition Programs

3. **Production of productive foods:** It is being achieved at the village level by:
   a. Establishing school gardens and orchard.
   b. Setting up poultry units.
   c. Production of fish in local tanks.
   d. Inshore fishery in selected centers in coastal areas.

The medical officer and their staffs in the primary health center will help impart nutrition to the people, who come to the center and subcenter for medical care.

Role of Other Agencies

Women's Organization

Women's organization has an important role to play as they are being entrusted with the feeding of preschool and school children. These organizations are being supplied utensils. For cooking and serving balanced diets. Training program and cooking demonstrations have been organized by this women's organization.

Balwadi

Under this program, a certain number of balwadis have to be organized in each block, where the preschool children can gather for reaction and lunch.

Youth Clubs

Youth clubs are encouraged to take plots of land for cultivation of vegetables, so that the youth team practices farming. This system also establishes a spirit of competition among the youths. Youth clubs are also encouraged to take up poultry units.

School Teachers

The success of the program for school gardens will depend upon the interest and leadership of the teacher. Therefore, the subject of nutrition has been included in the syllabus of teacher training courses.

Role of International Agencies

The international agencies responsible for this program are UNICEF, FAQ and WHO. The UNICEF also provides assistance for the production of textbooks, literature and visual education aids. The FAQ provides technical assistance for all the components of the program. WHO through its regional offices provides technical assistance in the field of health.

▶ INTEGRATED CHILD DEVELOPMENT SERVICES

The ICDS scheme was initiated by the Government of India under the Ministry of Social and Women's Welfare on October 2nd in 1975, in pursuance of the National Policy for children, which was recommended by the Srivastava Committee during the fifth five year plan (1974–1979). At present the most important scheme in the field of child welfare is the ICDS scheme. The ICDS scheme has been implemented in India since 1975. There are about 100 such workers in each ICDS project. According to the available statistics, there are over 5,320 ICDS blocks are functioning in India and 185 ICDS blocks are functioning in Karnataka. The ICDS staff order is given in Figure 28.1.

The selection criteria of an Anganwadi worker are as follows:

1. Educational qualification SSLC pass or fail.
2. Willing to serve for the community.

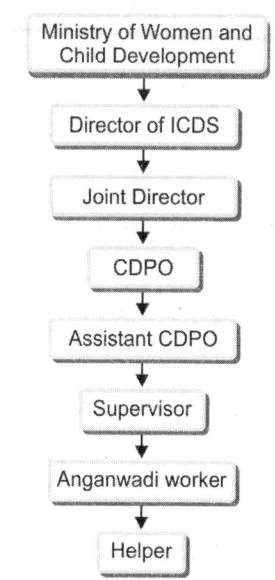

Fig. 28.1: Integrated Child Development Services (ICDS) staff order (CDPO, Community development program officer)

3. Belongs to the same community/culture.
4. In case of more volunteers from the same community. Village committee will select the candidate.

Objectives

1. To improve the nutritional and health status of children in the age group of 0–5 years.
2. To lay the foundation for proper psychological, physical and social development of the child.
3. To achieve effective coordination and implementation among the various departments working for the promotion of child development.
4. To reduce morbidity, mortality and malnutrition among 0–5 years' children and reproductive age mothers.
5. To enhance the capability of the mother and nutritional needs of the child through proper nutrition and health education. Packages of ICDS scheme:
   a. Supplementary nutrition.
   b. Immunization.
   c. Health check up.
   d. Medical referral services.
   e. Nutrition and health education for women.
   f. Non-formal education for 3–5 years children.

The primary health centers of the ICDS blocks have been strengthened by the following additional inputs:

1. One medical officer.
2. Two lady health visitors.
3. Eight Auxiliary Nursing and Midwifery (ANM) in rural blocks and four ANMs in urban and tribal projects.

Anganwadis were established as focal points for the delivery of ICDS services. Each village with a population of 1,000 has one Anganwadi.

The Anganwadi worker is the key person for the delivery of services at the Anganwadis. An Anganwadi worker has the following functions:

SECTION 3: Infant and Child Nutrition

1. Organizing supplementary nutrition feeding at the center.
2. Non-formal preschool education.
3. Primary medical care.
4. Health and nutrition education to women.
5. Assisting the PHC staff in the implementation of the health components of one ICDS, eliciting community support and maintaining records.

▶ MINIMUM NEED PROGRAM

Launched at the very outset of the fifth five year plans (1975–1980), the main aim of the program is to meet certain minimum needs of the people and thus raise their living standards.

The minimum needs identified under this program are:
- Nutrition
- Rural health
- Elementary education
- Rural water supply
- Adult education
- Rural roads
- Rural electrification
- Rural housing
- Environmental improvement of urban slums.

The modes of meeting the nutritional needs of the people and children are:

1. By extending nutritional support to 11 million eligible individuals.
2. By expanding the Special Nutrition Program for all the ICDS projects.
3. By consolidating the Mid-day Meal Program and links it with health, portable water and sanitation.

▶ TWENTY POINT PROGRAM

The Twenty Point Program (TPP) was launched in 1975 as an agenda for national action for promoting social justice and economic growth. In 1986, the program was modified.

The modified TPP has at least eight points concerning health in some way or the others as indicated below:
- Point 1 relates to rural poverty
- Point 7 relates to clean drinking water
- Point 8 relates to 'health for all'
- Point 9 relates to 'two-child' norm
- Point 10 relates to expansion of education
- Point 14 relates to housing
- Point 15 relates to improvement in slums
- Point 17 relates to protection of environments.

▶ CHILD SURVIVAL AND SAFE MOTHERHOOD PROGRAM

Every year over 27 million pregnancies take place in the country. All women need additional care during pregnancy. They need to eat and rest more than they did, when they were not pregnant. All women need to be advised on the preparations they must make for delivery. These women must be given periodic health check-ups so that maternal complications or risk factors are identified in time and treatment started early and the women are counseled to deliver in a hospital.

The program is introduced as part of the overall strategy for:
1. Reduction of infant mortality rate (IMR) to below 60/1,000 live births.
2. Child mortality to below 10/1,000 child population.
3. Reduction of percentage of low-birth-weight (LBW) babies to less than 10%.
4. Maternal mortality to below 2/1,000 live births by 2,000.
5. Perinatal mortality should be less than 35/1,000 live births.
6. Immunization coverage should be 100%.
7. Deliveries by trained personnel by 100%.
8. Antenatal care should be 100%.
9. Control of blindness should be less than 0.3%. The Child Survival and Safe Motherhood (CSSM) Program came into

SECTION 3: Infant and Child Nutrition

force in August 1992 and this is implemented with financial assistance from World Bank and UNICEF.

Objectives

1. Sustaining and strengthening the ongoing Universal Immunization Program.
2. Continuing oral rehydration therapy (ORT) program for children below the age of 5 years.
3. Introducing and expanding the program for control of acute respiratory infection for children below 5 years of age.
4. Universalizing the Vitamin 'A' Prophylaxis Program from 6 months to 5 years.
5. Iron and folic acid administration program to pregnant mother and children up to 5 years.
6. Improving newborn care and maternal care at the community level.

Components

1. Package consisting of Universal Immunization Program (UIP), ORT, prophylaxis, schemes and acute respiratory tract infections (ARTs) in all states and Union Territories.
2. Safe motherhood programs for six high maternal mortality rate (MMR) states of Assam, Bihar, Madhya Pradesh, Orissa, Rajasthan and Uttar Pradesh.

Two districts of Tamil Nadu had been taken up earlier under UNICEF-assisted pilot project. The CSSM project will be implemented in a phased manner.

Reproductive and Child Health Program

Reproductive and Child Health Program followed revisions in the CSSM Program as per recommendation made at the International Conference on Population and Development in Cairo in 1994 and was born in 1997.

The package of services offered by Reproductive and Child Health (RCH) Program.

Program addresses the needs that have emerged over years of implementing the Family Welfare Program. Unification of many women and child health areas will now enable health workers to move easily and completely understand service needs and deliver services accordingly. As opposed to the Family Welfare Program, the RCH Program aims to be more in tune with the ground realities concerning:
- Overall health needs of women and children
- Implementation needs of health workers
- Local demographic needs and conditions.

Program Components

The RCH was build on the success of the UIP and the CSSM Program. In addition, it will cover all aspects of women's reproductive health across their reproductive cycle, from puberty to menopause. In a nutshell, will cover the services offered under the CSSM and the Family Welfare Program as well as two new interventions, namely management of reproductive tract infections and adolescent reproductive health.

For children
- Essential newborn care
- Exclusive breastfeeding
- Immunization
- Appropriate management of ARI
- Vitamin A prophylaxis
- Treatment of anemia.

For mother
- Tetanus toxoid immunization
- Prevention and treatment of anemia
- Antenatal care and early identification of maternal complications
- Deliveries conducted by trained personnel
- Promotion of institutional deliveries
- Management of obstetrical emergencies
- Birth spacing.

SECTION 3: Infant and Child Nutrition

For eligible couples
- Prevention of unwanted pregnancy
- Safe abortion.

For reproductive tract infection (RTI)/sexually transmitted disease (STD)
- Prevention and treatment of RTI and STD
- RCH Program is a target-free program with voluntary participation of the community.

▶ **CONCLUSION**

Nurses play a key role in the care of their patients through various nutrition-related programs. A number of nutritional programs were initiated by the government of India. Various feeding programs and nutritional programs, which are implemented through various organizations can be used as nutrition education channels. Feeding programs under the family and child welfare departments, school feeding programs under the family and child welfare departments, school feeding programs, the composites programs for women and preschool children, the applied nutrition programs, world food programs and other state programs can be utilized for education purposes.

SECTION 4

Community Nutrition

SECTION 4

Community recruition

Chapter 29

Community Nutrition

▶ INTRODUCTION

The science of community nutrition is concerned with the nutritional requirements for the promotion, protection and maintenance of health in all the groups of population. Such knowledge is necessary in order to assess the nutritional adequacy of diets for growth of infants, children and adolescents; adults and during pregnancy and lactating women. The main target of nutritional improvement in the community is the family. The housewife is the gatekeeper to the consumption of foods in the family. In some families husband determines what food will reach the table. Harmful food taboos and dietary prejudices can be identified and corrected. Ignorance and illiteracy are the main causes of ill health in a country. Family dietary habits may lead to health problems.

▶ NUTRITIONAL NEEDS OF INDIVIDUALS

Nutritional needs of individuals is important to recognize that people's dietary needs change during their life span. A suitable balanced diet for a small child will not be suitable for an adult or older person, so needs must be taken into account when caring for different individuals.

Infancy (0–3 Years)

At birth, babies rely only on milk to meet their nutritional requirements. Breast milk is the ideal food for newborns because it contains nutrients for all the baby's needs in the right amounts. Although it is low in iron and copper, the baby has enough of these stored until it starts eating solid foods. In addition, breast milk provides immunity and is clean, readily available and does not have to be prepared. Some mothers are either unable or choose not to breastfeed and use formula milk, which is modified cow's milk. This must be made up to the right concentration to prevent damage to the immature kidneys. The equipment used must be sterilized to prevent infection.

Weaning should not be done before 4 months of age as doing it early may cause later obesity or allergies. Different foods can be introduced gradually such as cereals, then fruit, vegetables, egg yolk and finely minced meat. By about 12–18 months, the toddler should be eating the same food as the rest of the family, with no extra salt or sugar added. It is usually advised that until the age of 2 years, children should be given whole milk, but after this they can be given semi-skimmed milk. Skimmed milk should not be given until the age of 5. The amount of milk drunk will decrease as the child eats more and more solid food.

Nutritional Requirements

In early infancy most of the nutrient requirements are met by breast milk and weaning foods should start by 4–5 months.

Energy: The energy requirements of infants are much higher. Infants require 120 kcal/kg body weight.

Proteins: In an infant protein requirements are higher. In the initial months, the human milk provides the essential amino acids needed for growth.

The protein requirement of an infant is as follows:
1. In terms of milk proteins:
   a. 0–3 months 2.3 g/kg body weight.
   b. 3–6 months 1.8 g/kg body weight.
2. Partly vegetable proteins:
   a. 6–9 months 1.8 g/kg body weight.
   b. 9–12 months 1.5 g/kg body weight.

If the protein and calorie requirements are not met adequately, it could lead to protein calorie malnutrition.

Minerals: Rapid growth requires large quantities of minerals, especially calcium and phosphorus. Though mother's milk has less calcium it is better absorbed from breast milk. The intake of cow's milk leads to hypocalcemia due to its high phosphate content.

Vitamins: Vitamins are essential for the rapid growth of infant. Breast milk provides sufficient vitamins. Cow's milk is deficient in vitamins C and D.

Fats: About 35%–45% of calories are provided by fat in the initial stages of infancy. Supplementary foods provide fat in the later stages.

Carbohydrates: Lactose in human milk provides 25%–55% of calories.

Fluids: Water intake in full-term infants is 60 mL/kg body weight on day 1. It increases to 150–170 mL/kg by day 3–4. As weaning starts boiled, cooled water should be given along with fresh fruits and juices or porridges and gruels.

Supplementary foods for infants and toddlers: The first solid foods are introduced at 5–6 months of age. The foods given are cereals, cereal milk or cereal dahi preparations such as suji halwa, rice milk, upma, rice dal, khichdi, pongal, bread, rice flakes/poha, etc. Fruits such as ripe banana, mango, papaya, which are soft and pulpy are also given. Well-cooked non-fibrous vegetables such as ash gourd, potato, pumpkin are fed along with rice.

Most of the problems of food acceptance begin in the toddler stage. The child will show a remarkable decrease in appetite in the 2nd year as compared to the 1st year. So, it is important to give small portions of food and let the child enjoy the food. Allow the child some freedom to decide when he/she is satisfied. Allow some flexibility in choices and help the child to form good food habits.

Toddlers: Children can share family meals by the time they are 2 years old. A few alterations may be needed when the family makes highly spiced food. Toddler should not be given foods, which are too fatty or too sweet. Such foods may fill limited space, without providing the nutrients need. The child may be encouraged to eat sweets toward the end of the meal so that he/she may not eat these to the exclusion of other foods.

It is good to give appetizing beverages such as fruit juices and milk to the children. It is good to serve part of their milk needs in the form of soups, kheer, custard or ice cream. Fruits are ideal snacks. Crisp crackers or toast are liked and children can eat these without help, which helps to feel independent (Fig. 29.1).

Childhood (4–10 Years)

Children aged between 4 and 10 years of age tend to be very active and are growing fast. Although their energy requirements are not as high as adults', they need almost the same amount of some vitamins and minerals. Some children seem to have big appetites—this is not due to greed, but to the fact that they have high nutritional needs. During childhood, children should be encouraged to eat healthy meals consisting of meat, fish or eggs and potatoes, pasta or rice, with plenty of vegetables and fruit. They should not eat too many sweets, crisps, biscuits and fizzy drinks, as these can lead to obesity and tooth decay.

Diet for Preschool Children

Preschoolers have a very short span of attention and are easily distracted from eating. Their response to food is rather inconsistent. The muscle coordination is limited and eating behavior is generally messy. When opportunity is provided, the preschooler learns things faster by taking advantages of parents. Young children have extreme taste sensitivity and prefer mildly flavored foods.

Three times meal pattern along with midmorning and midafternoon snacks is best for extremely active children.

CHAPTER 29: Community Nutrition

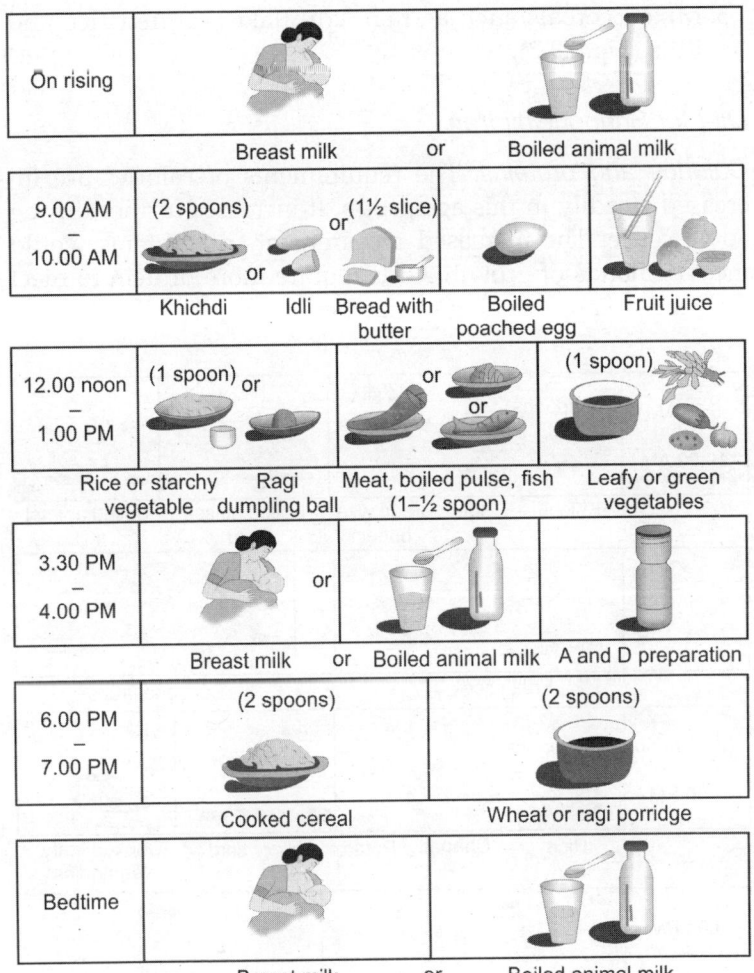

Fig. 29.1: Meal plans for 1- to 3-year-old children

Types of food suitable for a preschooler:
1. Fresh fruit juices.
2. Milk and milk beverages, curd, cheese pieces.
3. Fruit pieces like slices of apple, papaya, mango, sapota.
4. Boiled/raw vegetables, carrots, cucumber, potato, cauliflower, beans.

5. Mixed cereals such as ragi, cornflakes, puffed rice and idlis (Fig. 29.2).

Diet for School Children

Calories and proteins: The requirements of calories are increased steadily in this age group. It increases further during adolescence. The increased requirements of proteins would meet demands of growth. Girls require more protein to meet the needs of approaching menarche.

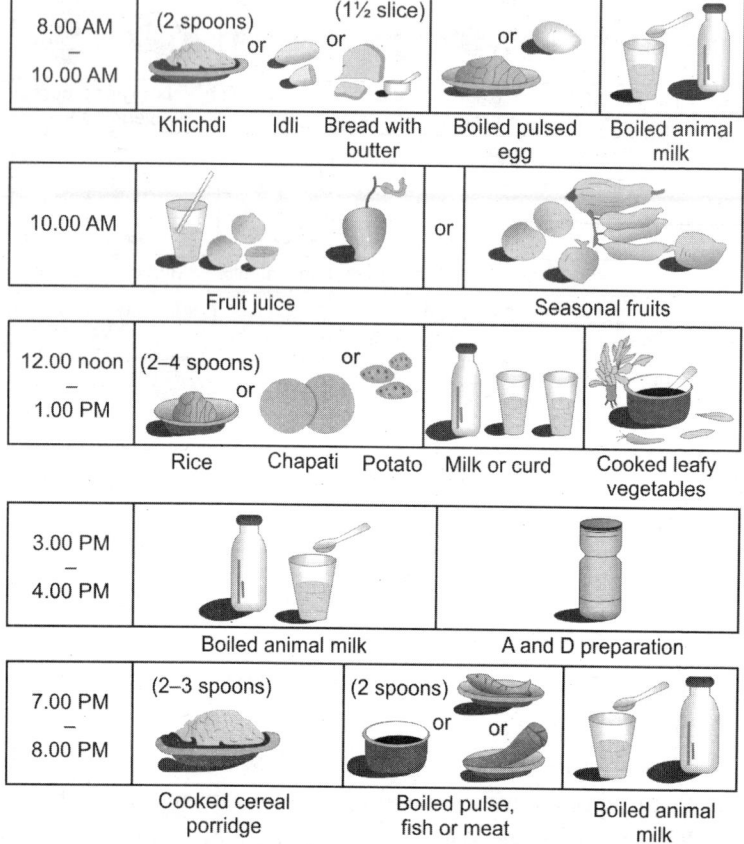

Fig. 29.2: Meal plans for 3- to 5-year-old children

Minerals: A 10 to 12-year-old children require more calcium than adults to meet skeletal growth. As the blood volume increases, there is an increased demand for iron.

Adolescence (11–18 Years)

The nutritional needs of adolescents are greater than for any other age group. This is because they have large appetites and are still growing. It is important that people in this age group are encouraged to eat sensibly at regular intervals and not to go through phases of overeating or starving themselves in order to lose weight. In addition to encouraging healthy eating, they should be advised to maintain a regular amount of physical activity. Again they should not eat too many sweets, crisps, biscuits and fizzy drinks.

Adolescent (12–16 Years)

Adolescent is the age of rapid growth and intense activity. Individual variation is marked in this age group. A number of physical, emotional and mental changes occur in this period of life. Girls mature between 11 and 13 years whereas major changes occur in boys between 13 and 15 years. It is normal for boys to eat a lot at this age especially if they are fond of outdoor sports.

Dietary Consideration for Teenagers

The transition phase from childhood to adulthood is known as adolescence with speeded physical, biochemical and emotional development. It is during this period that the final growth occurs.

There are many changes in the body due to hormones. Even boys and girls who had an excellent pattern of food intake are likely to succumb to strange imbalanced diets during adolescence. They feel independent and seek own identity and freedom to make their own decisions. Emotional difficulties often stem from feelings of social inadequacy or pressure of school work.

Meeting Food Needs of Adolescents

Adolescence is the age of group activities. Therefore, if nutrition education is introduced as a group activity, it may help in improving eating habit. Boys may need to consume a lot of energy rich foods. Girls must give special attention to foods rich in protein, iron and other nutrients necessary for synthesis and regeneration of red blood cells. Girls diet should include iron rich foods such as dals, leafy green vegetables, dried fruits, egg, liver and red meat (if acceptable).

It is important for adolescents to gain appropriate weight for their height and body build. Any deviation from normal indicates some feeding problem, which must be identified and corrected with the help of a dietitian. Checking a 3 days food intake record, may help in identifying the specific lack or excess and thus form the basis or a plan of action.

Adulthood (19–65 Years)

During adulthood, nutritional needs reduce with age. In general, adults need to eat a healthy diet consisting of complex carbohydrates such as bread, potatoes, rice or pasta, protein such as meat, eggs, cheese, fish, fruit and vegetables. Fatty and sugary foods should be kept to a minimum and adults should be advised to take physical activity on a regular basis. Alcohol intake should be limited as it contributes extra kilocalories to the diet.

Pregnancy and Breastfeeding

During pregnancy and breastfeeding a woman's nutritional needs are increased to provide nutrition for the growing baby, and for making breast milk after the baby is born. Although there is a belief that being pregnant means that a woman can 'eat for two', only about an extra 200 kcal are required in the last 3 months of the pregnancy and about 450–570 kcal during breastfeeding. This is to give the mother the energy she needs to carry the extra weight of the baby and to make breast milk. Women planning to become pregnant should be advised to eat a diet rich in folic acid to prevent damage to the fetus, particularly spina bifida.

Old Age (65 Years and Above)

Although, in general, there is no much difference in the energy needs of adults and older adults, as we age we become less mobile and our energy requirements decrease. Appetite also decreases, so it is important that older adults have a diet that provides concentrated sources of protein, vitamins and minerals. Gentle exercise should also be encouraged. Elderly people who live alone often cannot be bothered to cook a hot meal for one person, so they should be encouraged to eat foods that do not require much preparation, but are high in nutrients. Taste buds become less efficient in older people so they may require extra flavoring in their food.

Physiological Changes in Aging

Reduced BMR: Basal metabolic rate (BMR) is reduced in all tissues. BMR is highest in infants and then it goes on decreasing as age advances. Because of reduction of BMR in all organs, functions of all the organs are lowered to a certain extent.

Nervous system: There is decreased memory, decreased ability and rate of learning, decreased reaction time and dimness of vision. Due to arteriosclerosis and lack of vitamins, the mental faculty is depressed. This leads to lack of interest in living. Changes in behavior takes place due to lack of work, isolation and loneliness.

Gastrointestinal tract: There is reduction in secretion of most of the digestive juices and gastric acidity is also reduced. This leads to indigestion and affects absorption. In addition, there are certain changes in the intestinal mucosa, which cause reduced absorption of nutrients. The motility of gastrointestinal tract (GIT) is also reduced and there is tendency to develop constipation. Appetite is reduced due to lack of physical activity. Digestion is also affected, because of improper mastication due to lack of teeth/artificial dentures.

Cardiovascular system: As the age advances cholesterol is deposited in the inner walls of arteries. This leads to atherosclerosis. Atherosclerosis occurring in the arteries going to important organs (such as coronary arteries supplying the heart) causes decreased blood flow to these organs thereby decreasing their efficiency. Atherosclerosis in the vessels also increases the tendency of clot formation (thrombosis) in the vessels leading to almost complete blockage of blood flow, e.g. cerebral thrombosis, coronary thrombosis, etc.

Renal system: Overall functioning of the kidney is reduced.

Skin: As age advances, elasticity of the skin is reduced. Wrinkles appear.

Endocrine system: Activities of the endocrine glands such as thyroid, adrenal cortex and islets of Langerhans (pancreas) are diminished. Hormones of these glands are responsible for different metabolic activities in the cells so overall cellular metabolism is influenced to a considerable extent.

Nutritional Requirements

Diet of old people becomes imbalanced due to:

1. Often they live alone. They are reluctant to cook and also reluctant to go to a restaurant. The result is that they miss their meals.
2. In many, food intake is limited due to restriction in diet because of various diseases such as diabetes, hypertension and renal diseases. Therefore, certain foods are to be avoided.
3. There is constipation and worry about the falling health, which also reduces the appetite.
4. The teeth are lost due to decay. Many people use artificial teeth. Digestion is affected as there is improper mastication by artificial teeth.

Nutritional Requirements for Various Food Components

Calories: Because of reduction in BMR and restrictions in physical activity caloric requirement is reduced. Caloric intake is so adjusted that body weight remains constant preventing any tendency for obesity. But if there is loss of weight or emaciation, sufficient calories should be supplied to regain the normal weight.

Proteins: Due to decreased appetite and poor digestion, the food intake is generally inadequate to meet the protein requirements of old people. Deficiency of proteins leads to anemia, edema and lowered resistance. The daily intake of protein should be increased. It should be about 70 g/kg body weight. For non-vegetarians meat, fish and egg can be given, but there may be problem of chewing or mastication. So minced meat, half-boiled egg, milk and milk products should be given.

For vegetarians pulses are rich sources of proteins. If the diet is not able to provide sufficient proteins it should be given in the form of food supplements such as skimmed milk powder.

Fats: Older people tend to have high cholesterol levels. Fats are also difficult to digest. So in old age, daily intake above 40–50 g of fat is avoided. Half this quantity should be in the form of vegetable oils rich in essential fatty acids (EFAs) to reduce serum cholesterol level.

Carbohydrates: Old people tend to take cheaper readily available food, which does not require cooking, e.g. bread, biscuits, cakes, etc. Diet containing larger quantities of these substances, produces protein deficiency in old people. It also causes constipation, loss of appetite resulting in further malnutrition.

Minerals: Osteomalacia and osteoporosis are common in old age. Though exact reason is not known, osteoporosis is partly due to diminished intake and absorption of calcium. Osteomalacia is due to diminished vitamin D because of limited exposure to sunlight. The daily calcium intake should be increased to 0.8–1.0 g and iron intake 30–40 mg. For calcium supply the person should take at least half a liter milk and two eggs. Exposure to sunlight is essential for supply of vitamin D.

Vitamins: In old age, vitamin C deficiency is common in those who do not eat fruits and food is unbalanced. It is desirable that old people take one multivitamin tablet daily.

Fluids: Water intake should be liberal (more than 1.5 L) to ensure that the volume of water excreted is not less than 1.5 L/day. This will keep up the elimination of waste metabolic products such as urea, uric acid and creatinine. Old people are reluctant to take liquid as they have to urinate frequently, especially old people with diabetes and enlarged prostate. They should be advised to take sufficient liquid during day and refrain from drinking at night so that sleep is not disturbed.

Roughage: Old people have a tendency to constipate. They should therefore take sufficient amount of fiber in the form of fruits and vegetables in the diet.

Meal pattern: As far as possible, old people should take small frequent meals. They should take dinner early evening to prevent gaseous distribution and disturbance of sleep. Physical exertion after meals should be avoided especially in the people who have a poor coronary circulation.

Planning Diets for Adolescence

Adolescence is a stage of rapid growth and covers almost a span of 10 years. Individual variation is also great in this group. A number of physical changes and mental changes occur in this period of life. Girls mature between 11 and 14 years of age and boys between 13 and 16 years. The pattern of body water, lean body mass, bone and fat show noticeable differences between boys and girls.

As may be expected, the nutritional needs during this time very as rapid growth periods are tremendous. Anyone who has seen a teenager dieting during this period will attest to their voracious appetite. If plenty of foods are available, they will be eaten especially by boys. Unfortunately, enough of even a poor choice of foods will also satisfy the appetite, but will not supply the essential nutrients required for growth. The difference between poorly nourished and well-nourished becomes evident during this period. Normally, the poor diet is inadequate in both calories and calcium, but the adolescent boy may not show any obvious evidence of calcium deficiency, because of stunted growth resulting in decreased calcium requirements. Also, a deficient supply of calcium may lead to reduction in food intake and stunted growth. Occasionally, a fast growing adolescent may have an adequate calories supply combined with a deficiency of calcium and this results in poor skeletal growth and an uneven gait. Symptoms such as bowed legs and flat feet become exaggerated during this period. In the scarcity areas of Gujarat, feeding a good lunch was found to increase the weight of adolescent boys 4–6 kg, whereas younger children were found to show an increase of only 1–2 kg. Much of the difference in the physical stature between Indians and Westerners is due to slowing down of growth during this period.

Nutritional Requirements

The spurt in growth is earlier in for girls and a little later for boys. Therefore, the energy intake is higher for girls at 13–15 years and for boys at 16–18 years. Also the difference in energy intake between adolescent girls and boys is partly due to a lower metabolic rate in females as compared to males. The boys require 2,450 kcal at 13–15 years, while 2,640 kcal at 16–18 years of age. Adolescent girls require 2,060 kcal at 13–18 years of age. Protein intake for boys is significantly higher than girls due to a bigger stature of boys. At the end of growth period boys have one and a half times more lean mass as compared to girls. Girls have larger portions of fat deposits. Boys require 71 g and 79 g of protein at 13–15 years and 16–18 years of age respectively.

Since the bones grow in size and number, and mineralization continues even after full length is attained, the calcium requirements are higher during peak of growth and slightly lower thereafter for both boys and girls. Both the sexes require about 600 mg during 13–15 years and 500 mg during 16–18 years of age.

Iron need is higher than during childhood due to continuous increase in the blood volume. Adolescent boys require about 41–50 mg of iron at 13–18 years of age. Girls require 28 mg at 13–15 years and 30 mg at 16–18 years.

Requirement for vitamin A is the same as during childhood, i.e. both the sexes require 600 µg of retinol from 13–18 years of age. Thiamine, riboflavin and nicotinic acid requirements are recommended in relation to increased calories intake. The requirements of these vitamins are always higher for boys due to increased energy requirement. Vitamin C requirement is the same as during childhood, i.e. 40 mg. Dietary intake of vitamin D has been fixed at 200 IU for all the age groups, hence the requirement. 100 µg of folic acid has been recommended taking into account the bioavailability of food folates. Since vitamin B_{12} is present only in animal foods and Indian diets are basically vegetarian, dietary allowance of 1 µg has been recommended, which also takes into account cooking losses and the uncertainty about the extent of absorption of vitamin B_{12}. The requirement for vitamin B_6 is considered to be related to protein intake and adolescents require 2.0 mg daily.

Factors

The following points should be kept in mind while planning diets:
1. The planned diet should be well-balanced. With the increase in calcium requirement, extra milk can be provided, if possible. For an adolescent, from low socioeconomic status (SES), cheaper calcium rich sources should be provided like parched grains, whole grain cereals, pulses and green leafy vegetables. The diet should also contain sufficient energy sources to meet the increased energy requirements. Girls tend to be anemic as their iron requirement increases considerably. This increased iron requirement should be taken care of by providing green leafy vegetables, whole grain cereals and pulses and if possible, egg, meat, liver and fish.
2. Likes and dislikes should be considered.
3. Socioeconomic status of the family should be kept in mind. An adolescent from low SES may want to copy their classmates from high SES with respect to the purchase of high cost snacks. To avoid that, they should be given cheap yet attractive and nutritious snacks in tiffin.

4. There should be variety in terms of color, texture and flavor. The adolescents are more fussy, especially girls about eating at home. If meals are served attractive, it will encourage them to eat at home.
5. If tiffin is to be given it should be nutritionally balanced, more so if it is in place of a main meal.
6. Seasonal drinks like cold/soft drinks and tea/coffee may be included to make the day's diet interesting.
7. Satiety value of the diet should be taken care of especially for the boys. If they are still hungry extra salad can be provided.
8. The meals should be served in a pleasant atmosphere.
9. 'Snacking' in between meals is common amongst adolescents. Snacks should be wholesome and not only a source of energy but also proteins and other essential nutrients.

Adults

Adulthood represents the steady state in life when a person would have completed his/her growth in terms of body size. People at this age do not have to include nutrients for growth and strenuous activity of youth. The nutritional needs are for maintenance of body functions. The energy needs in adults are mainly to sustain body functions and activity. Adulthood also represents the productive stage of life. Therefore, it is important that the nutritional needs of an adult be met adequately so as to keep vitality and a positive attitude to life, which is essential for optimum productivity. A good diet fosters a vigorous maturity and can do much to delay the characteristics of old age. Inadequate amount of certain nutrients in the diet in earlier years, if continued at this age, may have serious repercussions. Therefore, good nutrition, as well as other health habits should be stressed.

Nutritional Needs

As mentioned earlier, the nutritional needs are mainly for maintenance of body functions, and to bear daily wear and tear. The requirements of different nutrients for adults and recommended dietary allowances for various nutrients cannot be given for any individual person. Indian Council of Medical Research (ICMR) has based the recommendations for adults in terms of reference of Indian man and women are discussed in Table 29.1.

Reference Indian man has been defined as "an adult man between 20 and 39 years of age, weighing 60 kg. He is free from disease and is physically fit for active work. On each working day, he is employed for 8 hours in occupation that usually involves moderate activity. While not at work, he spends 8 hours in bed, 4–6 hours in sitting moving about and 2 hours in walking, active recreation on household duties." For such a reference man, ICMR has taken a height of 163 cm.

Similarly, the reference Indian woman is defined as "an adult woman between 20 and 39 years of age, weighing 50 kg. She may be engaged for 8 hours in general household work, in light industry or in any other moderately active work. Apart from 8 hours in bed, she spends 4–6 hours in sitting or moving around (light activity) and 2 hours in walking, active recreation or household duties." For such a reference woman, ICMR has taken a height of 151 cm.

Energy: The energy need in adults is mainly to sustain body functions and activity. While planning meals for adults occupied in different occupations, consideration should be given to their energy requirements. Occupation of adults can generally be as follows.

Light work (sedentary work)

Men: Office workers, professionals like lawyers, doctors, accountants, teachers and architects.

Women: Office workers, housewives using mechanical appliances or servants, teachers and most other professionals.

Moderate work

Men: Most men in light industry, construction works (excluding heavy labor), many farm workers, shopkeepers.

CHAPTER 29: Community Nutrition

Table 29.1: Recommended allowances for Indians

Group	Particulars	Body Weight kg	Net energy kcal/day	Carbohydrate g/day	Protein g/day	Fat g/day	Calcium mg/day	Iron mg/day	Vitamin A	Thiamine mg/day	Riboflavin mg/day	Nicotonic acid mg/day	Pyridoxine mg/day	Ascorbic acid mg/day	Folic acid	Vitamin B_{12} µg/day
Man	Sedentary work	60	2,425		60	20	400	28	600	1.2	1.4	16	20	40	100	1
	Moderate work		2,875							1.4	1.6	18				
	Heavy work		3,800							1.6	1.9					
Woman	Sedentary work	50	1,875		50	20	400	30	600	0.9	1.1	12	20	40	100	1
	Moderate work		2,225							1.1	1.3	14				
	Heavy work		2,925							1.2	1.5	16	25	40	400	1
	Pregnant woman	50	+300		+15	30	1,000	38	600	0.2	0.2	+2				
	Lactation 0–6 month	50	+550		+25	45	1,000	30	950	0.3	4					
	6–12 month		+400		+18					0.2	0.2					
Infants	0–6 month	5.4	108 /kg		2.05		500		350	55	65	710	0.1	25	25	0.2
	6-12 month	8.6	98/kg		1.65					50	60	650	0.4			

Contd...

SECTION 4: Community Nutrition

Contd...

Group	Particulars	Body Weight kg	Net energy kcal/day	Carbohydrate g/day	Protein g/day	Fat g/day	Calcium mg/day	Iron mg/day	Vitamin A	Thiamine mg/day	Riboflavin mg/day	Nicotonic acid mg/day	Pyridoxine mg/day	Ascorbic acid mg/day	Folic acid	Vitamin B$_{12}$ µg/day
Children	1–3 year	12.2	1,240		22	25	400	12	400	0.6	0.7	8	0.9	40	30	0.2–1.0
	4–6 year	19.0	1,690		30			18	400	0.9	1.0	11	1.6		40	
	7–9 year	26.9	1,950		41			26	600	1.0	1.2	13			60	
Boys	10–12 year	35.4	2,190		54	22	600	34	600	1.1	1.3	15	1.6	40	70	0.2–1.0
Girls	10–12 year	31.5	1,970		57			19		1.0	1.2	13				
Boys	13–15 year	47.8	2,450		70	22	600	41	600	1.2	1.5	16	20	40	100	0.2–1.0
Girls	13–15 year	46.7	2,060		65			28		1.0	1.2	14				
Boys	16–18 year	57	2,640		78	22	500	50	500	1.3	1.6	17	2.0	40	100	0.2–1.0
Girls	16–18 year	49.9	2,010		83			30		1.0	1.2	16		40		0.2–1.0

Women: Workers in light industry, housewives without mechanical household appliances or servants, departmental store workers.

Heavy work (very active)

Men: Agricultural workers, laborers, soldiers or active service, mine and steel workers, athletes.

Women: Farm workers, dancers and athletes. In addition to physical activity and to the type and nature of non-occupational activities, the energy requirements of individuals also depends on factors such as body size and composition, age, sex and climate. Energy expenditure depending on body size and composition will be influenced by resting metabolism, the physical effort of moving the whole body, the work of standing of maintenance of posture and small movements of the limbs. Also, the total physical activity of an individual may be influenced by the quantity of adipose tissue in the body. The energy requirement of women is less than that of men, because they have a larger proportion of fat. The energy expenditure of adults may change with age because of changes in body weight or body composition (as in old age). It is generally recognized that the energy requirements of people in cold climates is more than that of those in hot climates.

Proteins: It is required by a normal adult for maintaining the tissue integrity, repairing and replacing the protein loss by wear and tear. An allowance of 1 g/kg body weight has recommended. Thus, the total daily allowance of protein of an average Indian man weighing 60 kg will be 60 g and for an average Indian woman weighing 50 kg will be 50 g.

Minerals: The recommended allowance of calcium for both men and women is 400 mg. The iron requirement is 30 mg for women and 28 mg for men. The women normally lose up to 2 mg of iron per day in the menstrual blood and thus iron deficiency anemia is more common among women.

Vitamins: Recommended allowances of vitamin A, ascorbic acid, folic acid and vitamin B_{12} are the same as for normal adult men and women, i.e. 600 μg of vitamin A in form of retinol or 2,400 μg in the form of B carotene; 40 mg of ascorbic acid; 100 μg of folic acid and 1μg of vitamin B_{12}. Thiamine, riboflavin and niacin requirements vary according to the energy requirements. For men, thiamine requirement varies from 1.2 to 1.6 mg/day for women 0.9–1.2 mg/day. Riboflavin for men varies from 1.4 to 1.9 mg/day and for women 1.2–1.5 mg/day. There is no variation in the requirement of vitamin D, which is 200 IU for all the age groups.

Factors

Factors to be kept in mind while planning diets:

1. The diet should be nutritionally balanced. Emphasis should be that each meal is nutritionally balanced. The day's nutritional needs of the individual should be divided almost equally in the three main meals, i.e. breakfast, lunch and dinner.
2. In case of persons going to office a nutritious, well-balanced, attractive and easy to carry packed lunch must be provided.
3. Careful attention should be given to the amount and type of fat to be included in the diet so as to reduce risk of hypertension/high blood pressure (BP) and heart diseases.
4. Traditions, customs and religious attitude of the person should be considered.
5. His/her likes and dislikes should be taken into consideration. If, however, a particular group is not liked, then its form can be, e.g. instead of milk, curds, paneer, custard, etc. may be given.
6. Variety in the food is a must, it should be provided in terms of color, texture and flavor.
7. The diet should be planned according to the socioeconomic status of the person. Selection of the foodstuffs should be such that they are purchased within the budget. If expensive foods cannot be afforded, then emphasis should be on cheap, yet, nutritious foodstuffs, e.g. peanuts, green leafy vegetables, etc.

8. Availability of time and energy of the person should be considered. If the plan is for a working woman/wife, then elaborate cooking can be avoided.
9. The planned menu should be according to the season. Seasonal vegetables and fruits should be selected as they are tastier, nutritious, cheaper and easily available. Seasonal drinks may be included to make the plan interesting.
10. The diet should be planned such that provides us sufficient satiety value. Adequate amounts of raw fruits and vegetable should be included to provide sufficient dietary fiber.
11. Meals should be served in a pleasant atmosphere.

Elderly

The process of aging brings about some physiological, psychological and immunological changes, which influence the nutritional requirements. There is a decrease in the water content and the lean body mass is accompanied by an increasing proportion of body fat. By 80, it is estimated that half of the muscle cell remain. There is a decrease in the number of functioning parenchymal cells. Such changes are particularly evident in tissues without generation capacity, such as brain, cartilage, heart, kidney and skeletal muscles. Specific functioning cells are replaced in part by non-specific fat and connective tissues. With time there is a decline in the number of functioning cells of various organs, so that their performance is reduced. Demineralization of bone has been observed commonly in aged persons. This condition is known as osteoporosis.

The sense of taste and smell are less acute in later years, so that some of the pleasure derived from food is lost. Loss of teeth due to increased decay of teeth and gums is common in aged persons. Consequently, these individuals eat more soft and carbohydrate rich foods that fail to provide adequate intake of essential nutrients such as calcium, proteins and vitamins.

Decreased secretion of saliva and decreased ability to digest starch has been observed in elderly. Gastric acidity decreases in a large percentage of old people. Peptic, tryptic, amylolytic and lipolytic activities of the digestive secretions are decreased.

The stomach empties rapidly in persons having hypoacidity of the stomach contents. Due to reduced mobility of gastrointestinal tract, there is more likelihood of abdominal distention from certain foods. Due to lesser cardiovascular sufficiency, digestion, absorption and distribution of nutrients are retarded.

Nutritional Requirements

Data regarding the nutritional requirements is given in Table 29.2. From 25 years of age the basal metabolism decreases about 2% for each decade. The decline in the basal metabolism is less in person who remains healthy and pursues vigorous activity in their later years. The lower metabolic rate and reduced activity in elderly stage reduces the energy requirement.

Table 29.2: Nutritional requirements for women

Nutrients	Indian reference women (sedentary work)	Pregnancy (second half)	Lactation
Calorie	1,875	+ 300	+ 550
Protein (g)	50	+ 15	+ 25
Calcium (mg)	400–500	1,000	1,000
Iron (mg)	30	38	38
Vitamin A (µg)	600	600	600
Vitamin D (µg)	2.5	10	10
Thiamine (mg/1,000 cal)	0.5	0.5	0.5
Riboflavin (mg/1,000 cal)	0.6	0.6	0.6
Niacin (mg/1,000 cal)	6.6	6.6	6.6
Ascorbic acid (mg/1,000 cal)	40	40	80
Folic acid (µg)	100	400	400
Vitamin B_{12} (µg)	1	1	1

Energy: The energy (calorie) intake should be adjusted to maintain the body weight constant in case of old people with normal body weight. In case of obese people, the calorie intake should be adjusted to reduce the body weight gradually to about normal level. In view of the tendency to eat less as a result of decreased appetite and poor digestive capacity, old people are likely to consume less protein and suffer from protein deficiency.

Proteins: Adequate intake of protein should be ensured. Since milk is a good source of protein besides vitamins and minerals, adequate quantities of milk should be consumed. The daily protein intake should be at least 1.0–1.4 g/kg body weight.

Fats: The diet should contain at least 50 g fats, as it is a concentrated source of energy. Half of this quantity should be in the form of vegetable oils, which are rich in EFAs.

Calcium and iron: Deficiencies occur frequently as absorption of these nutrients is less efficient than in normal adults. The calcium intake should not be less than 0.5 g and the iron intake is 28 mg. Since even mild anemia affects the health of old people due to less efficient circulation of blood, iron intake should be adequate to prevent anemia.

Vitamins: Mild deficiencies of several vitamins occur frequently among old people. It is, therefore, essential to ensure adequate intakes of all essential vitamins. If the diet consumed does not contain adequate amounts of all vitamins, a multivitamin tablet providing the daily requirements of different vitamins should be taken daily. Requirements of thiamine, riboflavin and niacin are based on energy requirements. Ascorbic acid requirement is 40 mg, folic acid, vitamin B_{12} and vitamin B_6 are required about 100 µg, 1.0 µg and 2.0 mg respectively. It is essential to include 400 IU of vitamin D daily as it will help in the absorption of calcium to prevent osteoporosis.

Fluids: The importance of adequate fluid intake so as to maintain the volume of urine excreted at a minimum of 1.5 L is not generally recognized. Water can be consumed as such or in the form of butter milk, fruit juices, porridge, soups, etc. during summer season. Adequate intake of soft unavoidable carbohydrate (roughage) in the form of non-fibrous vegetables and fruits should be ensured to avoid constipation. The senile intestinal mucosa does not tolerate fiber from mature vegetables and bran of cereals.

Factors

Factors to be kept in mind while planning diets:
1. The diet should be a nutritionally balanced and emphasis should be given on the adequate intake of protein, calcium, vitamin and fiber, which are liable to be deficient in most cases.
2. Since chewing may be a problem, the meals prepared should be soft and one or two liquid items may be given such as soup, dal or gruel so that swallowing becomes easy, salads can be grated. As such the food should be well-cooked. Chapati can be made thicker if chewing is a problem and if needed, they may be soaked in milk, soup or other liquid preparation.
3. An adequate intake of calcium should be ensured to compensate for its losses due to gradual demineralization of bones associated with aging.
4. With the advancement of age the capacity to digest and tolerate large meals offend decreases. Therefore, the quantity of food given at a time needs to be decreased. The number of meals may be increased as per individual's tolerance.
5. Soft unavoidable carbohydrates should be included in the diet to avoid constipation.
6. Excess consumption of sweet rich desserts should be cut to a minimum as they provide empty calories, but take away the appetite.
7. Calorie intake should be adjusted to keep the body weight constant in case of normal old people.
8. For poor appetite low bulk, concentrated calorie food, prepared and served in an appetizing way should be planned. These people may be given midmorning or mid afternoon snack.
9. Factors such as likes and dislikes, special needs, fear of new foods, food prejudices, lack of money, poor appetite should be given.

Nutrition in Pregnancy

Pregnancy and lactation are normal physiological processes. During pregnancy fetus draws its nourishments from the mother's diet. This increases the requirement of proteins, vitamins and minerals of the mother, as her body stores are used by the fetus (refer Table 29.2).

During the I trimester of pregnancy, the food intake is generally lowered, because of nausea and vomiting (morning sickness). During this period, frequent small easily digestible foods including fresh fruits, fruit juices and vegetables should be given.

Energy

The increase in calories trimester wise is as follows:
- I trimester 10 kcal/day
- II trimester 90 kcal/day
- III trimester 200 kcal/day.

The increase in energy is to support the growth of the fetus, placenta and maternal tissue, and for the increase in basal metabolic rate due to additional work of the growing fetus and the increase in maternal size.

Proteins

The normal protein requirement of an adult is 50 g/day. ICMR has increased the requirement during pregnancy by 15 g/day. The additional protein is for:
1. The transfer of amino acids from the mother to fetus.
2. Rapid growth of the fetus.
3. Formation of amniotic fluid and storage reserves during delivery, labor and lactation.
4. The enlargement of the uterus, placenta and mammary glands.
5. For increase in maternal circulating blood volume and subsequent demand for increased plasma protein.

Vitamins

Anemia due to B_{12} deficiency during pregnancy is not very common. Milk, fruits and vegetables can supply all necessary vitamins. Thus, when a good balanced diet is given, there is no need for vitamin supplements.

There is increased use for vitamin D to enhance the maternal calcium absorption and calcium metabolism in the fetus.

Vitamin K is of vital importance for the synthesis of prothrombin, which is necessary for normal coagulation of blood for preventing neonatal hemorrhage.

The water-soluble vitamins B complex and vitamin C must be supplied in adequate amounts. There is an increased requirement of folic acid for promoting fetal growth and to prevent macrocytic anemia during pregnancy. Deficiency of iron puts additional stress on folate metabolism.

Minerals

An increased intake of calcium by mother is very essential not only for the calcification of fetal bones but also for protection of calcium reserves of the mother to meet the large demands during lactation. Use of vitamin D and calcium supplements reduce muscular cramps during pregnancy.

Iron

During pregnancy, there is also an increased requirement of iron due to the following:
1. Iron is necessary for the growth of fetus and placenta.
2. It is necessary for the promotion of hemoglobin as there is 40%–50% increase in the maternal blood volume.
3. To replace the maternal iron losses.
4. To achieve high levels of hemoglobin in the infants, this is stored in the liver for 3–6 months. Iron must be transfused to uterus of the mother during gestation.

Fats

Fats must be provided according to the normal requirements.

Nutritional Requirements During Lactation

Milk is secreted by the mother for feeding the baby. Therefore, during lactation nutritional requirements are increased.

Calories

Mother requires total amount of about 13,000 kcal during lactation period of 6 months. Mother needs additional 700–750 kcal daily to convert food energy into milk.

Proteins

Daily milk produced is about 850–1,000 mL during lactation. Human milk contains about 1% protein and thus there is daily excretion of 8–10 g of protein. Therefore, lactating woman should take about 20–25 g of extra protein daily. In vegetarians 2–3 cups of milk and milk products will supply this need.

Non-vegetarians should take one average helping of either meat, chicken, egg or fish daily. In addition, two cups of milk should also be taken as extra.

▶ CONCLUSION

The role of nurse has changed with the current preventive healthcare focus and emphasis upon wellness and with the expanding responsibilities the nurses are assuring in the care of their patients in the hospitals as well as in primary health care centers. The nurse must follow an epidemiologic approach while taking numerical histories and developing care plans for patients and family with nutritional inadequacies.

Chapter 30

Nutritional Problems and Policies

▶ INTRODUCTION

Only a small portion of India's population is able to achieve balanced and nutritious food, the remaining population is suffering from malnutrition. Higher-income group faces ailments caused by overnutritious diet, while lower-income group has to suffer from the problems caused by undernutrition. Major reasons of higher maternal mortality rate are malnutrition and anemia. Malnutrition is the main cause of improper growth and development in 90% of school going children.

▶ FACTORS AFFECTING NUTRITIONAL STATUS

Factors that affect nutritional status are given in Figure 30.1.

Nutritional problems can be divided into two groups:
1. Susceptibility of individuals.
2. Environmental factors.

Susceptibility of Individuals

If we take a group of people, some individuals may be more susceptible to malnutrition than others. The vulnerable groups include infants and preschool children, pregnant women, the elderly and the sick. During these stages, the nutritional demands are tremendously increased or need special attention (Fig. 30.2).

Environmental Factors

Poverty and ignorance are the leading causes of malnutrition throughout the world. Lack of available food is the main cause

CHAPTER 30: Nutritional Problems and Policies

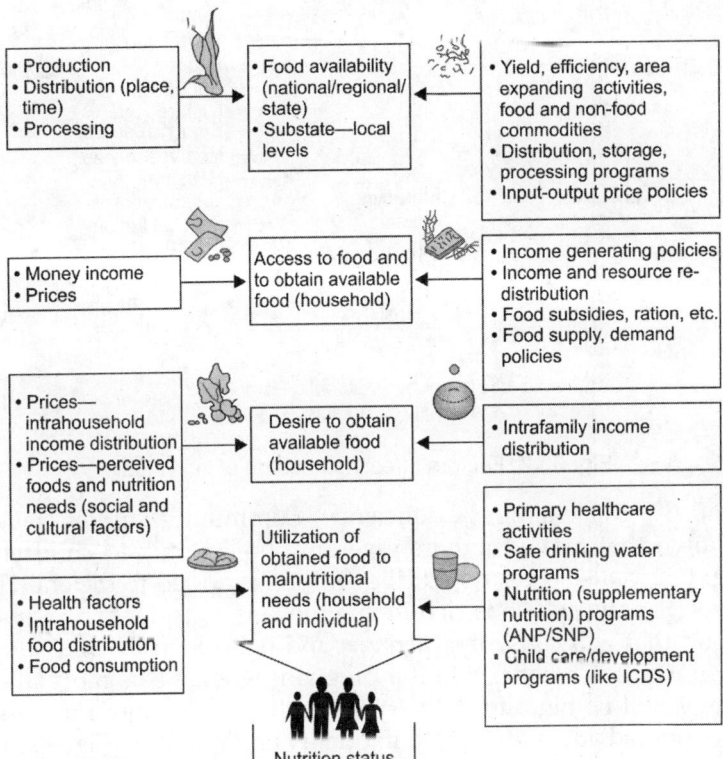

Fig. 30.1: Factors affecting the nutritional status (ANP, applied nutrition program; ICDS, Integrated Child Development Service; SNP, special nutrition program)

of malnutrition in the underdeveloped and developing countries. Other environmental factors include population explosion, insufficient food production, unequal distribution of food, urbanization, cultural factors, lack of education, misinformation and faddism.

▶ STEPS TO SOLVE NUTRITIONAL PROBLEMS

Common Nutritional Problem

A survey in South India has revealed that about 1% children aged 1–5 years showed signs of kwashiorkor, 2% marasmus

SECTION 4: Community Nutrition

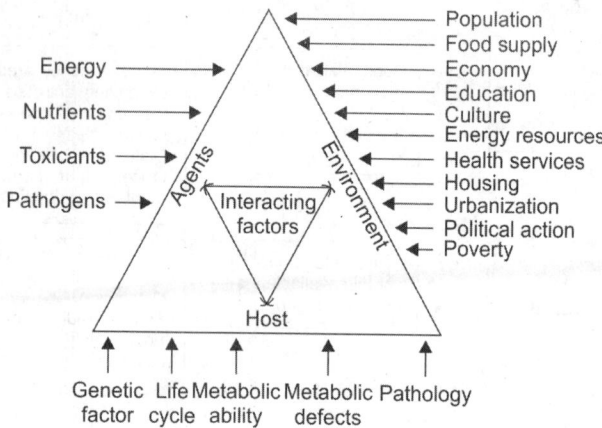

Fig. 30.2: Factors affecting nutrition of individual

and 3%–5% vitamin A deficiency. Community studies have shown that many mothers give only breast milk to children up to 2 years. Thus, no additional food is added to the child's diet. Papaya, which is rich in vitamin A is considered as a hot food that will cause miscarriage, and is avoided by pregnant women. It is a belief that if a pregnant woman eats more, the baby will be big and delivery difficult, so expectant mothers are not fed adequately both in quality and quantity (Fig. 30.3).

▶ NUTRITIONAL DEFICIENCY

Nutritional deficiencies can be broadly classified in two major categories:
1. Macronutrient deficiencies.
2. Micronutrient deficiencies.

Macronutrient Deficiencies

Protein-energy Malnutrition

Protein-energy malnutrition (PEM) is caused due to the deficiency of protein and energy in the diet, and is the most important nutritional deficiency of public health concern. It can affect people of different age groups, especially children.

CHAPTER 30: Nutritional Problems and Policies

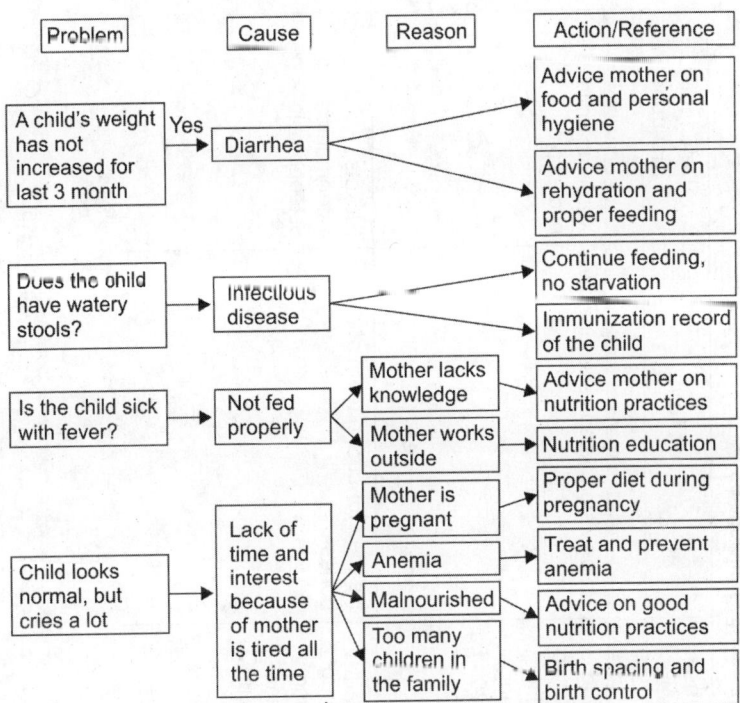

Fig. 30.3: Steps to solve nutritional problems

Forms of PEM: The PEM has two forms, kwashiorkor and marasmus. They are the two facets of the same disease and the third one is the mixed PEM, where the symptoms of kwashiorkor and marasmus both are observed at the same time (Table 30.1).

Kwashiorkor

It was discovered by Dr Cicely Williams in the 1930s and called 'kwashiorkor'. This is 'the disease, the deposed baby gets when the next one is born'. Normally, in developing countries they are breastfed for almost 2 years or may be longer. After the arrival of the new baby, the older child is put on high-carbohydrate and low-protein diet. The symptom start becoming evident in 3–4 months after the child has been weaned. It occurs mostly in the age group of 1–3 years.

Table 30.1: Vitamin deficiencies

Name	Sources	Recommended daily allowance	Functions	Deficiency diseases
Fat-soluble vitamins				
Retinal (vitamin A)	Fish liver oils, butter, milk, kidneys and muscles of meat; beta carotene is present in yellow fruits and leafy green vegetables	Adults: 750 µg Children: 300 µg Women during pregnancy and lactation: 1,200 µg	Helps vision, keeps skin healthy	Xerophthalmia, nyctalopia
Cholecalciferol 'sunshine' vitamin (vitamin D)	Eggs, butter, fatty fish, fish liver oils; human exposed year round to bright sunlight, do not require dietary vitamin D	Adult: 5 µg Children: 10 µg Women during pregnancy and lactation: 10 µg	Needed for strong teeth and bones	Rickets, osteomalacia, osteoporosis

Contd...

Contd...

Name	Sources	Recommended daily allowance	Functions	Deficiency diseases
Tocopherol (vitamin E)	Green leafy vegetables—spinach cabbage, alfalfa, putrefied fish meal, liver, eggs and cheese	Male: 15 IU Female: 12 IU	Keeps skin and RBCs healthy; antioxidant prevents oxidation of vitamin A and unsaturated fatty acids	Muscular weakness, creatinuria and fragile RBCs
Coagulation vitamin (vitamin K)	Green leafy vegetables—spinach, cabbage, alfalfa putrefied fish meal, fish liver oils, liver, eggs and cheese	Adult: 50–100 µg Children: 1 µg/kg	Needed for blood clotting; Essential for the synthesis of clotting factors including prothrombin by liver	Retarded/Delayed blood clotting

Contd...

Contd...

Name	Sources	Recommended daily allowance	Functions	Deficiency diseases
Water-soluble vitamin				
B complex vitamin Thiamine (vitamin B_1)	Lean meats, legumes and whole grains	1–15 mg/day	Needed for healthy nerves	Beriberi, a disorder of the nervous system with dependent edema involving the trunk and extremities
Riboflavin (vitamin B_2)	Liver, dried yeast, egg, whole milk, milk powder, fish, whole cereals, legumes and green leafy vegetables	Adult: 1.5 mg During pregnancy and lactation: 1.72 mg	Yellow crystalline compound helps cells use energy in foods FMN and FAD are coenzymes required for oxidation reaction in metabolism	Inflammation and breakdown of tissue around the mouth, tongue and nose, wound healing is impaired

Contd...

Contd...

Name	Sources	Recommended daily allowance	Functions	Deficiency diseases
Niacin, formerly known as nicotinic acid (vitamin B_3)	Liver, kidney, heart, yeast, peanuts and wheat germ, amino acid tryptophan can supply much of body's need of niacin	Adult: 20 mg Pregnancy: 22 mg Lactation: 25 mg	Helps cells use energy in food; niacinamide along with thiamine and riboflavin, serves as a coenzyme in tissue oxidation; it functions in the mitochondria in the form of NAD^+ and $NADP^+$	Pellagra, a disorder of the nervous system and skin rashes and glossitis
Folic acid (vitamin B_3)	Liver, kidney and fresh leafy vegetables, cauliflower	Male: 200 µg Female: 180 µg	In reactions involving transfer of methyl groups as in the synthesis of hemoglobin, nucleic acids and methionine	Megaloblastic anemia and gastrointestinal disturbances
Biotin (vitamin B_7)	Liver, egg yolk, kidney, yeast and milk	200–300 µg	As a coenzyme for carboxylation reactions in the formation of fatty acids	Delay dermatitis, muscle pains, nausea and depression

Co.ntd...

Contd...

Name	Sources	Recommended daily allowance	Functions	Deficiency diseases
Pyridoxine (vitamin B_6)	Yeast, liver, egg yolk and the germs of the various grains and seeds, less in milk and leafy vegetables	Male: 2–0 mg Female: 1.6 mg	Pyridoxal phosphate and pyridoxamine serve as coenzymes for decarboxylation of amino acids; takes part in the reactions occurring in gray matter of the CNS. Pyridoxine is involved in the absorption of zinc by the intestine	Epileptic seizures
Pantothenic acid (vitamin B_5)	Egg yolk, yeast, kidney lean meats, skimmed milk, sweet potatoes and molasses	4–7 mg	One of the constituents of coenzyme A (CoA), which is involved in the metabolism of carbohydrates, fats and proteins, and in the synthesis of cholesterol	Normally there is no deficiency as the RDA is easily met with an ordinary diet

Contd...

Contd...

Name	Sources	Recommended daily allowance	Functions	Deficiency diseases
Cobalamin (antipernicious anemia factor) (vitamin B_{12})	Liver, kidney, fish, eggs, milk, oysters and clams, it contains the element cobalt (4.35%)	20 µg	In the transfer of methyl groups, maintenance of the myelin sheath, synthesis of nucleic acids and hemoglobin, and metabolism of carbohydrates and lipids	Pernicious anemia, similar to folic acid deficiency
Ascorbic acid (vitamin C)	Amla, guava gooseberry, orange, lemons lime, papaya, tomatoes, green chilies, green leafy vegetables	50 g/day	Tissue healing increased, resistance to infection, antioxidant	Scurvy, poor wound healing, bleeding gums, mucous membranes, loose teeth

Symptoms

1. **Edema:** It may be slight or gross depends partially on the amount of salt and water and the diet. It may be on the whole body including the face, but mostly on the lower limbs.
2. **Growth failure:** It is the initial symptom. The weight of the child with kwashiorkor will be less as compared to their normal years. Sometimes the edema may mask the actual weight and show relatively higher weight. The weight of the child may be less than 80% of the normal weight for age.
3. **Mental changes:** This could be the most serious consequence of PEM. Mental development may be arrested. The child may lose interest, become irritable and apathetic, and prefer to stay in one position.
4. **Hair changes:** The hair becomes sparse, soft and thin, it loses its healthy sheen. Negro children lose their characteristic curl. There might be pigmentation with diffused patches. These changes are often observed in Negro than in Asian children. Hair may be easily plucked with no pain at all.
5. **Skin changes:** Dermatosis is often observed in many cases. Initially the skin becomes thick as if varnished then it peels off and looks like 'flaky paint,' which leaves bleeding patches or cause shallow ulceration. In severe cases, desquamated part of the child's body resembles burns. Usually lower limbs, buttocks and perineum are most affected, but the ulceration can also appear over pressure points and deep cracks in skin folds.
6. **Moon face:** Edema causes moon face. The cheeks may be swollen due to accumulation of fluid and fatty tissue.
7. **Micronutrient deficiency:** Minerals and vitamin deficiencies are quite common in PEM. Some degree of anemia is commonly encountered. Vitamin A deficiency is common in kwashiorkor. Vitamin B complex deficiency is also seen in many cases.
8. **Fluid and electrolyte imbalance:** The presence of edema explains this symptom. The extracellular fluid volume increases in PEM.

9. **Infection:** In the presence of infections such as measles, gastroenteritis or some other infection, the prekwashiorkor child rapidly advances to kwashiorkor. There may be lower respiratory tract infection besides diarrhea or dysentery.

Nutritional marasmus

The age of the children plays an important role in determining, whether severe PEM is nutritional marasmus or kwashiorkor. Marasmus mostly develops in children up to 2 years. This could occur either due to failure of breastfeeding or not carried on for long enough time and suitable weaning foods were not available or the cultural feeding practices did not allow them.

Symptoms
1. **Severe growth retardation:** The child looks dry and shrunken, and there is little or no subcutaneous fat in the body. The weight of the child is much below the normal for age. If the disease continues for a long period of time, the length of the child will be less. The weight of marasmic children may be generally below 60% of the normal standard.
2. **Extreme emaciation:** Muscles are weak and lack of subcutaneous fat makes the child look as skin and bone. The characteristic features include old man's or monkey face, lose and hanging skin folds, especially over the buttocks.
3. **Absolute weakness:** Marasmic child may have no strength or may be so weak that they do not have the energy to even cry.
4. Unlike kwashiorkor, edema is absent.
5. There are no skin and hair changes.

Causes
1. Inadequate supply of breast milk to meet the nutritional requirements of the infant.
2. Breastfeeding is not accompanied by supplementary foods after the age of 6 months.
3. Inadequate infant formulas may have substituted for breastfeeding. Because the commercial infant formulas are expensive, they may be diluted and prepared in unsanitary

conditions; with the result, they provide neither sufficient calories nor proteins to meet the infant's needs.
4. Lack of knowledge and ignorance play an important role in the development of the disease.

Marasmic-kwashiorkor

In areas where PEM is common, the patients show the symptoms of both marasmus and kwashiorkor. In this condition, the marasmic child may develop edema and kwashiorkor child loses edema. The symptoms of marasmic-kwashiorkor include extreme muscle wasting, 'skin and bones' appearance loose and hanging skin, edema, weakness and old man's or monkey's face appearance.

Prevention and treatment of PEM: These are as follows:
1. Maintain a growth chart at home. Due to lack of knowledge, most mothers are unable to recognize the changes. Regular monitoring of weight helps detect the malnutrition and the seriousness of the disease may be reduced.
2. Use of oral rehydration therapy helps prevent dehydration caused by diarrhea. The rehydration solutions can be prepared at home by adding sugar and salt and water. It can be given at home and the child can be saved from dehydration.
3. Breastfeeding must be encouraged. It must be done exclusively for 6 months and thereafter, supplementary foods may be introduced along with breastfeeds. These foods must be prepared in sanitary conditions to avoid any infection.
4. Infants and children must be immunized at prescribed age.

Micronutrient Deficiencies

Micronutrient deficiency such as vitamin A, iron and iodine affect a large population. Although these are required in small amounts, these play crucial role in normal metabolism as well as other body functions; micronutrient deficiencies commonly encountered among Indian population are vitamin A deficiencies; iron deficiency anemia (IDA), iodine deficiency disorder and zinc deficiency (Table 30.2).

CHAPTER 30: Nutritional Problems and Policies

Table 30.2: Mineral deficiencies

Elements	Metabolic functions	Deficiency manifestations
Macrominerals or trace elements		
Sodium	Principal extracellular cation, buffer constituent, water and acid-base balance, cell membrane permeability	Dehydration, acidosis, excess leads to edema and hypertension
Potassium	Principal intracellular cation, buffer constituent, water and acid-base balance, neuromuscular irritability	Muscle weakness, paralysis and mental confusion, acidosis
Chloride	Principal extracellular anion electrolyte, osmotic balance and acid-base balance, gastric HCl formation	Deficiency secondary to vomiting and diarrhea
Calcium	Constituent of bone and teeth, blood clotting, regulation of nerve, muscle and hormone function	Tetany, muscle cramps, convulsions, osteoporosis, rickets
Phosphorus	Constituent of bone and teeth, nucleic acids and NAD, FAD ATP, etc. required for energy metabolism	Growth retardation skeletal deformities, muscle weakness, cardiac arrhythmia
Magnesium	Cofactor for phosphate transferring enzymes, constituent of bones and teeth, muscle contraction, nerve transmission	Muscle spasms, tetany, confusions, osteoporosis, rickets
Sulfur	Constituent of proteins, bile acid, glycosaminoglycans, vitamins like thiamine, lipoic acid, involved in detoxification reactions	Unknown
Microminerals or trace elements		
Chromium	Potentiate the effect of insulin	Impaired glucose metabolism

Contd...

Contd...

Elements	Metabolic functions	Deficiency manifestations
Cobalt	Constituent of vitamin B_{12}	Macrocytic anemia
Copper	Constituent of oxidase enzymes, e.g. tyrosinase, cytochrome oxidase, ferroxidase and ceruloplasmin, iron absorption and mobilization	Microcytic hypochromic anemia, depigmentation of skin, hair Excessive deposition in liver in Wilson's disease
Fluoride	Constituent of bone and teeth, strengthens bone and teeth	Dental caries
Iodine	Constituent of thyroid hormones (T_3 and T_4).	Microcytic anemia
Manganese	Cofactor for number of enzymes, e.g. arginase, carboxylase, kinases, etc.	Not well-defined
Molybdenum	Constituent of xanthine oxidase, sulfite oxidase and aldehyde oxidase	Xanthinuria
Selenium	Antioxidant, cofactor for glutathione peroxidase, protects cell against membrane lipid peroxidation	Cardiomyopathy
Zinc	Cofactor for enzymes in DNA, RNA and protein synthesis, constituent of insulin, carbonic anhydrase, carboxypeptidase, LDA, alcohol dehydrogenase, alkaline phosphatase, etc.	Growth failure, impaired wound healing defects in taste and smell, loss of appetite

Iron-deficiency Anemia

Iron-deficiency anemia is widespread throughout the world. It is the most common micronutrient deficiency both in developed and developing countries. It is the second most prevalent nutritional deficiency in the world after protein-energy deficiency. IDA generally occurs in preschool children, adolescents

CHAPTER 30: Nutritional Problems and Policies

and women of childbearing age. It is also seen in people of low-economic status.

Anemia is a condition in which there is reduced total circulating hemoglobin. Due to this oxygen carrying capacity of the blood is diminished. Anemia is diagnosed, when the hemoglobin level is below 12 mg/dL in adult women and below 13 mg/dL in adult men. Anemia is mostly caused due to iron deficiency, but other causes are folate, vitamin B_{12} and protein deficiency.

Causes

1. Deficient intake of iron in the diet during the stages of increased demand:
   a. Infancy-blood volume rapidly expands.
   b. Adolescence—rapid growth spurt and onset of menses in girls.
   c. During pregnancy and lactation.
2. Impaired absorption of iron:
   a. As in celiac disease, diarrhea and pellagra.
   b. Reduced acid medium in the stomach.
   c. Antacid therapy in chronic renal disease neutralizes the acid content.
3. Blood loss:
   a. Due to accidental bleeding.
   b. Chronic disease such as peptic ulcer, tuberculosis, hiatal hernia and bleeding piles.
   c. Heavy menstrual losses.
   d. Too frequent blood donation.
   e. Presence of parasites.
4. Nutritional deficiency:
   a. Severe protein depletion.
   b. Protein-energy malnutrition.
   c. Poverty and ignorance.

Symptoms

1. Paleness of conjunctiva, tongue and soft palate due to reduced hemoglobin level.

2. Breathlessness because of oxygen-carrying capacity of hemoglobin is reduced.
3. Finger nails become thin and bend upward 'spoon shaped', which is known as 'koilonychia'.
4. In severe anemia, especially in pregnancy swelling of feet occurs.

Treatment

The primary emphasis for the treatment of IDA is on the supplements of iron salts, such as fersolate, ferrous sulfate, gluconate or fumarate. Initially some people find difficult to tolerate the supplement due to its side effects, but gradually become adjusted to it. Therefore, it is advised to take the medication after meals.

The IDA can be prevented by supplementation to vulnerable groups, fortification of food, dietary modification, nutrition education and proper healthcare facilities.

Zinc Deficiency

Zinc deficiency is frequently seen in preschool children in developing countries. Prolonged diarrheal conditions are the important causes of growth retardation and death. This condition is mostly associated with zinc deficiency.

Functions

1. It is an integral part of many enzymes, which belong to a large group known as metalloenzymes, such as carbonic anhydrase, lactic dehydrogenase, alkaline phosphatase, carboxypeptidase, aminopeptidase and so on.
2. It acts as a cofactor in the synthesis of DNA and RNA.
3. It mobilizes vitamin A from the liver to maintain normal levels.
4. It enhances the action of follicle-stimulating hormone and luteinizing hormone.
5. It is essential for normal immune functions.
6. Helps in the stabilization of membrane structure.

7. It is essential for spermatogenesis and normal testicular functions.

Clinical problems

Several clinical manifestations associated with zinc deficiency include growth retardation, hypogonadism in males, poor appetite, mental lethargy, delayed wound healing, increased susceptibility to infections, skin lesions, loss of hair, altered taste and smell, hypogeusia and dysgeusia. Zinc deficiency can occur in several disease conditions such as malabsorption, kidney disease, pancreatic insufficiency, sickle cell anemia, inflammatory bowel disease and chronic liver disease.

The severity of zinc deficiency varies at different ages:

1. **Infants:** Diarrhea is quite prominent in infants up to 2 months of age. Zinc deficiency in early stages of life leads to cognitive function impairment, behavioral changes, mood changes and memory impairment.
2. **Preschool children:** Frequent skin problems are observed, but mood changes, gastrointestinal disturbances and anorexia becomes less frequent as the child grows
3. **School-going children:** Hair loss (alopecia), growth retardation, inflammation of eyelids and conjunctiva, and frequent infection are commonly seen in school-going children.
4. **Elderly:** Older persons with chronic illness in aging and non-healing ulcers are particularly vulnerable to zinc deficiency. As a result, they often suffer from recurrent infections due to reduced immune function.
5. **Pregnancy:** Zinc deficiency during pregnancy may lead to intrauterine growth retardation—low birth weight, poor fetal neurobehavioral development and increased neonatal morbidity. The infant may be delivered preterm and the mother may develop pregnancy-induced hypertension.

Sources of zinc

1. Highest concentration in animal foods, such as organ meats, flesh of beef, pork, poultry, fish and shellfish.
2. Relatively high concentration in nuts, seeds, legumes and whole grain cereals.

3. Lesser amounts in eggs, milk and milk products.
4. Lower in tubers, refined cereals, fruits and vegetables.

Deficiency

Zinc deficiency is not of a public health concern; however, some experts in the field suggest the supplementation of zinc especially to children.

▶ NATIONAL NUTRITIONAL POLICY

Severity of Nutritional Problems

Nutrition affects growth and development of the person. There is a wide gap in food production and food consumption. Severity of nutrition problem can be predicted from the following estimates:

1. Approximately 27% of the population is still living below poverty line.
2. As many as 46% children below 3 years of age suffer from underweight.
3. About 38% of these children are stunted and 19% are wasted.
4. Majority of rural and tribal children below 5 years of age suffer from malnutrition.
5. Roughly 79% under 3 years children and almost 58% of the expectant mothers in the third trimester of pregnancy suffer from anemia as reported in National Family and Health Survey (NFHS-III), which is higher than previous findings in NFHS-II.
6. Anemia in men was 24% (NFHS-III).
7. Nutritional blindness affects children in India 7 million/year results mainly from the deficiency of vitamin A, couples with PEM. Prevalence of conjunctival xerosis and Bitot's spot was observed as high as 7.8% among slum children, followed by industrial labor (6.3%).
8. Prevalence of low-birth-weight babies in India ranged between 26% and 57% in the urban slums and 35% and 41% in rural areas.

CHAPTER 30: Nutritional Problems and Policies

9. In large parts of India, the rainy months are the worst months for the rural and landless poor. There are regions in the country, which are almost every year affected by famines, droughts and floods.
10. About 33% of the women and 28% of the men suffer from low body mass index (BMI).
11. There is a problem of overnutrition in certain areas and certain groups of people in the country, which have a serious health effects. About 15% of the women and 12% of the men were obese (NFHS-III).
12. Almost universal deficiency of zinc in pregnant mothers in developing countries (Caulfield et al 1998).

Policy Goals

The National Nutrition Policy was adopted in 1993 with the following goals:

1. Reduction in the incidence of moderate and severe malnutrition and stunted growth among children.
2. Reduction in the incidence of low birth weight to less than 10%.
3. Elimination of blindness due to vitamin A deficiency.
4. Reduction in the iron deficiency anemia among pregnant women to 25%.
5. Universal iodization of salt for reduction of iodine deficiency disorders to below the endemic level.
6. Special emphasis to geriatric nutrition.
7. Annual production of 250 million tons of food grain.
8. Improving household food security through poverty alleviation programs.
9. Promoting appropriate diets and healthy lifestyle. 'Malnutrition Free India' is the vision for National Nutrition Policy for the next decade as visioned by 11th Plan.

Interventions

Direct Intervention (Short Term)

1. Nutrition intervention for special vulnerable groups: Program for 0–6 year children, mothers and adolescent girls, e.g. Integrated Child Development Service (ICDS).
2. Fortification of essential foods: Salt with iodine and/or iron, bread with iron, vitamin A and fat with vitamin A.
3. Popularization of low cost nutritious food.
4. Control of micronutrient deficiency amongst vulnerable groups, e.g. Vitamin A Prophylaxis Program, National Nutritional Anemia Prophylaxis Program.

Indirect Policy Instruments

Long-term institutional and structural changes are:

1. Food security: To ensure aggregate food security and availability of 215 kg/capita/year of food grains need to be attained.
2. Improvement of dietary pattern through production and demonstration.
3. Policies for effecting income transfers, so as to improve the entitlement package of the rural and urban poor.
4. Improving the purchasing power, e.g. Integrated Rural Development Program (IRDP), Jawahar Rozgar Yojana, Nehru Rozgar Yojana and Development of Women and Children in Rural Area (DWCRA), where 100 days job to laborers are provided.
5. Public distribution system.
6. Land reforms.
7. Health and Family Welfare, e.g. 'Health for All by 2000 AD' Program.
8. Basic health and nutrition knowledge.
9. Prevention of food adulteration.
10. Nutrition surveillance: National Nutrition Monitoring Bureau (NNMB) and National Institute of Nutrition (NIN) will be responsible for nutritional surveillance.

11. Monitoring of nutrition programs.
12. Research.
13. Equal remuneration.
14. Communication: Department of Women and Child Development have well-established communication division and Ministry of Information and Broadcasting have been involved.
15. Minimum wage administration.
16. Community and participation.
17. Education and literacy.
18. Improvement of the status of women.
19. Intersectoral coordination.

This policy have been implemented and administered by several ministries and departments of the Government of India and governmental and non-governmental organizations (NGOs). A National Plan of Action on Nutrition (NPAN) was formulated in 1995 with sectoral commitments to be undertaken by 14 nutrition-related ministries and departments, viz. agriculture, food production, civil supplies, public distribution, education, forestry, information and broadcasting, health and family welfare, labor, rural development, urban development, women and child development, etc. There is an Interministerial Coordination Committee, a National Nutrition Council for policy coordination, review and direction at the national level. Nutrition situation has been monitored by NIN, National Institute of Health and Family Welfare, Central Health Education Bureau and other agencies and NGOs. The Department of Women and Child Development, is the nodal agency, responsible for implementation of the National Nutrition Policy.

National Nutrition Mission (NNM), which has been set up in 2002, with an overall responsibilities of eliminating/reducing both macro- and micro-nutritional deficiencies in the country. As part of the efforts of NNM, a new program to combat undernutrition among adolescent girls and expectant and nursing mothers is being launched by the Department of Women and Child Development on pilot basis during 2002–2003—covering two most backward district in each of the major states and most populous districts in rest of the smaller states. Under this pilot program, food grains are supplied free of cost through targeted public distribution system (PDS) directly to identified families with under/malnourished persons (Planning Commission, 2002). Under this mission all the department must work forward to meet the goal of the policy in the next decade.

Constraints of National Nutrition Policy

1. Malnutrition is still to be focused as a national problem.
2. Nutrition neither have the status of a separate ministry nor even a department and all existing departments have their own mandates.
3. Nutrition is not seen as an explicit goal by the concerned sectors.
4. Nutrition is invariably seen as synonymous with feeding.
5. State level actions on nutrition policy instruments depend on directions supported by resource allocations.

In this mission mode approach following actions is recommended:

1. Malnutrition to be viewed as impediment to national development at highest level.
2. Silent emergency of malnutrition to be fought on war footing.
3. Sustained political commitment needed.
4. A high-level standing interagency coordination mechanism must be created at center and state levels to direct macro- and micro-levels strategies.
5. Social sector—nutrition, health, education women and child development must receive higher budgetary allocations.
6. The problem of malnutrition must be made visible at different levels. There must be concentrated nutrition awareness, advocacy, communication and capacity building in respect of both the community and functionaries at various levels.

7. The health sector should include nutrition in all spheres of its activities, viz. medical education, training, primary health care, surveillance, etc.

▶ OBESITY

Obesity may be defined as abnormal growth of the adipose tissues due to an enlargement of fat cell size (hypertrophic obesity) or an increase in fat cell number (hyperplastic obesity) or combination of both. Obesity is perhaps the most prevalent form of malnutrition in both developed and developing countries.

The connection between severe obesity and premature death from diabetes, hypertension and coronary heart diseases is well-established.

Factors Contributing to Obesity

1. **Age and sex:** Obesity can occur at any age in either sex. The incidence is higher in persons, who lead sedentary lives.
2. **Economic status:** It is more common among high-income groups as they consume excess food and do less physical work than those of low-income groups.
3. **Physical activity:** It is very common in those who lead sedentary lives with increase of transport and advanced technology, the proportion of people, who lead sedentary lives has been increasing.
4. **Proneness to obesity:** Recent investigations have shown that some persons are more prone to gain weight. They have usually large proportion of adipose tissue cells as compared with normal persons. These cells are filled with fat, when excess food is consumed.
5. **Genetic factors:** There is genetic component in the etiology of obesity.
6. **Eating habits:** Eating habits are established very early in life, e.g. eating between meals, preference to sweets, fried foods, fast foods, etc.

It has been calculated that a child, whose energy requirements is 2,000 kcal/day and who consumes 100 kcal/day extra will gain about 5 kg weight per year.

7. **Endocrine factors:** These may be involved in occasional cases, e.g. Cushing's syndrome, deficiency of growth hormone, thyroid insufficiency, etc.

Assessment of Obesity

Visual Inspection

Visual inspection is a simple method of assessing obesity though not scientific. Deposition of fat on certain parts of the body giving it a particular most often resembles an apple or pear.

Standard Weight for Height Measurement

Standard weight for height measurement is the best method and can be used by lay persons. Both underweight and overweight persons are detected with the help of this chart.

▶ CONCLUSION

Nutritional problems are the result of multiple factors, all the patients have a genetic core and together with the influence of past life experiences may make them more susceptible to problems. The factors influencing nutrition are biological, psychological, sociocultural and environmental factors. The nurse within any healthcare setting should assume responsibility for provision of optimal nutrition and nutrition counseling for patients. Preventive health teaching should be initiated during first visit and referral to appropriate community resources helps the patient to maintain a preventive approach to health care.

Chapter 31

Community Nutrition Programs

▶ INTRODUCTION

Everyday 799 million people in developing countries and about 18% of the world's population–go hungry. In South Asia, one person in four goes hungry and in Sub-Saharan Africa the share is as high as one in three. Around 175 million children under 5 are estimated to be underweight, a third of preschool children are stunted, 16% of newborn babies weigh less than 2.5 kg and 243 million adults are severely malnourished. 2 billion women and children are anemic, 250 million children suffer from vitamin A deficiency and 2 billion people are at risk from iodine deficiency (Micronutrient Initiative 1998). Malnutrition has different levels of causation. It is strongly linked with poverty; poor children are more likely to be underweight at birth and less likely to receive energy-rich complementary food (Brown et al, 1998) and iodized salt (UNICEF 1998). In India, nutrition affects growth and development of a person. That is why food security has been a major goal of development policy in India since the beginning of planning. There was acute starvation and shortage of food at the time of independence of the country. The major public health problems were chronic energy malnutrition, kwashiorkor, marasmus and micronutrient deficiencies such as goiter, beriberi, blindness due to vitamin A deficiency and anemia.

▶ NUTRITION PROGRAMS

The Government of India has launched various nutrition programs to benefit for mothers and children, and to tackle major problems of malnutrition prevailing in India. Lack of nutrients will lead to decrease in work output, physical intolerance and increase in mortality and morbidity particularly among the pregnant women, lactating mothers and children up to 5 years forming the vulnerable group of the population.

Vertical Nutrition Programs

Programs operating at national levels are called vertical programs such as Integrated Child Development Service (ICDS), Vitamin A Prophylaxis Programs, Iodine Deficiency Disorder Control Programs, etc.

Horizontal Nutrition Programs

Programs operating at state level and integrated with primary health centers are horizontal programs, e.g. Balwadi Nutrition Programs and Tamil Nadu Integrated Nutrition Programs, etc.

Most of the nutrition programs do not have much impact, particularly on the mortality of the vulnerable group. The reasons are as follows:

1. Poor community participation.
2. Negligence of the nutrition.
3. Poor implementation of the programs.
4. Old stock supplies.
5. Unaware of the programs by the people.

The Government of India have initiated several large scale supplementary feeding programs and programs aimed at overcoming specific deficiency diseases through various ministries to the combat malnutrition including Ministry of Health and Family Welfare, Ministry of Social Welfare and Ministry of Education. The major factors leading to malnutrition in India include inadequate intake of calories and proteins, deficiency of certain micronutrients (such as iron, vitamin A, calcium and iodine), maldistribution of essential food commodities, low purchasing power, lack of knowledge about balanced nutrition and limited access to healthcare facilities. The vicious cycle of poverty, malnutrition and ill health has to be combated through the integrated efforts of socioeconomic development, better nutrition is widely lacking, especially amongst those who live below.

They are direct and indirect interventions programs as described below.

Interventions

Direct

1. Department of Women and Child Development:
   a. Integrated Child Development Services Scheme.
   b. Nutrition Program for Adolescent Girls.
   c. Nutrition Advocacy and Awareness General Programs for Food and Nutrition Board (FNB).
   d. Follow-up action on National Nutrition Policy 1993.
2. Ministry of Health and Family Welfare:
   a. Iron and folic acid (IFA) supplementation for pregnant women.
   b. Vitamin A supplementation for children of 9–36 months age groups.
   c. National Iodine deficiency Disorder Control Program.
3. Department of Elementary Education and Literacy:
   a. Mid-day Meal (MDM) for primary school children.

Indirect

1. Department of agriculture and cooperation:
   a. Increased food production.
   b. Horticulture interventions.
2. Food and public distribution:
   a. Targeted public distribution system.
   b. Antyodaya anna yojana.
   c. Annapurna scheme.
3. Rural and urban development:
   a. Food for work program.
   b. Poverty alleviation program.

    c. Safe drinking water and sanitation program.
    d. National Rural Employment Guarantee Scheme.
4. Ministry of Health:
    a. National Rural Health Mission (NRHM).
    b. Integrated Management of Neonatal and Childhood Illnesses (IMNCI).
    c. Various public health measures.
5. Department of Elementary Education and Literacy:
    a. Sarva Shiksha Abhiyan.
    b. Adult Literacy Program.
6. Department of Women and Child Development:
    a. Various women's welfare and support programs.

History

A number of programs were implemented in the past from time to time with minor successes or failures. Some of these are mentioned below.

Special Nutrition Program

Special Nutrition Program (SNP) was launched in the country in 1970–71. It provided supplementary feeding of about 300 calories and 10 g of protein to preschool children and about 500 calories and 25 g of protein to expectant and nursing mothers for 6 days a week. This program was operated under minimum need program. The program was taken up in rural areas inhabited predominantly by lower socioeconomic groups in tribal and urban slums. Fund for nutrition component of ICDS Program was shared with SNP budget.

Balwadi Nutrition Program

Fund for the supplementary feeding of Balwadi Nutrition Program was given by the Central Government, which was launched in 1970–71 through voluntary organizations. It had provided 300 cal/child/day and 10 g protein/child/day for 270 days a year.

CHAPTER 31: Community Nutrition Programs

Applied Nutrition Program

Applied Nutrition Program (ANP) was introduced as a pilot scheme in Orissa in 1963, which later on extended to Tamil Nadu and Uttar Pradesh with the objectives of:
1. Promoting production of protective food such as vegetables and fruits.
2. Ensures their consumption by pregnant and nursing mothers and children.

During 1973, it was extended to all the state of the country. The nutritional education was the main focus and efforts were directed to teach rural communities through demonstration, how to produce food for their consumption through their own efforts. The beneficiaries were children between 2 and 6 years and pregnant and lactating mothers. Nutrition worth 25 paise/child/day and 50 paise/woman/day was provided for 52 days in a year. No definite nutrient content had been specified. The idea was to provide better seeds and encourage kitchen gardens, poultry farming, beehive keeping, etc. But this program did not produce any impact. The community kitchens and school gardens could not function properly due to lack of suitable land, irrigation facilities and low financial investment.

Tamil Nadu Integrated Nutrition Program

Tamil Nadu Integrated Nutrition Program (TINP) was started in 1980 targeting 6–36 months old children; and pregnant and lactating women.

The objectives of TINP were:
1. To reduce malnutrition up to 50% among children under 4 years of age.
2. To reduce infant mortality by 25%.
3. To reduce vitamin A deficiency in the children under 5 year from about 27%–5%.
4. To reduce anemia in pregnant and nursing women from about 55%–20%.

The project had four major components:
1. Nutrition services.
2. Health services.
3. Communication.
4. Monitoring and evaluation.

The projects were assisted by World Bank and with the goal of universalization of ICDS, all the TINP blocks were converted into ICDS blocks.

Wheat Based Supplementary Nutrition Program

A centrally sponsored program was introduced in 1986, but now transferred to the State Sector. This program follows the norms of SNP or of the nutrition component of the ICDS. Central assistance for the program consist of supply of free wheat and supportive costs for other ingredients, cooking, transport, etc.

▶ CURRENT NUTRITIONAL DEFICIENCY STATUS

A wide gap is there in food production and food consumption. The achievement of macro food grain security at the national level did not percolate own to household and the level of chronic food insecurity in India is still high. Many aspects of life and development are reflected in this one statistic—including the income and education of parents, the prevalence of disease, the availability of clean water, efficacy of health services, infant feeding practices, access to food and care, food and dietary habits, the health and nutritional status of mothers and more broadly, the position of women in society. According to National Family Health Survey (NFHS) in 2005–06, 46% of children below 3 years of age were underweight, 38% were stunted and 19% were wasted that are lower than Sub-Saharan Africa.

Approximately, 26.1% of the population is still living below poverty line. Undernourishment is higher among rural than urban children. The proportion of underweight children in urban areas was 36% as against 49% in rural areas. Similarly, levels of stunting and wasting are higher in rural than in urban areas.

It is estimated that 2.2 million children are afflicted with cretinism, and about 6.6 million are mildly retarded and suffer from motor handicaps. It is also estimated that iodine deficiency accounts for 90,000 still births and neonatal deaths. Nutritional blindness affects 7 million children in India per year resulting mainly from the deficiency of vitamin A, couples with protein-energy malnutrition (PEM). Prevalence of conjunctival xerosis and Bitot's spot was observed to be as high as 7.8% among slum children, followed by industrial labor (6.3%). Prevalence of low-birth-weight babies in India ranged between 26% and 57% in the urban slums, and 35% and 41% in rural areas. About 40% of the adults in rural area and 50% of the tribal adults are suffering from chronic energy deficiency. There is a problem of overnutrition in certain areas and certain groups of people in the country, which have serious health effects.

▶ FIVE YEAR PLANS ON NUTRITIONAL ASPECTS

10th Five Year Plan

Initiatives of 10th Five Year Plan to have paradigm shift:

1. Household food security to nutritional security for family and individuals.
2. Untargeted food supplementation in vulnerable group to screening of all persons to identify various grade of undernutrition and appropriate management.
3. Lack of focused interventions on prevention of overnutrition to promotion of appropriate lifestyle and dietary intakes for prevention and management of overnutrition and obesity.
4. Integration of various sectors to support the nutrition program for better output.

SECTION 4: Community Nutrition

11th Five Year Plan

National Nutrition Goals for 11th Five Year Plan:
1. Reduce the prevalence of underweight in children less than 5 years to 20%.
2. Eradicate the prevalence of severe undernutrition in children less than 5 years.
3. First hour breastfeeding rates to increase to 80%.
4. Exclusive breastfeeding rates to increase to 90%.
5. Complementary feeding rate at 6 months to increase to 90%.
6. Reduce prevalence of anemia in high-risk groups (infants, preschool children, adolescent girls, pregnant and lactating women) to 25%.
7. Eliminate vitamin A deficiency in children less than 5 years as a public health problem and reduce subclinical deficiency of vitamin A in children by 50%.
8. Reduce prevalence of iodine deficiency disorders to less than 5%.

▶ INTEGRATED CHILD DEVELOPMENT SERVICE

Integrated Child Development Service scheme was launched on 2nd October, 1975 (5th Five Year Plan) in pursuance of the National Policy for Children in 33 experimental blocks. The network consists of 5,659 projects in rural and urban slum pockets. Now, the goal is universalization of ICDS throughout the country.

The primary responsibility for the implementation of the program is with the Department of Women and Child Development, Ministry of Human Resources Development at the center and the nodal departments at the state, which may be social welfare, rural development, tribal welfare, health and family welfare or women and child development (Fig. 31.1).

Beneficiaries

1. Children below 6 years.
2. Pregnant and lactating women.

CHAPTER 31: Community Nutrition Programs

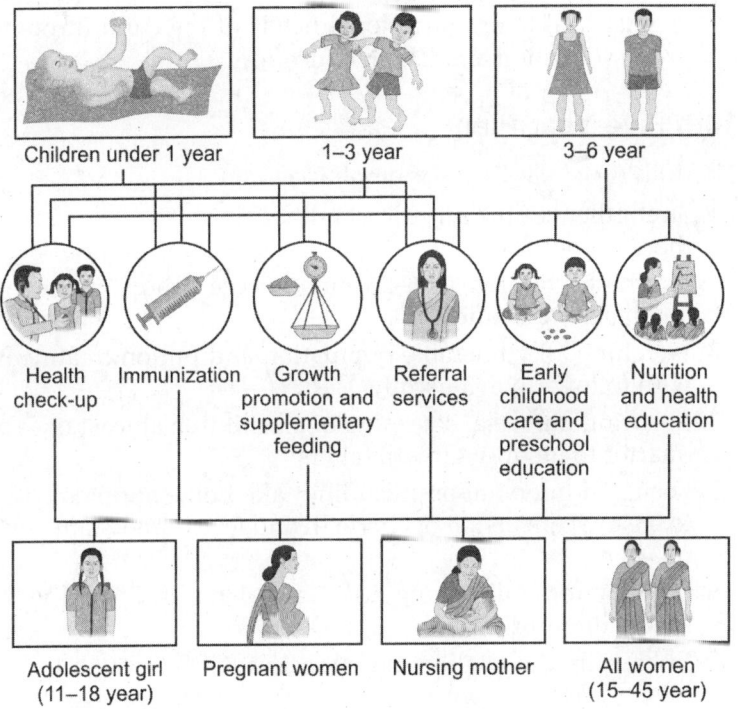

Fig. 31.1: Health and nutritional needs for children and women

3. Women in the age group of 15–45 years.
4. Adolescent girls in selected blocks.

Objectives

1. To improve the nutritional and health status of preschool children in the age group of 0–6 years.
2. To lay the foundation of proper psychological development of the child.
3. To reduce the incidence of mortality, morbidity, malnutrition and school dropout.
4. To achieve effective coordination of policy and implementation amongst the various departments to promote child development.

5. To enhance the capability of the mother to look after the normal health and nutritional needs of the child through proper nutrition and health education.

10th Five Year Plan

The 10th Five Year Plan has emphasized on:
1. Strengthening the nutrition and health component so that there is appropriate intrafamilial distribution of food.
2. Reaching children in 6–36 months age group, pregnant and lactating women.
3. Weighing all vulnerable population and put on treatment with follow-up in 3 months.
4. Ensuring universal screening of all children at least once a quarter to identify growth falters.
5. Focus on intervention including take home supplements, to ensure conversion of Grade III and IV to Grade II in next quarter.
6. Looking for and treating health problems associated with severe undernutrition.
7. Enhancing the quality and impact of ICDS through training and supervision.
8. Intersectoral coordination for nutrition action.
9. Creating nutrition awareness.
10. Establishing reliable monitoring and evaluation.

11th Five Year Plan

1. Overall objective is to reduce child malnutrition through strengthening of ICDS services.
2. Wheat flour fortified with iron, vitamin A, folic acid should be supplied.
3. The calories and protein norms for children in age group of 6 months to 6 years need to be enhanced to 500 cal/child/day and 10 g protein/child/day from the existing 300 calories and 8–10 g protein. Severely malnourished children in this age group need to be given 600 calories and 20 g protein/child/day. Financial norms for normal children for supplementary food per day should be enhanced to

₹ 4/- while for severely malnourished children to ₹ 10/-. For a severely malnourished child, nutrient dense food 5 6 times a day is recommended.

4. Similarly, for pregnant and lactating mothers 500 calories and 20 g protein with a financial norm of ₹ 4/- beneficiary/day is recommended.
5. Flexibility to districts to provide nutritionally dense supplementary food to ICDS beneficiaries in the form of cereal-pulse combination, supplemented with vegetables and fruits or micronutrients was also considered necessary. Fortification of supplementary food with soybean flour in the range of 5%–10% should be made compulsory.
6. A performance appraisal system for Anganwadi workers (AWWs) may be introduced. There shall be reward and disincentive mechanism for effective delivery of services. An accreditation system, to grade Anganwadi centers (AWCs), with defined quality standards need to be looked into.
7. Observation of monthly nutrition and health education days, celebration of mother and children related functions will make AWCs socially more active.
8. Regular and 100% weighing of babies, implementation of standardized mother and child growth charts will facilitate mothers to monitor the health of the child.

▶ MID-DAY MEAL PROGRAM

One of the pioneers of the scheme is the Madras Presidency that started providing cooked meals to children in corporation schools in the Madras city in 1923. The program was introduced in a large scale in 1960s under the Chief Ministership of K Kamaraj Nadar. But the first major thrust came in 1982, when the Chief Minister of Tamil Nadu, Dr Ramachandran MG, decided to universalize the scheme for all children in government schools in primary classes. Later, the program was expanded to cover all children up to class 10. Tamil Nadu's Mid-day Meal Program is among the best known in the country. Several other states of India also have had MDM Programs. The most notable among them is Gujarat that has had it since the late 1980s. Kerala started providing cooked meals in schools since 1995 and so did Madhya Pradesh and Odisha in small pockets. On 28th November, 2001, the Supreme Court of India gave a landmark direction, which made it obligatory for the government to provide cooked meals to all children in all government and government assisted primary schools. The direction was resisted vigorously by state governments initially, but the program has become almost universal by 2005. Neither a child that is hungry, nor a child that is ill can be expected to learn. There are about 150 million children officially enrolled in nearly 800,000 schools throughout the country. Relatively high overhead costs of school coupled with poor school infrastructure, lack of structure, lack of teachers and teacher absenteeism are the most often cited reasons for low levels of schooling in the country (probe 1996).

Aims

Realizing this need the National Program of Nutritional Support to primary education, popularly known as MDM Scheme was formally launched on 15 August 1995, with the aim of improving in three areas:

1. School attendance.
2. Reduced dropouts.
3. A beneficial impact on children's nutrition.

Beside these, MDM could be a valuable means of imparting health and nutrition education not only to children but also to the parents and the community. MDM could also create employment opportunities for poor women of the village. Majority of cooks engaged in the programs could be women, most of them coming from underprivileged backgrounds. MDM has been effective in improving enrolment rates, particularly of girls (Dreze and Goyal, 2003). From October 2002, the program has been extended to children studying in government supported schools.

Recommendations of Nursing Foundation of India

Following recommendations are made in a report by Nutrition Foundation of India:

1. Each MDM should provide roughly a third of the daily nutrient requirement (350–500 kcal depending on the age of the child). The meal should contain a part from cereals, a good quality of vegetables, particularly, dark green leafy vegetables to combat micronutrient deficiencies.
2. Meal should be of hygienic quality that demands monitoring of the raw material and cooked preparation by trained personnel.
3. In urban areas a centralized kitchen should be set up and meal should be prepared, transported and served hygienically. This model was adopted by Chennai and Naandi Foundation in Hyderabad and ISKON group in Bangalore. In rural areas self, help groups and Panchayat should be involved.
4. Convergence of synergistic activities: School health services, environmental sanitation and safe water supply, sensitization of teachers, involvement and networking of professional bodies and communities.

▶ NATIONAL NUTRITIONAL ANEMIA PROGRAM

Anemia Among Children

Anemia is a serious concern for young children as it can adversely affect cognitive performance, behavioral and motor development, coordination language development and scholastic achievement as well increase morbidity from infectious.

Hemoglobin (Hb) levels are classified into three categories:
1. Mild (10.0–10.9 g/dL).
2. Moderate (8.0–9.9 g/dL).
3. Severe (less than 8.0 g/dL).

The proportion of anemic children of 6–35 months has risen from 74% in 1998–99 to 79% in 2005–06. The increase is noticed in both rural and urban areas, though the increase is higher in rural than in urban areas.

The level of anemia among children of 6–35 months varies from 56% in Kerala and 59% in Himachal Pradesh, 85% in Uttar Pradesh and 88% in Bihar. The levels of anemia are also higher among rural than urban children. And the rural-urban differential has widened from 4% points in 1998–99 to 8% points in 2005–06.

Available studies on prevalence of nutritional anemia in India shows that 65% infant and children, 60% 1–6 years of age, 88% adolescent girls (3.3% have Hb < 7 g/dL; severe anemia) and 85% pregnant women (9.9% severe anemia) having anemia (Table 31.1).

Table 31.1: Percentage of iron deficiency anemia in different age group

Sl No	Iron deficiency anemia	Percentage
1.	Children (6–35 month)	79 (NFHS*-3)
	a. 6–11 month	71.7–80
	b. 12–23 month	77.7–78
	c. 24–35 month	72
	d. < 6 month–6 year (< 11 g/dL)	70
	e. 5–11 year	73
2.	Adolescent girls < 12 g/dL	52–88
	a. Mild anemia	34
	b. Moderate anemia	15.7
	c. Severe anemia	1.8
3.	Adolescent girls in urban slum of Delhi	46.6
4.	Pregnant and lactating women (< 11g/dL)	58 (NFHS-3) 81.7 (ICMR†)
5.	Women 15–49 year even married	56 (NFHS-3)
6.	Adult male (< 13 g/dL)	24 (NFHS-3)

*NFHS, National Family Health Survey; †ICMR, Indian Council of Medical Research.

Anemia in Adult

Prevalence of anemia was marginally higher in lactating women as compared to pregnancy. The commonest is iron deficiency anemia.

The program was launched in 1970 to prevent nutritional anemia in mothers and children. Under, this program, the expected and nursing mothers as well as acceptors of family planning are given one tablet of iron and folic acid containing 60 mg elementary iron, which was raised to 100 mg elementary iron, however, folic acid content remained same (0.5 mg of folic acid) and children in the age group of 1–5 years are given one tablet of iron containing 20 mg elementary iron (60 mg of ferrous sulfate and 0.1 mg of folic acid) daily for a period of 100 days.

This program is being taken up by Maternal and Child Health (MCH) Division of Ministry of Health and Family Welfare. Now, it is a part of Reproductive and Child Health (RCH) Program. But this program has failed to make any impact in India. Experiences from other countries in controlling moderately severe anemia have suggested that long-term measures such as fortification of food items such as milk, cereal, sugar and salt with iron are beneficial interventions. India has also identified fortification of salt with iron as a useful measure to control anemia. Pilot project of salt fortification with iron has been started in Tamil Nadu. Nutrition education is needed to improve dietary intakes in family for receiving needed macro and micronutrients as protein, iron and vitamins such as folic acid, B_{12}, C, etc. for Hb synthesis is important. Nutritional Anemia Control Program should be comprehensive and incorporate nutrition education through school health, and ICDS infrastructure to promote regular intake of iron, folic acid rich foods, to promote intake of food, which helps in absorption of iron and folic acid and adequate intake of food.

Iron supplementation can be risky for children living with high-malarial areas and can lead to severe illness and death. As India has many high-malarial states where prophylactic iron may be risky, an alternative policy is required in such areas. According to another research study conducted in Teheran revealed that the expectant mothers should not unnecessarily be given iron pills unless anemic, as it may cause development of high blood pressure and hence, small gestation age babies.

SECTION 4: Community Nutrition

▶ SPECIAL NUTRITION PROGRAM

Special Nutrition Program was launched in 1970, as a crash program to provide supplementary nutrition to children below 6 years of age and pregnant and lactating mothers. The socially and economically handicapped are to be reached through this program, as well as those in slums, drought prone and flood affected areas. It is now envisaged that the SNP should include some of the components of the ICDS, in order to render it more effective, properly selected target groups of mothers and children are to be supported with basic health inputs, including nutrition and health education.

Objectives

Objectives of the program are to improve the nutritional status of pregnant and lactating mothers, and children below 6 years of age in the weakest sections and most vulnerable areas. The objectives are now to include a reduction in mortality and morbidity in children below 6 years, enhance the capacity of mothers to look after the daily health and nutritional needs of children, and to strengthen the supportive services.

The main activities of the program are:
1. To provide supplementary nutrition.
2. To provide health services including supply of vitamin A solution and iron and folic acid tablets (since 1976).

This program is for the nutritional benefit of children below 6 years of age, pregnant and nursing mothers, and in operation in urban slums, tribal areas and backward rural areas. The supplementary food supplies about 30 kcal/child/day and 10–12 g protein/child/day. The beneficiary mothers receive daily 500 kcal and 25 g of proteins, this supplement is provided to them for about 300 days in a year. This program is gradually merged into ICDS.

The major objective of the program is to prevent anemia. The specific objectives as identified from general description of the program are as follows:

1. To assess the baseline prevalence of nutritional anemia in mothers and young children through estimation of Hb levels.
2. To put the mothers and children with low Hb levels (less than 10 g% and less than 8 g%) on antianemic treatment.
3. To put the mothers with Hb levels more than 10 g/dL and children with more than 8 g/dL on the prophylaxis program.
4. To monitor continuously the quality of the tablets, distributions and consumption, and to assess periodically the Hb levels of the beneficiaries.
5. To negative mothers, through relevant education, to consume the iron-folic acid (IFA) tablets and to give the same to their children.

▶ NATIONAL GOITER CONTROL PROGRAM

Government of India, realizing the magnitude of endemic goiter, launched the National Goiter Control Program (NGCP) in 1962. It aimed at replacement of ordinary salt by iodized salt, particularly in goiter endemic regions. Surveys indicated that the problem of the goiter and iodine deficiency disorders was more widespread than it was thought earlier, with nearly 145 million people estimated to be living in known endemic areas of the country. As a result, the program started in 1986 with objective to replace the entire edible salt by iodized salt in a phased manner by 1992.

Objectives

1. Initial survey to assess the magnitude of the iodine deficiency disorders.
2. Supply of iodized salt in place of common salt to the entire country by 1992.
3. Repeat surveys to assess the importance of iodized salt after 5 years.

Accordingly, the program has been implemented and shown some progress, but reveals strengthening of NGCP. Areas requiring strengthening of the NGCP related to:
1. Irregular distribution of iodized salt for varying periods.
2. Lack of supportive supervision for the quality of iodized salt distributed.
3. Failure of lifting of the allotted quotas of iodized salt by wholesale agents for further distribution to retailers.
4. Poor interpersonal relationship between salt dealers and food inspectors, the implementation of prevention of food adulteration (PFA) act.
5. Coordination between department of food and civil supply, health and wholesale dealers.

▶ NATIONAL PROGRAM FOR PROPHYLAXIS AGAINST BLINDNESS DUE TO VITAMIN A DEFICIENCY

National program for prophylaxis against blindness due to vitamin 'A' deficiency was launched in 1970 under Ministry of Health as a part of MCH program. Studies have shown that in the southern and eastern parts of the country, about 30%–50% preschool children have eye problems as a result of vitamin 'A' deficiency. It is estimated that 2% of the total blindness in India is caused by vitamin 'A' deficiencies.

The specific objective of the program is reduction of diseases and prevention of blindness due to vitamin deficiency. An evaluation of the program has shown that in areas, where it has been implemented well there was significant reduction in the prevalence of signs of vitamin 'A' deficiency. The reason for coverage has been inadequate supplies of vitamin 'A' and adoption of clinic approach instead of house-to-house visit for the distribution. As a part of RCH program [earlier Child Survival and Safe Motherhood (CSSM)] attention is now focused upon children up to 3 years of age.

CHAPTER 31: Community Nutrition Programs

▶ BALWADI NUTRITION PROGRAM

The Balwadi Nutrition Program was started in 1970–71 or the preschool child as it is operated through Balwadis and daycare centers, and is under the charge of the Social Welfare Department. The objective of the program is to supply one fourth of the calorie requirements and half of the protein requirements of the preschool child, as a measure to improve the nutritional status. It is to be a supplement to what the child receives at home. As far as possible, locally available foodstuff is to be utilized. Children belonging to the lower socioeconomic group would be selected. Community involvement would be encouraged.

The nutrition supplement providing 300 cal/day and 10 g protein/day/child for 270 days a year is provided in Balwadis or daycare centers, where some non-formal education of the preschool child is given. It is envisaged that package including basic health components are to be included as in the ICDS.

This program is directed by the Ministry of Social Welfare through several voluntary organizations. Balwadi is managed by bal sevikas assisted by helper, coordination committees at the center, state, district and block along with the community are to ensure regular supply of resources and effective management.

▶ APPLIED NUTRITION PROGRAM

Applied nutrition program in improvement of nutritional status depends largely upon awareness and knowledge as well as availability of food. The rest expanded program of nutrition started in India in 1960. It was started first in Odisha and Andhra Pradesh and extended in 1960 to Tamil Nadu and in 1962 to Uttar Pradesh. In 1963, the ANP was extended to the whole country through the Government of India, along with aid from UNICEF with the active participation of the states.

The program was launched in 1963 to combat malnutrition in vulnerable groups, particularly mothers and children in rural area. The program was basically education oriented program, operate at the village and family level.

SECTION 4: Community Nutrition

Main Objectives

1. People should conscious of their nutritional needs.
2. To increase the production of nutritious foods and its consumptions.
3. To provide supplementary nutrition to vulnerable groups through locally produced foods.

Main Components of Applied Nutrition Program

1. Production of protective foods.
2. Training of functionaries involved in the production of these foods.
3. Nutrition education and demonstration (demonstration of improved technique of cooking and feeding were also used).

The program is coordinated by the Ministry of Rural Reconstruction. At the state level, the Panchayati Raj and Community Development are generally in charge of the program. In the field, block development officer is in charge of the program.

Activities of Applied Nutrition Program

1. Kitchen gardens, school gardens and community gardens are set up to promote the concept of a balanced diet, as well as to increase production.
2. Fishery units and poultry units are set up to give employment, added income and more production of food (poultry farming, beehives keeping, etc.).
3. Providing better seeds as well as well-breed cattle.
4. Supplementary feeding through local food production was given to vulnerable pregnant and lactating mother and children.

▶ WORLD FOOD PROGRAM

World Food Program (WFP) is the world's largest international food aid organization, serving in 84 countries, working with the goal of achieving. "A world in which every man, woman and child has access at all times to the food needed for an active and healthy life. Without food, there can be no sustainable peace, no democracy and no development." Founded in 1963 as the food aid arm of the United Nation after the Rome Declaration on World Food Security in 1996, WFP is committed to achieve the goal of reducing half the number, who are without adequate access to food by 2015.

World Food Program in India

Nearly half of the world's hungry reside in India. Despite a substantial increase in food grain production since the independence in 1947, India is still classified as low-income and food deficit country. Around 35% of India's population is considered food insecure, consuming less than 80% of minimum energy requirements. However, National Sample Survey Organization claimed it has reduced to 27%. Without adequate nutrition, a person may be unable to perform work productively or a child may be unable to learn school lessons to their capacity or a mother may give birth to a child with permanent impaired brain development.

World Food Program Goals and Objectives in India

1. Improve nutrition and quality of life for the most vulnerable population at critical times in their lives.
2. Make sustainable improvements in household food security for the poorest, especially for women and child, and invest funds in development for long-term security.
3. Strengthen channels for locally produced food grains and support local entrepreneurship.
4. Advocate for ecological-restoration through participatory methods and development.

Beneficiaries

1. Poor women, particularly mothers and children at risk.
2. Poor forest-dependent population.

Over the years, more than 70 development projects of WFP have included supplementary feeding supported forestry, livestock and dairy development, irrigation and rural development activities. A blend of precooked maize and soy fortified with micronutrients called corn-soy blend (CSB) has been developed in India in the name of Indiamix, distributed through existing infrastructure of the ICDS projects. The Indiamix project is operational in Rajasthan, Uttar Pradesh, Odisha, Madhya Pradesh, Gujarat, Kerala, Assam and Bihar.

Nutritive Value of Indiamix

Indiamix is precooked, nutritious commodity, appropriate for both on the spot feeding and take home rations made from wheat (75%) and full-fat soybean (25%) or alternatively, maize (40%) and wheat (40%) and full-fat soybean (20%) and has the nutritive values providing 80%–90% of recommended dietary allowance (RDA) of a child for iron and vitamin A.

Activities Under World Food Program

Helping women (Table 31.2) to gain better access for food, education and involvement in community decisions are the activities under WEPs. It works in many directions MCH care access to maternal and child health care; improving child survival, 'food for work' program in collaboration with forest department; providing food in emergencies, access to health services, potable water and sanitation; proper caring practices for young children, education particularly girls and women; supporting generation of biogas, protection of forest through mass awareness and active participation; irrigations, income generating

Table 31.2: Nutritional requirements of women

Nutrients	Amount/100 g
Protein	20 g
Fat	6 g
Crude fiber	2 g
Carbohydrate	60 g
Energy	390 kcal
Calcium	191 mg
Iron	15 mg
Vitamin A	1,454 µg

projects, creating market by local manufacturing of Indiamix and effective program implementation.

▶ CONCLUSION

Community nutrition programs in India organized through various ministries have initiated large scale supplementary feeding programs and programs aimed at overcoming specific deficiency diseases. The community nutrition programs are vitamin A prophylaxis program, prophylaxis against anemia, iodine deficiency disorder control, special nutrition program, balwadi nutrition program, integrated child development scheme and mid-day meal program. Community health nurses play as bridge between community residents and healthcare system. Because of frequent and extended contact with patients in the community, nurses have excellent opportunities to provide information and counseling about the importance of nutrition preventing illness and promoting health.

Chapter 32

Community Nutritional Rehabilitation

▶ INTRODUCTION

Nutrition rehabilitation center is being incorporated into primary health care (PHC) program as nutrition education was utilized to teach mothers, how to prepare weaning diets from locally available foodstuffs. It also served as a center for the prevention of malnutrition and diarrheal diseases.

▶ REHABILITATION FOR PROTEIN-ENERGY MALNUTRITION CHILDREN

As soon as children are able to take normal food and infection is under control, it is economical for medical services to discharge them to a center where their nutritional rehabilitation can be supervised. Follow-up studies done at the Institute of Child Health and Hospital for Children at Chennai revealed that one third of the children who had been treated in hospital for protein-energy malnutrition (PEM) were dead within a year from the disease for which they had been successfully treated and still others were malnourished. Causes can be attributed to poverty or failure to involve parents; particularly mother in treatment and recovery. The concept of nutritional rehabilitation is based on practical nutritional training for mothers in which they learn by feeding their children back to health, under supervision and using local foods.

Residential Units

In residential units, mothers are admitted with their children. Under the guidance of nutrition demonstrator they work as a

CHAPTER 32: Community Nutritional Rehabilitation

group, and prepare a suitable therapeutic diet with available foods and feed their children.

Day Care Centers

In day care centers, mothers help in cooking and feeding in 1 or 2 days a week, though the children attend daily. It therefore takes longer time for mothers to appreciate to the essential messages about better feeding.

Domiciliary Rehabilitation

Domiciliary rehabilitation is done at home and is more personal, as nutritional advice and help is given on one-to-one basis by a nutrition demonstrator or specially trained health worker.

Successful nutritional rehabilitation requires detailed knowledge about local foods, cooking and feeding practices. Based on this knowledge, a diet should be designed, which can be practiced even by poor families. Mothers who take active part in preparation of food and feeding their children and watching them recovering to their health and vitality are more likely to retain ideas, and continue with a similar regime at home.

Suggested Diet During Convalescence

1. Increasing the quantity of existing food (like idli, rice, chapati).
2. Increasing the number of meals to satisfy calorie and protein requirement.
3. Addition of oil or ghee 1–2 tablespoon to increase calories without increasing bulk.
4. Consumption of sugar can be increased to increase calories in the diet.
5. The child can be given cereals and pulses mixture.
6. If the patient can afford milk, egg and skimmed milk can be included in the diet.

Low Cost Recipes for Children Recovering from PEM

1. Ragi, green gram, jaggery—puttu.
2. Ragi, Bengal gram, wheat—puttu.
3. Bengal gram, milk, jaggery—payasam.
4. Rice, Bengal gram—porridge.
5. Red gram, spinach dal.
6. Wheat rava, green gram dal, vegetables—upma.
7. Malted wheat, green gram and groundnut powder (can be made as chapati; gruel or laddu with jaggery).
8. Rice, green gram dal—pongal, khichdi.
9. Idli with sugar.

Concentrated Food Supplements

For rapid replacement of lost tissues and to catch up with growth, children need a high-energy diet with ample protein. It is often difficult when the energy density of the family is low. Malnourished children need supplements of vegetable oil to increase the energy density. Concentrated food like malted cereals, in combination with pulses can be given. If the child can afford, commercial weaning mixes or egg custard can be given.

▶ COMMUNITY NUTRITION TRAINING

In most developing countries, the majority of the population—the rural population especially, does not receives even the most basic health care or any nutritional advice. Malnutrition is not merely one of the greatest public health problems in the world today. It is both, a result and a cause of social and economic underdevelopment. The root of the problem is in the home to solve it. The family must be helped to learn better habits of nutrition and must be served by better health care. Community health worker is the responsible person at the family level.

CHAPTER 32: Community Nutritional Rehabilitation

Community Health Workers' Nutrition Tasks

The tasks can be grouped into eight main categories namely:
1. Getting to know the community needs.
2. Measuring and monitoring the growth and nutrition of children.
3. Promoting breastfeeding.
4. Giving nutritional service on feeding infants and young children.
5. Giving nutritional advice to mothers.
6. Identifying, managing and preventing nutritional deficiencies.
7. Providing nutritional care during common infections.
8. Conveying nutritional messages to the community.

Need for Change in Nutrition Training

The training in nutrition that the community health worker receives commonly suffers from three main defects:
1. The nutrition trainers are often professionals from different disciplines (doctors, nutritionists and nurses). This often leads to the training being biased toward the profession of the trainer and being aimed at too high level of learning.
2. The training is based mainly on lecturers, during which the trainees remain passive listeners. There is no exchange of ideas between them and the lecturer would help them remember the information, he/she is attempting to pass on. Thus, lecturing is not always the best method of conveying information to the trainees.
3. There is a lack of simple training material designed specifically to teach community health workers about how to perform certain tasks. Most manuals on nutrition concentrate on technical aspects of the subject. They do not specify the tasks the trainees will be expected to perform. They do not explain how the training should be conducted so that the trainees learn the necessary skills. And they do

not indicate how to check whether the trainees in fact, have learned those skills.

Purpose of Guidelines

To improve nutrition in that area by leaving in a practical way, the most important things one will need to know and do.

Main Considerations

1. The training should be directed to the performance of specific tasks (nutritional problems in that area).
2. The community health workers should be trained to perform a limited number of practical tasks for the improvement of health and nutrition.
3. To be fully effective, training requires the maximum participation by the trainers also. This can be achieved by what is called 'teaching-learning method'.
4. It is very important for the trainers to have strong motivation to learn their job and to serve the community.
5. The training should be given near the community in which a trainee will be working later.
6. The trainees will have to acquire certain knowledge and skills that may not seem to be directly related to the technical aspects of nutrition. This is because the whole community must participate as much as possible in solving their own problems by organizing and motivating groups.
7. The duration of the training will depend upon the educational background of the trainees, on how many tasks they will be expected to perform and on how complicated these are.
8. Training is not necessarily completed in a set period of time or at the end of the formal training course. Refresher training at regular intervals will increase the effectiveness of community health workers.

Learning Objectives

1. Collect information that will help to show the nutritional and nutrition-related problems, and needs of the community.

CHAPTER 32: Community Nutritional Rehabilitation

2. Decide, which social groups, families and individuals are at special risk of nutritional problems. Help should be given for target population:
   a. Antenatal mothers.
   b. Postnatal mothers.
   c. Children.
3. Identify people and the organizations in the community, which can help with the nutrition-related problems, and prepare a list of what they can do, how they can help and how to build an understanding with them.
4. Identify the nutritional problems and with the help of the supervisor, plan the actions to deal with these problems.
5. Decide, which people are seriously ill and they should be referred to the nearest health center and medical supervisor.

Health workers need to know the following:
1. Getting to know the community and its needs.
2. Actually felt trends with respect to nutrition.
3. Growth and development of child.
4. Grading of malnutrition.
5. Additional information about each child.
6. Information about the community.
7. Economic status and education.
8. Land tenure (who owns the land).
9. Working women.
10. Food availability.
11. Food distribution within the family.
12. Beliefs about foods.
13. Resource persons.

A community health worker cannot solve all problems of the community:
1. She must select those problems that she can do something about.
2. Measuring and monitoring the growth and nutrition of children.

3. Promotion of breastfeeding.
4. Nutritional advice on the feeding of infants and young children.
5. Nutritional care of mothers.
6. Identification, management and prevention of common nutritional deficiencies.
7. Nutritional care during diarrhea and other common infections.
8. Conveying nutrition messages to the community.
9. Solving nutritional problems in the community:
   a. Understand that a number of activities are generally necessary to solve one nutritional problem, because nutritional problems often have many causes.
   b. Identify the major causes of malnutrition in a child, select the causes that one can deal with and carry out appropriate tasks to find solution those causes.
   c. Convince parents that regular weighing of children is necessary to know the actions that are required at different ages, so that the child grows well.

Training Strategy

All supervisory functionaries of the project receive institutionalized job training, after the supplementation of training. A small, but significant feature of the manpower development strategy consists of joint training, review sessions and coordination workshops. Joint training of community nutrition workers (CNWs) with multipurpose health worker (female) (MPHW) (F) was organized and coordination training was organized during the last 10 days of the CNW basic training program. These sessions provided an opportunity to understand each other's role and to coordinate activities.

Two Types of Nutrition Programs

1. Programs operating at national levels also called vertical nutritional programs, e.g. Integrated Child Development Services (ICDS), Vitamin A Prophylaxis Program, etc.

CHAPTER 32: Community Nutritional Rehabilitation

2. Programs operating at state level also called horizontal nutritional program [Chief Minister Noon-Meal Program (CMNMP) and Tamil Nadu Integrated Nutrition Project (TINP), etc.]:
   a. Mid-day supplementation for schoolchildren—1955.
   b. Applied Nutrition Programs—1950.
   c. Supplementary nutritional program—1960.
   d. Anemia Prophylaxis Program—1992.
   e. Goiter Prophylaxis Program.
   f. Vitamin A prophylaxis scheme.
   g. ICDS—1976.
   h. TINP-Phase I—1980–89.
   i. CMNMP—1982.

▶ NUTRITION EDUCATION

Nutrition education is essential to the community because, a number of factors influence the food habits such as sociocultural practices, educational and economic level of community and availability of food in a geographical area. Once the food habits are established, they are handed down from generation to generation and such habits are based on false idea and ignorance.

Educating people regarding nutrition is important. In nutrition education, the primary aim is to remove prejudices and to import good dietary habits. People are ignorant about balanced diets; they should be educated about the nutritive value of food, storage, preparation, cooking, serving and eating the food. Traditional beliefs, religious beliefs, food fads and geographic factors are changing food habits.

Traditional Belief

Consumption of papaya fruit by pregnant woman is believed to lead to abortion. Dal is not given to mother, which will produce flatus to mother and indigestion to baby.

Religious Belief

Muslims are forbidden from eating pork while Hindus are forbidden from eating beef.

Geographic Factors

Soil, climate, water resources and local agricultural practice comes under geographic factors. The type of food that can be grown in the locality the food that can be practiced in that locality is the staple food. Because of all these reasons, nutrition education is important. Nutrition education on good nutrition is necessary in improving dietary habits, helps them to select right foodstuff within their economy. Nutrition education must be given in simple words and in a language, which is easily understood by people. Success of nutrition education will depend on whether people have understood the importance of it and have started practicing on the new ideas given to them.

Importance of Nutrition Education

Nutrition education is an important tool to improve the nutrition of the community in the developing countries:

1. Nutrition education gives the knowledge in right direction and corrects faulty practices.
2. It educates people to make best use of their limited income.
3. It educates people to make wise food choices for health and well-being of the family members.
4. It tells about the appropriate eating habits.
5. If the whole family is given nutrition education, the nutritional status of the whole family will improve with the result of this, the coming generation will be born with good nutritional status and the problem of malnutrition can be decreased to a great extent.

Approaches to Nutritional Education

Food is one of the important and basic biological needs of man. Food is the foundation for good health. It is essential for life,

CHAPTER 32: Community Nutritional Rehabilitation

growth and repair of human body, regulation of body mechanism and production of energy for work. Nutritional education is essential part in community development.

Objectives and Need for Nutritional Education

1. To educate the individual, the family and community about the food sources, food and their nutritive values, proper methods of cooking, balanced diet and requirements of energy.
2. To educate the individual, the family and community about food selection, preparation, purchase and storage.
3. To provide information about food substitutes, changes and modification in diet.
4. To educate the effects of various cooking methods on the nutrients.
5. To provide information about the importance of various nutrients and their required amount.
6. To inform about various signs and symptoms of nutritional deficiencies, and early detection of disease condition.
7. To explain about the importance of food hygiene.
8. To understand the nutritional requirements of the vulnerable group (children, pregnancy, lactation and old age).
9. To provide health education to avoid bad habits, prejudices, idiosyncrasies and wrong motions regarding diet.
10. To educate various methods and techniques of prevention and control of nutritional deficiencies.

Implications of Nutrition Education

1. Promote traditional diets and eating patterns with their positive aspects.
2. Encourage the use of easily and locally available fruits and vegetables.
3. Encourage cooking methods that require less fat.
4. Observe and respect religious and cultural food restrictions.

5. Promote healthy eating habits for the whole family rather than an individual.
6. Identify the target groups that are vulnerable such as young children, pregnant and lactating women and the elderly.
7. Local members of the community, such as health workers, mothers may be involved.
8. The health workers need to have thorough knowledge of nutrition and health issues.
9. Nutrition education material such as leaflets, posters or audiovisual samples must be prepared in local language.
10. The health workers must be fluent in local language to communicate effectively.

Methods of Nutrition Education

1. Individual nutrition education: During pregnancy, lactation and to the mothers of malnourished children, nutrition education in their homes is more effective.
2. Group nutrition education: Community program for the entire families in the community are given in particular place and information are given by cooking demonstration, which is more useful in learning.
3. The following techniques can be used to make nutrition education more effective, e.g. role playing drama on nutrition, puppet show, music and folk dance, posters, pictures, tape recorder, computer, television and films about nutrition.

Nutrition education can be organized during:
1. Home visit.
2. School health programs.
3. Organization of special clinics, e.g. antenatal clinic, under five clinic, postnatal clinic and preschool clinic, etc.
4. Special community health programs and health camps.
5. The indoor and the outdoor clinics with patients and their attendants.
6. In ladies club meetings, during nutrition demonstration.

CHAPTER 32: Community Nutritional Rehabilitation

Principles of Nutrition Education

It is difficult to change the dietary habits of person. Hence, the nurse should be aware about her role and responsibilities, while imparting nutrition education. For this, the nurse should observe the following principles:

1. The following factors are important in nutrition education:
   a. The educational level of the individual or the community.
   b. Culture, religion, dietary habits and idiosyncrasies.
   c. Local availability of foodstuff.
   d. Cleanliness of house and surroundings.
2. The individual should be given sufficient time to adopt new ideas and habits.
3. Any changes or suggestions regarding diet should be made according to the individual's practices, religion and culture.
4. The individuals/patients should be made familiar with the importance and objectives of nutrition education.
5. The local names should be used for the foodstuff and the education should be imparted in day to-day language.
6. The persons should be encouraged to ask question to satisfy their queries regarding nutrition.
7. Nutrition education should be combined with reproductive and child health.
8. The food articles, which are not within the purchasing power of the individual or which are not consumed by them should not be advised to be included in the diet.

Responsibilities of Nurse in Nutrition Education/Teaching

1. Assessing the health status of the individual/the family/the community.
2. Making an early diagnosis of nutritional diseases and deficiencies and their treatment.
3. Paying special attention to nutrition of the vulnerable groups, e.g. children, pregnant and lactating women and poor class people and to check adulteration.

4. Telling the importance of kitchen garden (village shak vatika).
5. Imparting applied nutrition education using modem and attractive techniques.

▶ FOOD AND NUTRITION BOARD

The Food and Nutrition Board was formed in 1964 under the Ministry of Agriculture to bring variety in the dietary habits with the dual objective of reducing the demand of food grains and to make the individual diet more nutritious. In April 1993, the board was brought under the Women and Child Development Department in accordance with the National Nutrition Policy.

▶ ACTIVITIES OF FOOD AND NUTRITION BOARD

1. Education and training in nutrition:
   a. Nutrition demonstration programs.
   b. Training in domestic preservation of fruits and vegetables.
   c. Integrated nutrition education.
   d. To observe world nutrition week (1–7 September).
   e. To observe world food day (16 October).
   f. To observe world breastfeeding week (1–7 August).
2. Development and enhancement of nutritive foods:
   a. Assessment of regularity and quality of supplementary food in Anganwadi.
   b. To encourage production of nutritious foods in the community.
   c. Fortification of food:
      i. To fortify milk with vitamin A.
      ii. To fortify salt with iodine.
   d. Food analysis.
   e. Research and development.

CHAPTER 32: Community Nutritional Rehabilitation

f. National nutrition policy and implementation:
  i. Constitution of a standing committee for implementation of national nutrition program.
  ii. Activities for control of micronutritional deficiencies.
  iii. Nutritional surveillance.
  iv. Planning of district level diet and nutritional programs and their implementation.

▶ NUTRITION SOCIETY OF INDIA

The Nutrition Society of India (NSI) was established in 1967, is an organization dedicated to keep abreast of the latest developments in the basic and applied aspects of science of nutrition. The society continues to analyze issues related to the diverse aspects of nutrition. The society activities involve scientists, programs and policy makers throughout the country and abroad who are working in the field. Through its annual conference, the society provides a forum for new ideas, encourages innovations, recognizes important research findings, increases awareness of the latest survey data and promotes action programs.

▶ FOOD AND AGRICULTURAL ORGANIZATION

Food and Agricultural Organization (FAO) is one of the specialized agencies of the United Nations formally formed in 1945 with headquarters in Rome. It was the first United Nations organization specialized agency created to look after several areas of world cooperation. The FAO's primary aim is to increase agriculture production to keep pace with growing population in the world (Fig. 32.1).

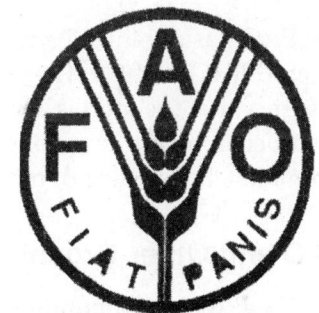

Fig. 32.1: Logo of Food and Agricultural Organization

Chief Aims

1. To increase the efficiency of farming, fisheries and forestry.
2. To improve the condition of rural people.
3. To ensure that the food is consumed by the people who need it in sufficient quantities and in right proportions.
4. To develop and maintain a better state of nutrition throughout the world.
5. To help nations raise their living standards.

Functions of FAO

1. To help nations raise their living standards.
2. To improve nutrition level of people of all countries.
3. To secure improvement of production and distributions of all food and agricultural products.
4. To improve the conditions of rural populations.

The main activity of this agency is to promote production of food to keep pace with the rising world population. The joint World Health Organization (WHO)/FAO expert committee provides the base for many cooperative activities, such as nutritional surveys, training courses, seminars and the coordination or related research programs.

Objectives of FAO

The FAO has organized a world Freedom From Hunger Campaign (FFHC) in 1960. The primary objective of FAO is toward ensuring that the food is consumed by the people who need it in sufficient quantities and in right proportions to develop and maintain a better state of nutrition throughout the world.

FAO and Other Organizations

1. The FAO is collaborating with other international agencies such as United Nations Children's Fund (UNICEF), WHO in applied nutritional program.

2. The joint WHO/FAO expert committee has provided the basis for many cooperative activities—nutritional surveys, training courses, seminars and the coordination of research programs on brucellosis and other zoonoses.

▶ COOPERATIVE FOR ASSISTANCE AND RELIEF EVERYWHERE

Cooperative for Assistance and Relief Everywhere (CARE) was founded in North America in 1945. It is one of the world's largest independent non-profit, non-sectarian international relief and developmental organization. CARE provides emergency aid and long-term development assistance.

The CARE began its operation in India in 1950. Till the end of 1980s, the primary objective of CARE India was to provide food for children in the age group of 6–11 years. From mid 1980s, CARE India focused its food support in the ICDS program and in development programs in the areas of health and income supplementation.

CARE India has given help in the field of medicine, literacy, vocational training and agriculture. It also helps schools by providing garden tools, pumps and improved seeds to grow more food. It also provides mobile medical vans, X-ray machines, diagnostic equipments, eyeglasses and frames, medical books, medicine and vitamins.

▶ NATIONAL INSTITUTE OF NUTRITION, HYDERABAD

National Institute of Nutrition (NIN) set up under Indian Council of Medical Research (ICMR) (Fig. 32.2), is the premier research institution of the country. It has published many research publications including 'the nutritive value of Indian foods'. This handbook provides detailed information on the nutrients composition of a wide range of common Indian foods. Up-to-date information on nutritional requirement and recommended dietary allowances and guidelines for formulation of nutritionally rich diets are also provided by NIN for the benefit of health professionals and informed public. The data on nutrient composition of foods given are based mainly on Indian research work carried out at the NIN, Hyderabad itself.

Vision

"To achieve optimal nutrition of vulnerable segments of population such as women of reproductive age, children, adolescent girls and elderly by 2020." —**NIN website.**

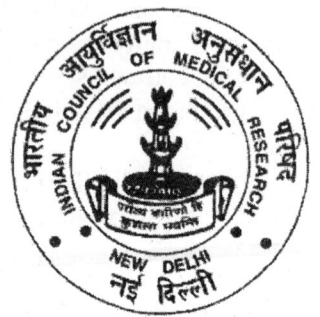

Fig. 32.2: Logo of Indian Council of Medical Research

Mission

"To enable food and nutrition security conducive to good health, growth and development and increase productivity through dedicated research, so as to achieve the national nutrition goals set by the Government of India in the National Nutrition Policy."—**NIN website.**

Objectives

1. To identify various dietary and nutrition problems prevalent among different segments of the population.
2. To continuously monitor food and nutrition situation of the country.
3. To evaluate effective methods of management and prevention of nutritional problems.
4. To conduct operational research connected with planning and implementation of national nutrition programs.
5. To dovetail the nutrition research with other health programs of the government.
6. Human resource development in the field of nutrition.

7. To disseminate nutrition information.
8. To advice governments relating to nutrition.

▶ CENTRAL FOOD TECHNOLOGICAL RESEARCH INSTITUTE, MYSORE

Central Food Technological Research Institute (CFTRI) (Fig. 32.3) is situated in Mysore. It came into existence during 1950. A network of its founders and inspiring and dedicated scientists had the great vision to pursue in-depth research and development in the areas of food science and technology. The Bengal famine of 1943 and the ravages of the 2nd World War made the Government of India realize that the key to food security was in the right intervention of science and technology to conserve, preserve, process and distribute the available food resources. CFTRI was declared open on 21st October 1950 as the next step.

Through the decades, since then, CFTRI has produced and provided scores of technology solutions that have given a powerful thrust to the development of indigenous food industries and played a notable role in the socioeconomic transformation of the nation.

Technology Milestones of CFTRI

1. Formation of infant food using buffalo's milk.
2. Extraction of the plant protein for the nutrition base for a new class of food supplements–energy food, Indian multipurpose food, milestone and several weaning foods.
3. Improvement in the efficiency of process for handling, drying and willing of staple cereals.

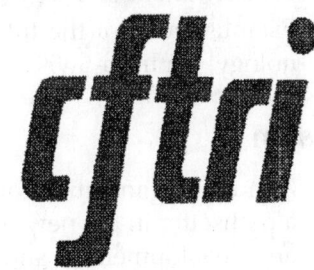

Fig. 32.3: Logo of Central Food Technological Research Institute

4. Design and fabrication of energy efficient and cost-effective equipment for milling food grains and pulses.
5. Refinement of millets and production of diversified millet products with enhanced nutritive value.
6. Efficient methods for parboiling paddy.
7. Formulation of products for preparing traditional Indian snacks.
8. Production of spice and oil resins by indigenous technology.
9. Fermentation and drying of cocoa mass, cocoa butter and cocoa powder by indigenous technology.

Support Area Milestones

1. Establishment of the International Food Technology Training Center (IFTTC) in collaboration with FAO—the nucleus of an internationally referred center of excellence in advanced knowledge in foods.
2. Selection by the United Nations University (UNU) as an associated institution.
3. Recognition by the University of Mysore for postgraduate studies and research in food technology, food science and allied disciplines.
4. Adoption by the National Information System for Science and Technology (NISSAT) as a sectoral information center (NICFOS) for food science and technology in India.
5. Establishment of a state-of-the-art pilot plant.
6. Establishment of the International school of milling technology: An Indo-Swiss venture ISO 9001 certification.

Vision

1. A model organization for scientific industrial research and a pathsetter in the new paradigm of self-financed research and development (R and D) in the country.
2. A global platform providing competitive R and D and high quality science-based technical services across the world.

CHAPTER 32: Community Nutritional Rehabilitation

3. A vital source of science and technology for national social mission, which provide a human face to the organization endeavors.

Mission

1. Generate and apply knowledge of food science and food technology for optimal conservation and utilization of the nation's resources.
2. Integrate scientific and technological knowledge into conventional and traditional systems, and local and regional realities.
3. Add value and utility to Agro Resources through R and D and contribute to sustain development, food security and food safety.
4. Aid and promote the development of food industry through interdisciplinary, innovative and state-of-the-art solutions.
5. Set national standards for food quality and spread food quality consciousness all around.
6. Sustain leadership in long-term strategic research and technology development.
7. Integrate the food supply chain from the cultivator to the consumer so that cultivators get optimal returns from processing and consumers get the food that they want, when they want, where they want, in whatever form they want and at affordable cost.
8. Build and bolster bonds with nodal agencies from the global to the grassroots level, particularly in the area of multilevel human resources development.
9. Develop new knowledge continuously, to address contemporary challenges and answer future emergencies.

▶ NATIONAL INSTITUTE OF PUBLIC COOPERATION AND CHILD DEVELOPMENT

National Institute of Public Cooperation and Child Development (NIPCCD) is a premier organization devoted to promotion of voluntary action research, training and documentation in the field of women and child development. It was established in New Delhi in the year 1966 under Societies Registration Act of 1860. It functions under the aegis of the Ministry of Women and Child Development. The institute has four regional centers, at Guwahati (1978), Bangalore (1980), Lucknow (1982) and Indore (2001) to cater to the specific needs of the country. This institute trains the functionaries of the ICDS program.

The Ministry of Women and Child Development has designated it as the nodal institute for imparting training for two important issues of child rights and prevention of trafficking of women and children for South Asian Association for Regional Cooperation (SAARC) countries.

The institute was recognized by UNICEF in 1985 for its expertise and performance. It was awarded the Maurice Pate Award for its outstanding contribution in the field of child development.

Vision

The vision of the institute is to become regional center of excellence and knowledge in the fields of women rights and child development. This institute envisions itself as an umbrella organization that will facilitate and stimulate exchanges between field experiences and academic research.

Mission

The institute shares the belief that human progress and overall development is fundamentally rooted in the progress of women and children, and in the realization of their rights. Working with this conviction, the strategic mission of NIPCCD is defined as:

1. Developing into an organization with a strong civil society orientation, while retaining characteristic advantages of technical institutions.

CHAPTER 32: Community Nutritional Rehabilitation

2. Forging strategic alliance with premier training institutes in other countries.
3. Intensification of collaborative ventures in the areas of training, research and documentation.
4. Acquiring flexibility in offering a broad spectrum of training opportunities that meet the changing demands in the context of issues related to women and children at national, regional and international level.
5. Integrating selected programs of the institute into the professional training system, though accreditation of these programs by the All India Council of Technical Education (AICTE) and other accrediting institutions.

▶ CONCLUSION

The WHO has traditionally focused on the vast magnitude of the many forms of nutritional deficiency along with their associated mortality and morbidity in infants, young children and mothers. Poor nutrition contributes to one out of two deaths (53%) associated with infectious diseases among children aged under five in developing countries. Undernutrition among pregnant women in developing countries leads to one out of six infants born with low birth weight. This is not only a risk factor for neonatal retardation, poor health, blindness and premature death. One out of three people in developing countries are affected by vitamin and mineral deficiencies, and therefore more subject to infection, birth defects and impaired physical and psycho-intellectual developments. Community nutrition rehabilitation play vital role in preventing nutrition-related health problems.

SECTION 5

Appendix

▶ BEVERAGES

Beverages are drinks used for the purpose of relieving thirst and including fluid in the day's diet. They contain nutrients and are also stimulants. Beverages can play an important role in providing essential nutrients. All beverages contain water, which supports proper hydration (Fig. A.1). Many 100% fruit and vegetable juices are also a good source of vitamin C, folate and potassium, while milk and some fortified juices provide calcium. Other beverages are formulated to meet specific nutritional needs. There are also new discoveries, such as research suggesting that the polyphenols found in some juices may have potential health benefits.

Nutritional Significance

Most beverages contain a great deal of water. This does not add many nutrients to the diet, but it does play an important role in maintaining body balance by preventing dehydration. Beverages are not usually consumed for their food value, but many, particularly the fruit drinks, contain quite a high percentage

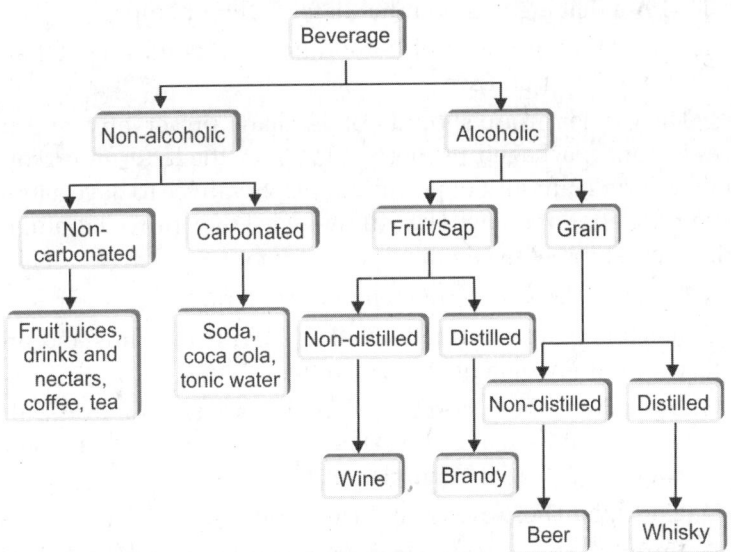

Fig. A.1: Classification of beverage

of sugar and therefore add to the energy content of the diet. Additionally fruit juices provide a supply of vitamins and minerals.

Certain drinks contain artificial flavorings and colorings. The use of such additives is governed by legal requirements and it is vital to keep to these regulations in order to protect the consumer from any undesirable side-effects. For example, some coloring agents are thought to cause hyperactivity in children and are therefore to be avoided. Alcoholic drinks are judged in terms of flavor and the stimulant effect they produce. In many countries alcohol production is strictly controlled by government agencies and it may be difficult to obtain the necessary permits to produce these beverages legally.

Non-alcoholic Beverages

A wide range of drinks can be manufactured, which contain as the base material either pulped fruit or juice. Many are drunk as a pure fruit juice without the addition of other ingredients, whereas others are diluted with sugar syrup. For simplicity, fruit drinks can be divided into two groups:

1. Those that are drunk immediately after opening.
2. Those that are used little by little from bottles, which are stored between uses.

The former group should not need any preservative if processed and packaged properly. However the latter must contain a certain amount of permitted preservatives to have a long shelf-life after opening. The following list may prove helpful in distinguishing between the different types of drink:

1. **Juices:** These are pure fruit juice with nothing added.
2. **Nectars:** These normally contain 30% fruit solids and are drunk immediately after opening.
3. **Squashes:** These normally contain at least 25% fruit pulp mixed with sugar syrup. They are diluted, to taste, with water and may contain preservatives.
4. **Cordials:** These are crystal-clear squashes.
5. **Syrups:** These are concentrated juices, which are clear. They normally have high sugar content.

Each of the above products is preserved by its natural acidity and by pasteurization. Some drinks (syrups and squashes) also contain a high concentration of sugar, which helps to preserve them.

Tea

Tea is obtained from the leaves and flowers of tea bush. The kind of tea obtained is determined by the manufacturing process and treatment. It is a stimulating and refreshing drink. The principle flavor components of tea are caffeine, tannin yielding compounds and small amounts of essential oils. Caffeine provides the stimulating effect, tannin the color, body and taste to the extract and the essential oils contribute the characteristic aroma.

Tea can be prepared by introducing tea leaves into boiling water in a kettle or by pouring boiling water over tea leaves in a preheated teapot and letting it steep. The time of steeping depends on the strength of the beverage desired and quantity of tea leaves used. To prepare good tea one teaspoonful of tea leaves for one cup is ideal. The tea should be brewed only for 5 minutes and strained. If it is kept for more than 5 minutes it will give a bitter taste. Milk and sugar should be added to individual taste.

Teas come in many varieties including herbal, caffeinated, iced, sweet, instant and ready to drink. Like coffee, tea does not provide calories, carbohydrates, protein or fat. Teas, particularly green and black, are good sources of flavonoids, substances believed to have antioxidant properties.

Coffee

Coffee is prepared from the beans of the coffee plant. Caffeine and flavoring substances such as tannins determine the quality of the end products. It is available in many varieties including caffeinated, decaffeinated, brewed, roasted, instant, flavored, iced and ready-to-drink.

1. Plain coffee and espresso do not provide calories, but can contain trace amounts of vitamins and minerals primarily

from the water used in brewing. However, cream, milk, sugar or other popular flavorings like chocolate and syrups commonly added to coffee can contribute significant calories. While a 355 mL cup of coffee contains zero calories, the same size mocha latte coffee provides about 340 calories.

2. Coffee also contains caffeine. Depending on how it is brewed, a 236 mL serving of regular drip coffee provides about 104–192 mg of caffeine. A 44 mL 'shot' of espresso contains about 30–100 mg. Even decaffeinated coffee contains a small amount of caffeine, about 2–4 mg per 240 mL serving.

3. Polyphenols, substances believed to have antioxidant properties, are found in coffee and may be beneficial to health. However, studies examining the health benefits of coffee have found mixed results.

Fruit Beverages

Fruit beverages are obtained by extracting the juice from fruits such as orange, grape, pineapple, lemon, tomato, etc. These juices are an excellent source of vitamins, minerals and energy depending on the fruit used. Fruit juices are not only refreshing, they are nutritious and increase fluid intake. Fruit squashes are prepared by combining sugar syrup and fruit juice. They have a long shelf life and can be readily mixed with water to obtain an instant refreshing drink.

Fruit pulp can be combined with milk and sugar to form milk shakes, e.g. apple, mango, sapota, etc.

100% juice: As follows:

1. The Dietary Guidelines recommend Americans consume nine servings (about 1 L) of fruits and vegetables a day. Fruit and vegetable juices can count toward intake, as long as the majority of fruit and vegetable servings come from whole foods.

2. Most 100% juices are a natural source of potassium, folate and antioxidants, including vitamin C and beta-carotene.

Many fruit and vegetable juices are also a source of phytochemicals, substances found in plants that may have health-protective effects. And, because juices are derived from fruit, they naturally contain fructose, a simple sugar found in fruit that provides carbohydrates and calories (energy).

3. Juices are available in many varieties including fresh-squeezed, pulp-free, home-squeezed, not-from-concentrate, concentrate, flavor blends, fortified and those that contain functional ingredients, such as plant sterols.

Juice drinks: It contain fruit juice, but at levels less than 100%. Some contain 50% fruit juice or more, while others contain 5% or less. Manufacturers are required to label the percent of real fruit juice in the product. The nutrient content of juice drinks depends on how much 100% juice is used in the product and on whether any nutrients are added.

Milk Beverages

Milk beverages are prepared by the addition of different flavors, viz. strawberry, pista, cardamom and chocolate to milk. They enhance the flavor of milk and thereby increase its consumption particularly by young children. Milk beverages are a good source of protein, calcium and vitamin A and B. Milk shakes are prepared by mixing fruit pulp with milk and sugar. Milk can be mixed with egg to prepare eggnog, which is a nourishing drink with a creamy consistency.

1. Milk is available in many varieties, including whole milk, 2% milk, 1% milk, skim milk, flavored, powdered, lactose-free, evaporated, condensed and buttermilk.
2. Milk is an excellent source of calcium and good source of other essential nutrients, including vitamin D, potassium, vitamin B_{12}, riboflavin, phosphorus and protein.
3. About 240 mL glass of milk contains 300 mg of calcium or about one-third of the daily recommended calcium intake for adults under the age of 50. In US, cow's milk is uniformly fortified with vitamin D to a level of 25% of the daily value per 240 mL serving.

4. The fat content of milk significantly affects its caloric level. In US, whole milk provides about 144 calories and 8–9 g of fat per 240 mL serving. The same size serving of 2% milk contains about half as much fat (about 5 g) and 120 calories per 240 mL serving. Skim milk is virtually fat-free and contains about 88 calories per 240 mL serving.

Soy-based Beverages

Many soy-based beverages contain an array of nutrients including protein, carbohydrates, potassium, B vitamins, iron, phosphorus and trace amounts of sodium and magnesium. Many are also fortified with nutrients, most commonly vitamin A, calcium and vitamin D, while some also have added riboflavin, zinc and vitamin B_{12}. Soy contains fairly high levels of phytochemicals including isoflavones and phytosterols.

Carbonated

Carbonated non-alcoholic beverages are those beverages that are generally sweetened, flavored, acidified and colored. The chief ingredient is water and this may be to the extent of 92%. The beverage contains 8%–14% of sugar, which contributes to the sweetness, calorie and body of the drink. Artificial sweeteners such as saccharin are also used. Carbon dioxide is added to produce the tingling effect, sparkle and effervescence of carbonated beverages.

Nutritionally, it is an empty food since it provides only calories and no other nutrients. A bottle of an aerated beverage (180 mL) gives 70 kcal of energy.

Phosphoric acid, citric acid, fumaric acid and tartaric acid, which are added to enhance the flavor, makes the drink acidic. It is therefore not recommended for patients suffering from acidity and ulcers. Saccharin, which is a suspected carcinogen is also present in aerated drinks. Children should not be encouraged to consume carbonated beverages since they have no food value and depress the appetite (Fig. A.2, Tables A.1 and A.2).

Soft drinks

Soft drinks are non-alcoholic carbonated beverages containing flavorings, sweeteners and other ingredients. Depending on the sweetener used, soft drinks may or may not contain calories. Soft drinks include regular, diet, low-calorie, mid-calorie, flavored, caffeinated and caffeine-free drinks. Soft drinks are carbonated by adding carbon dioxide into a beverage solution under pressure. Opening a soft-drink container releases the carbon dioxide in the form of bubbles. These bubbles intensify the flavor of the beverage.

Most regular and mid-calorie carbonated soft drinks are sweetened with high-fructose corn syrup (HFCS), a calorie-containing carbohydrate that provides 4 cal/g. A 355 mL serving of regular cola-type soft drinks contain about 140 calories, or 11 calories per 29 mL. Mid-calorie cola-type soft drinks generally contain about half that much. Diet soft drinks contain virtually no calories and are flavored with low- and no-calorie sweeteners, including acesulfame potassium, aspartame,

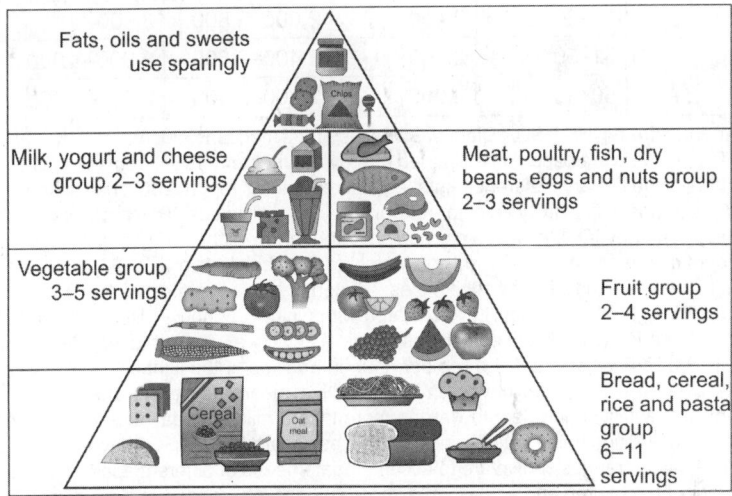

Fig. A.2: Food pyramid

saccharin and sucralose. Learn more about sweeteners. Soft drinks also contain small amounts of sodium, primarily from the water used in the soft drink plus nutritionally insignificant amounts of potassium and phosphorus.

Table A.1: Estimated calorie requirements (in kcal) fro each gender and age groups at three levels of physical activity*

Gender	Age (years)	Activity level		
		Sedentary[†]	Moderately active[‡]	Active[§]
Child	2–3	1,000	1,000–1,400[ǁ]	1,000–1,400[ǁ]
Female	4–8	1,200	1,400–1,600	1,400–1,800
	9–13	1,600	1,600–2,000	1,800–2,200
	14–18	1,800	2,000	2,400
	19–30	2 000	2,000–2,200	2,400
	31–50	1,800	2,000	2,200
	50+	1,600	1,800	2,000–2,200
Male	4–8	1,400	1,400–1,600	1,600–2,000
	9–13	1,800	1,800–2,200	2,000–2,600
	14–18	2,200	2,400–2,800	2,800–3,200
	19–30	2,400	2,600–2,800	3,000
	31–50	2,200	2,400–2,600	2,800–3,000
	50+	2,000	2,200–2,400	2,400–2,800

Adapted from HHS/USDA Dietary Guidelines for Americans, 2005.
*These levels are based on estimated energy requirement (EER) from the Institute of Medicine Dietary Reference. Intakes macronutrients report, 2002, calculated by gender, age and activity level for reference-sized individuals. 'Reference size', as determined by IOM, is based on median height and weight for ages up to age 18 years of age and median height and weight for that height to give a BMI of 21.5 for adult females and 22.5 for adult males; [†]Sedentary means a lifestyle that includes only the light physical activity associated with typical day-to-day life; [‡]Moderately active means a lifestyle that includes physical activity equivalent to walking about 1.5–3 miles per day at 3–4 miles per hour, in addition to the light physical activity associated with typical day-to-day life; [§]Active means a lifestyle that includes physical activity equivalent to walking more than 3 miles per day at 3–4 miles per hour, in addition to the light physical activity associated with typical day-to-day life; [ǁ]The calorie ranges shown are to accommodate needs of different ages within the group. For children and adolescents, more calories are needed at older ages. For adults, fewer calories are needed at older ages.

Table A.2: Calorie chart of commonly used Indian food

Snacks	Name	Quantity	Calories	Name	Quantity	Calories	Meat/Poultry
	Burger	1 piece	325	Chicken	1 cup	220	
	Pizza	1 portion	375	Tandoori chicken	2 pieces	450	
	Samosa/ Kachori	1 piece	256	Mutton (boiled)	1 cup	100	
	Pakoda	1 piece	200	Fish (boiled)	1 cup	100	
	Potato chips	10 pieces	110	Crab	1 cup	33	
	Dahi vada	1 piece	364	Egg (fried)	1 piece	100	
	French fries	10 pieces	235	Omelette	1 serving	110	
Fruits	Name	Quantity	Calories	Name	Quantity	Calories	Bread/Rice
	Apple	100 g	56	Bread	1 slice	60	
	Banana	100 g	95	Chapati	1 piece	100	
	Mango	100 g	70	Paratha	1 piece	280	
	Orange	100 g	53	Rice	100 g	325	
	Chikoo	100 g	94	Wheat flour	100 g	341	
	Papaya	100 g	32	Maize flour	100 g	355	
	Peach	100 g	50	Vegetable oil	1 tablespoon	130	

Contd...

SECTION 5: Appendix

Vegetables	Name	Quantity	Calories	Sweets/Miscellaneous	Name	Quantity	Calories
	Potato	100 g	97		Barfi	1 piece	100
	Peas	100 g	93		Gulab jamun	1 piece	100
	Cauliflower	100 g	30		Jalebi	1 piece	200
	Cabbage	100 g	45		Rasgulla	1 piece	150
	Carrot	100 g	48		Sugar	1 tablespoon	60
	Mushroom	100 g	18		Honey	1 tablespoon	30
	Onion	100 g	50		Jam	1 tablespoon	100
Milk and milk products	Name	Quantity	Calories	**Drinks/Beverages**	Name	Quantity	Calories
	Milk	1 cup	100		Cold drinks	1 bottle	95
	Skimmed milk	1 cup	45		Orange juice	1 glass	95
	Curd	1 cup	60		Apple juice	1 glass	95
	Butter	1 tablespoon	120		Beer	1 glass	100
	Cheese	1 cup	164		Whisky	1 peg	75
	Ice cream	1 scoop	114		Rum	1 peg	75
	Ghee	100 g	910		Tea/Coffee	1 cup	35

Contd...

Malted Beverages

Malted beverages are also known as Amylase Rich Foods (ARF). This is prepared by steeping whole grain like ragi or wheat in 2–3 times its volume of water. The excess water is drained and the moist seed is germinated for 24–48 hours till sprouts appear. The grains are sun-dried and roasted to remove moisture. Sprouts are removed and the grains are milled and powdered. The malt is cooked with water or milk to prepare a nutritious beverage.

The ARF is rich in enzyme amylase. The germination process activates the enzymes of the resting grain and facilitates the conversion of cereal starch to fermentable sugars. Hydrolysis of cereal proteins also takes place.

Traditional Beverages

Neera: It is a sweet drink from the fresh sap of palm.

Tendor coconut water: This is a refreshing drink obtained from coconut. Potassium, ascorbic acid and many vitamins of the B group are present in coconut water. Apart from this, the water also contains traces of calcium, phosphorus and iron.

Sugarcane juice: This is extracted from sugarcane contains 12%–15% sugar. The cane juice is acidic and in addition to sugar contains minerals and vitamins such as the B-group.

Soups

Soups are prepared with vegetables, pulses, poultry and meat. The food, which is to be used for making soup is cooked thoroughly in plenty of water. Clear soups are prepared using only the water in which the food is cooked, while cream soups are prepared by adding milk and white sauce to the water. Soups provide us with a variety of nutrients depending on the ingredients used. Soups also enhance appetite and add color to the meal. It is usually served at the beginning of a meal.

PREVIOUS YEARS QUESTION PAPERS

▶ NUTRITION AND DIETETICS—SEPTEMBER 2012

Long Essay

1. a. Define malnutrition.
   b. Explain various methods of nutritional assessment.
2. a. What are the fat-soluble vitamins?
   b. Discuss the sources, functions and deficiency of vitamin A and D.

Short Essay

1. High-calorie diet.
2. Methods of cooking.
3. Factors affecting meal planning.
4. Functions of protein.

Short Answers

1. Food adulteration.
2. Basal metabolic rate (BMR).
3. Weaning.
4. Balanced diet.
5. FAO.

▶ NUTRITION AND DIETETICS—MARCH 2012

Long Essay

1. a. Define community nutrition.
   b. Explain the need of community nutrition programs.
2. a. What are the nutritional needs of pregnant women?
   b. Plan a menu for a patient with diabetes.

Short Essay

1. Deficiencies of vitamins.
2. Bodybuilding food.

3. Undernutrition.
4. Planning diet for lactating mother.

Short Answers

1. Steaming.
2. Food preservation.
3. Vegetable soup.
4. Balanced diet.
5. Functions of vitamin B_{12}.

▶ NUTRITION AND DIETETICS—AUGUST 2011

Long Essay

1. a. Define dietetics.
   b. Explain the dietary management of hypertension.
2. a. Discuss the importance of nutritional education.
   b. Explain the role of a nurse in nutritional education.

Short Essay

1. Milk hygiene.
2. Preservation of food.
3. Functions of carbohydrate.
4. Baby-friendly Hospital Initiative (BFHI).

Short Answers

1. Grilling.
2. Phrynoderma.
3. Kwashiorkor.
4. Sources of iron.
5. Obesity.

▶ NUTRITION AND DIETETICS—FEBRUARY 2011

Long Essay

1. Discuss in detail about the importance of nutrition in health.
2. Discuss the balanced diet and dietary requirements for adolescent girls.

Short Essay

1. Composition of breast milk and cow's milk.
2. Therapeutic diet for hepatic disorders.
3. Prevention of nutritional anemia.
4. Methods of nutritional education for community.

Short Answers

1. Calorie requirements for toddler, preschooler and school age.
2. Iodine deficiency disorders.
3. Low-cost protein rich food.
4. Scurvy.
5. Permit Extension Act.

▶ NUTRITION AND DIETETICS—AUGUST 2010

Long Essay

1. Explain in detail the guidelines in planning diet to meet the nutritional needs of an elderly person.
2. Describe the methods of assessing the nutritional status in an individual and community.

Short Essay

1. Methods of preservation of food.
2. Advantages of school lunch program.

3. Vitamin A deficiency.
4. Therapeutic diet for renal disorders.

Short Answers

1. Protein requirements for infants.
2. Rich dietary sources of calcium.
3. Niacin deficiency.
4. Pasteurization of milk.
5. Exclusive breastfeeding

▶ NUTRITION AND DIETETICS—FEBRUARY 2010

Long Essay

1. Discuss on various deficiency diseases and methods to prevent them.
2. Explain in detail the methods of nutritional education in community and hospital.

Short Essay

1. Methods of cooking.
2. Preparation of weaning diet.
3. Problems in feeding the infant.
4. Nutritional needs of elderly people.

Short Answers

1. Vitamin A prophylaxis.
2. Undernutrition.
3. Balanced diet.
4. Overweight.
5. Preservation of nutrition.

GLOSSARY

▶ NUTRITION

1. **Absorption:** The process by which nutrients and other substances are transferred from the digestive system into the blood for transport throughout the body.
2. **Antioxidants:** Vitamins (C, E and plant forms of A or beta carotene) that are thought to inactivate 'activated oxygen molecules' sometimes called 'free radicals'. Free radicals are naturally created by human cells, but are also caused by environmental factors such as smoke and radiation. Free radicals may cause cell damage that leads to diseases of various kinds. If antioxidant vitamins work, they would inactivate the free radicals before they do their damage.
3. **Balanced diet:** It is a diet that contains carbohydrate, proteins, fats, minerals, vitamins and water in correct proportions and quality adequate for correct requirement as well as for the need in future emergencies.
4. **Basal metabolic rate (BMR):** The minimum number of calories needed to maintain vital functions, such as breathing and keeping the heart beating.
5. **Body mass index (BMI):** A formula that uses weight and height to estimate body fat, and gauge health risks due to carrying too much weight. The BMI is the only one factor in determining a person's health risk. A BMI in the 'healthy' range does not necessarily mean that everyone are fit and healthy.
6. **Calorie:** The scientific definition of a calorie is a unit of energy, for heat in particular. 1 calorie is the amount of heat that increases the temperature of 1 kg of water by 1°C.
7. **Essential nutrients:** The nutrients, which are essential to humans. The body cannot manufacture an essential nutrient by itself. One needs to get it from the diet.
8. **Fiber:** A carbohydrate found in plants that cannot be digested. Fiber comes in two forms such as soluble and insoluble. Soluble fibers are found in beans, fruit and oats, dissolves in water. Insoluble fibers are found in whole

grains and vegetables, does not dissolve in water. Both types of fiber help with digestion, lower cholesterol, and help control blood sugar.

9. **Healthy diets:** Recommended by the United States Department of Agriculture (USDA) in its dietary guidelines as a diet that emphasizes fruits, vegetables, whole grains, low-fat milk products, lean meats and protein from beans, eggs and nuts, and is low in saturated fats, trans fats, salts and sugars.
10. **Kilocalorie:** The amount of energy taken to raise the temperature of 1 kg of water 1° on a centigrade (Celsius) thermometer at sea level.
11. **Malaise:** A vague uneasy feeling of body weakness, distress or discomfort, often marking the onset of and persisting throughout a disease.
12. **Malnutrition:** It refers to the physical effects of a dietary intake, which is inadequate in quantity and/or quality. It has been defined as a pathological state resulting from a relative or absolute deficiency or excess of one or more essential nutrients.
13. **Marasmus:** A condition that results from general malnutrition of both calories and proteins. It is due to continued restriction of energy intake, it occurs due to early weaning.
14. **Mastication:** Chewing, tearing or grinding food with the teeth, while it becomes mixed with saliva.
15. **Mayonnaise:** A stable emulsion of vegetable oil and egg yolk, flavored with vinegar or lemon juice, eaten with cold salads.
16. **Metabolism:** It is the general name given to the changes, which takes place in nutrients from the time of their absorption until they have reached the end products of the various processes through which they pass.
17. **Milk-alkali syndrome:** A condition of alkalosis caused by the excessive ingestion of milk, antacid medications containing calcium or other sources of absorbable alkaline substances.

18. **Monounsaturated fatty acids (MUFA):** These fatty acids have only one double bond in their molecule. They typically remain liquid at extremely low temperatures. MUFA are found in vegetable oils. They lower the total blood cholesterol by reducing low-density lipoprotein (LDL) cholesterol and increasing high-density lipoprotein (HDL) cholesterol. Nut, canola, olive oils are high in monounsaturated fats.
19. **Nutraceuticals:** It refers to any substance that may be considered a food or part of a food and provides medical or health benefits, including the prevention and treatment of diseases.
20. **Nutrition:** It is the process by which food is used by the body to produce energy and heat, maintain body function and structure and promote growth.
21. **Recommended daily allowance (RDA):** The minimum amount of a specific nutrient that should be included in the daily diet to meet current health needs.

▶ DIETETICS

1. **Anorexia:** Loss of appetite.
2. **Dyspepsia:** Indigestion, a feeling of fullness, discomfort, nausea and anorexia.
3. **Dysphasia:** Difficulty in swallowing.
4. **Food allergy:** Also referred to as food sensitivity. An immunologically mediated adverse reaction related to the chemical composition of foods and their additives resulting from antigen-antibody combination.
5. **Food exchanges:** These are used to bring variety to the diet and to suit the family's economic capacity. Foods approximately containing the same calorie and protein values are grouped together, so that any item in that group can be chosen, while formulating the daily menu. Food exchanges are specifically useful for patients with diabetes.
6. **Food poisoning:** Any of a large group of toxic processes that result from the ingestion of a food contaminated by

toxic substances or by bacteria that contain toxins. Kinds of food poisoning include phallic food poisoning, mushroom poisoning and shellfish poisoning.
7. **Gluconeogenesis:** Formation of glucose or glycogen from non-carbohydrate sources such as glycerol and glucogenic amino acids.
8. **Glycemic index:** The measurement of the ability of food items to raise the blood glucose. It is calculated for individual food items and calculates the level of glycemia by comparing the carbohydrate content in foods per gram.
9. **Glycosylated hemoglobin (HbA):** A compound formed in the red blood cells by the irreversible reaction of hemoglobin A with glucose. The glycosylated hemoglobin concentration indicates the average blood glucose level over the previous 6–8 weeks.
10. **Low-oxalate diet:** A diet, which excludes consumption of foods that are rich in oxalates such as beans, chocolate, cocoa, potatoes, spinach, tea and tomatoes (chemicals found in plant foods). This diet is prescribed for patients with urinary calculi composed of oxalate.
11. **Nausea:** A sensation of sickness with inclination to vomit.
12. **Nutrients:** Constituents of food, e.g. carbohydrates, proteins, fats, minerals, vitamins and water.
13. **Obesity:** The generalized accumulation of excess adipose tissue in the body resulting in an increase of more than 20% of the desirable weight (ideal body weight). Obesity results when there is positive energy balance where the intake of calories (from food) is more than the expenditure of calories (physical activity).
14. **Oliguric phase:** The early phase of acute renal failure when urine volume is reduced.
15. **Parenteral nutrition:** The administration of nutrients by a route other than the alimentary canal, such as subcutaneously, intravenously, intramuscularly or intradermally. The parenteral fluids usually consist of physiologic saline solution with glucose, amino acids, electrolytes, vitamins and medications.

16. **Polydipsia:** Excessive thirst due to loss of body fluids, especially from the urine, as seen in diabetes mellitus.
17. **Polyphagia:**
    a. Swallowing abnormally large amounts of food at a meal.
    b. Excessive appetite as in diabetes mellitus.
18. **Polyuria:** Excessive secretion and discharge of urine as seen in diabetes mellitus.
19. **Regurgitation:** Backflow, e.g. backflow of partly digested food into the mouth from the stomach.
20. **Self-monitoring:** An important component of behavior modification in weight management. It includes maintaining a daily record of the place and time of food intake as well as accompanying thoughts and feelings, which stimulate food intake. It helps to identify physical and emotional settings in which eating occurs.
21. **Soft diet:** A diet that is soft in texture, low in residue, easily digested and well tolerated. It provides the essential nutrients in the form of semisolid foods, such as eggs, cheese, custards and puddings, pureed vegetables, ground beef and lamb, fowl, fish, mashed, boiled or baked potatoes, soft-cooked cereals and breads.
22. **Therapeutic diet:** Normal diet, which is modified to meet the altered requirements resulting from disease or injury; diet used in the treatment of a disease.
23. **Vomiting:** Expulsion of stomach contents via esophagus and the mouth.

▶ INFANT AND CHILD NUTRITION

1. **Angular stomatitis:** Characterized by inflammation at the corners of the mouth. It is a sign of riboflavin (vitamin B_2) deficiency.
2. **Anthropometric status:** The growth status of an individual's body measurements in relation to population reference values.
3. **Anthropometry:** It is the use of body measurements such as weight, height and midupper arm circumference (MUAC),

in combination with age and sex to gauge growth or failure to grow.
4. **Ariboflavinosis:** Clinical condition resulting from a deficiency in riboflavin (vitamin B_2). Clinical signs include the presence of angular stomatitis.
5. **Artificial feeding:** The feeding of infants with only a breast milk substitute.
6. **Beriberi:** Caused by thiamine (vitamin B_1) deficiency. There are many clinically recognizable syndromes including wet beriberi (which affects the cardiovascular system), dry beriberi (which affects the nervous system) and infantile beriberi [which affects infants breastfed by women with thiamine (vitamin B_1) deficiency].
7. **Breast milk substitutes:** Any food being marketed or otherwise represented as a partial or total replacement for breast milk, whether or not it is suitable for that purpose.
8. **Commercial infant formula:** A breast milk substitute formulated industrially in accordance with applicable Codex Alimentarius standards to satisfy the nutritional requirements of infants during the 1st month of life up to the introduction of complementary foods.
9. **Complementary food:** Any food, whether manufactured or locally prepared, used as a complement to breast milk or to a breast milk substitute.
10. **Counseling:** A way of working with people so that you understand their feelings and help them to develop confidence and decide what to do.
11. **Cup feeding:** Feeding an infant from an open cup without a lid, whatever is in the cup.
12. **Demand feeding:** Feeding a baby whenever he/she shows that he/she is ready, both day and night. This is also called `unrestricted' or `baby-led' feeding or feeding on cue.
13. **Exclusive breastfeeding:** Infant receives only breast milk (including breast milk that has been expressed or from a wet nurse) and nothing else, except for oral rehydration salts (ORS), medicines, vitamins and minerals.

14. **Expressed breast milk:** Milk that has been removed from the breasts manually or by using a pump.
15. **Formula:** Artificial milk for babies made out of a variety of products including sugar, animal milk, soybean and vegetable oils. They are usually in powder form to mix with water.
16. **Fortified foods:** These are foods that have certain nutrients added to improve their nutritional quality.
17. **Partial breastfeeding:** Infant receives other liquids or solids in addition to breast milk before 6 months of age.
18. **Predominant breastfeeding:** Infant receives certain liquids (water and water-based drinks, fruit juice), ritual fluids and ORS, vitamins, minerals, medicines in addition to breast milk.
19. **Responsive feeding:** Feeding infants directly and assisting older children when they feed themselves, being sensitive to their hunger and satiety cues.
20. **Rooming-in:** A baby staying in the same room as his/her mother.
21. **Severe acute malnutrition (SAM):** Malnutrition defined by a very low weight-for-height Z-score (WHZ below 3 z scores of the median WHO growth standards), MUAC less than 115 mm, by visible severe wasting or by the presence of nutritional edema.
22. **Undernourished:** A classification that indicates undernutrition such as stunting, underweight or wasting.
23. **Undernutrition:** A consequence of a deficiency in nutrient intake and/or absorption in the body. The different forms of undernutrition that can appear isolated or in combination are acute malnutrition (bilateral pitting edema and/or wasting), chronic malnutrition (stunting), underweight (combined form of wasting and stunting) and micronutrient deficiencies.
24. **Underweight:** A composite form of undernutrition including elements of stunting and wasting and is defined by a weight-for-age z-score (WAZ) below two standard deviations of the median (WHO standards). This indicator

is commonly used in growth monitoring and promotion (GMP) and child health and nutrition programs aimed at the prevention and treatment of undernutrition.
25. **Young child:** A person from the age of more than 12 months up to the age of 36 months.

▶ COMMUNITY NUTRITION

1. **Acupuncture:** A technique for insertion of special needles into particular parts of the body for the treatment of disease, relief of pain or production of anesthesia.
2. **AWW:** Anganwadi worker.
3. **CARE:** Cooperative for Assistance and Relief Everywhere.
4. **CFTRE:** Central Food Technology and Research Institute, Mysore.
5. **Diet therapy:** Use of food as an agent in effecting recovery from illness, prevention of disease and maintenance of health.
6. **FDTRC:** Food and Drug Toxicology Research Center, an additional centre of National Institute of Nutrition (NIN) along the NCLAS and NNMB.
7. **Gout:** A form of metabolic disorder in which sodium biurate is deposited in the cartilages of the joints; the big toe is characteristically involved and becomes acutely painful and swollen.
8. **Homeopathy:** A method of treating disease by prescribing minute doses of drugs, which in maximum dose, would produce symptoms of the disease; first adopted by Hahnemann.
9. **IAAH:** International Alliance Against Hunger, launched on World Food Day 16th October, 2003.
10. **ICDS:** Integrated Child Development Scheme.
11. **IDD:** Iodine deficiency disorder.
12. **MDSM:** Mid-day School Meal Scheme.

13. **NCLAS:** National Center for Laboratory Animal Sciences.
14. **NIPCCD:** National Institute of Public Cooperation and Child Development.
15. **NNMB:** National Nutrition Monitoring Bureau.
16. **Nutritional homeostasis:** A balanced state of available nutrients to the body tissues.
17. **Obesity:** Abnormal growth of the adipose tissues due to an enlargement of fat cell size (hypertrophic obesity) or an increase in fat cell number (hyperplastic obesity) or combination of both.
18. **Yoga:** A system of physical exercises and breathing control.

Index

A

Absorption 15, 74, 113, 116
   and excretion 113
   and utilization 68
   transport and storage 74, 78, 84,
     86, 89, 93, 96, 98, 102, 104, 105
Acid 368, 515t
   and alkali-producing food 327t
Adulteration
   concept 183
   definition 183
Alcohol 317
Alkali 327, 368
Amino acids 52, 54t
   sources 54t
Anemia 146, 563, 565
   control program 487
Angina pectoris 329
Antioxidants 271
Appetite 347
Applied nutrition program 487, 555, 569
   activities 570
Artificial feeding
   disadvantages 415
   methods 415
Ascites 303
Atherosclerosis 329

B

Baby-led weaning 443
Bacterial food poisoning 173, 173t
   common types 173
   prevention 174
Balanced diet 134
   elements 150t
   planning 165
Balwadi 489
   Nutrition Program 485, 554, 569
Basal metabolic rate 32, 33, 34t
Beriberi 109, 147

Beverage
   classification 599f
Blanching 203
Blood
   clotting 116
   sugar
     regulation 46
Body
   mass index 32
   size 36
   weight 309t
Bodybuilding food 22, 25
Breastfeeding
   advantages 411
   contraindication 410
   factors influencing 409
   important precautions 407
   methods 406, 406f
   policy 413
   technique 405
Bromelain 273
Bureau of Indian Standards 194

C

Calcium
   functions 115
   importance 118
Caloric values 31
   of nutrients 31t
Calorie 525, 607, 608
   chart of commonly used Indian
     food 607t
Carbohydrate 40, 278, 289, 296, 298,
   317, 323
   classification 41f
   digestion and absorption 44
   functions 42
   modified diets 255
   requirements 47
   sources 41t
Care digestible diet 281

Cereals 26
Child Nutrition Programs 484
Child Survival and Safe Motherhood
 Program 493
Chloride imbalance 131
Chlorine 131
Cholelithiasis 301
Cholestasis 303
Chromium 133
Cirrhosis of liver 297
Climate 36
Cold storage 216
Coma
 hepatic 299
Community nutrition 499
 programs 551
 rehabilitation 574
 training 576
Constipation 286
 causes 287
Consumer protection 194
Continuous tube feeding guidelines 477t
Cooking
 different methods 199
 methods 198
  combination 209
 objectives 198
Copper 132
Coronary heart disease 147, 329
Current nutritional deficiency
 status 556
Cutaneous tests 338
Cyanocobalamin 103

D

Day care centers 575
Deficiency
 diseases 530t, 531t, 535t
 effects 71, 77, 95, 97
 manifestations 539t, 540t
Degenerative Bright's disease 321
Dehydration 369
 causes and effects 369
 prevention 370
Dementia 98
Dermatitis 97
Detoxification function 43
Dexterity 348
Diabetes mellitus 48, 255, 306
Diabetic diet 242, 311

Diarrhea 97, 285
Diet 238
 and cancer 20
 and chronic diseases 20
 and dental diseases 20
 and diet therapy 21
 and mental health 21
 and nutrition 19
 and skeletal diseases 20
 high-protein 241
 in anemia 242
 in bleeding ulcer
  modification 292
 in sickness 236
 low
  calorie 240
  fat 241, 259
 plan for pre- and post-operative
  surgery 271
 principles 297, 310, 316,
  321, 330
 therapy
  allergy 334
  cardiovascular disorders 329
  endocrine and metabolic
   disorders 306
  gastrointestinal disorders 284
  liver diseases 294
  respiratory disorder 343
  urinary disorders 320
 therapy
  in different types of fever 275
  in fevers 274
  meaning 231
  principles 231
Dietary
 considerations 286, 288
  for teenagers 505
 counseling 315
 data collection 465
 fiber 312
 guidelines 291, 344
 history 337
 management 289, 290, 295, 298,
  300, 309, 316, 320, 322, 324,
  327, 331, 343
  in cardiovascular disorders 330
 modifications 249, 300
 requirements 398
 restriction for liver diseases 302
Digestion 14, 44, 67, 279

Index

Disaccharides 42
Dry
  beriberi 91
  heat methods 204
Drying method of preservation 220
Dumping syndrome 257

E

Edema 303
Electrolyte 286, 370
  imbalance 371
  regulation 371
Elimination diet
  role 340
Encephalopathy
  hepatic 302
Endocrine glands
  secretion 36
Energy-yielding foods 21, 25
Enteral
  feeding
    methods 474
  tube placement 472f
Enzyme activation 115
Essential fatty acids
  functions 67

F

FAO
  functions 588
  objectives 588
Fat 278, 289, 290, 296, 298, 302, 309, 316, 330, 332, 525
  controlled diets 258
  metabolism 43
  modified diets 258
  soluble vitamins 73
Fatty
  acids 65
  liver 304
Feeding
  artificial 414, 414t
  bottle 416
  complementary 422
  content 435
  cup 419
  fortifying 435
  intervals 279

intolerance
  management 436
  katori and spoon 418
  methods 434
Fever
  causes 276
  in children
    causes 277
  of short duration 275
  low grade 277
Financial resources 143
Fluids 268, 278, 285, 289, 317, 320, 323, 325
  and electrolytes 366
  modified diets 262
Fluoride 126
  deficiency and excess 127
Folic acid 101, 515t, 516t
Food
  adulteration 182
  Act
    prevention 192
  and health 185
  meaning 184
  allergy 149
  diagnosis 337
  and agricultural organization 587
  and nutrition board 586
    activities 586
  availability 143
  budget
    factors affecting 164
    importance 164
  classification 24
  contamination
    sources 171, 171f
  definition 182
  exchange 311
  expenditure 164
  fads and fallacies 156
  fiber content 312
  functions 21
  guide pyramid 237f
  hygiene 168
    basic rules 176
    sanitation 168
  intolerance 340
  laws and standards 192

poisoning 172
preservation
    methods 213
preservation
    principles 213
pyramid 605f
safety 179, 180
    Act 1990 179
sanitation
    principles 170
spoilage 212
    causes 212
Foodborne disease 172
Foodstuffs and climate
    availability 156
Freeze-drying 216
Fruit
    beverages 602
    juices 223

G

Gastric gavage 359, 360
Gastrointestinal tract 16f
    functioning 348
Gastrojejunostomy feeding 362
Gastrostomy feeding tube
    placement 473f
Gavage feeding 419
Glomerulonephritis 320
Glucose
    formation 46
    maintenance 42
Gout 315
Green leafy vegetables 28
Healthy balanced diet
    components 138

H

Hemochromatosis 304
High fever 277
Human milk 405t
Hydrogenation 70
Hygiene 168
    control 176
Hypercalcemia 383
Hyperkalemia 379
Hypermagnesemia 387
Hypernatremia 374

Hyperphosphatemia 391
Hypertension 331
Hyperthyroidism 314
Hypervitaminosis 78
Hypocalcemia 380
Hypokalemia 377
Hypomagnesemia 385
Hyponatremia 372
Hypophosphatemia 389
Hypothyroidism 314

I

Ideal body weight
    calculation 308
Infant
    feeding technique 424f
    nutritional assessment 456f
    weight measurement
    technique 459f
Infantile beriberi 92
Infective hepatitis 295
Intermittent fever 276
Iodine 124
Iron 120, 515t, 516t, 524
    deficiency anemia 540, 564

J

Jaundice 295
Joint diseases 315

K

Kilocalorie modifications 251
Kitchen appliances
    different types 198
Kwashiorkor 63t

L

Lactation 520t
Lactose intolerance 148, 258
Liquid diet 240
Logo of
    Central Food Technological
    Research Institute 591f
    Food and Agricultural
    Organization 587f

Index

Indian Council of Medical Research 590f
Low temperatures
    uses 217

M

Machine drying 216
Macronutrient 39
    deficiencies 528
Malnutrition 145, 480
    assessment 481
    causes 480
    effects 481
Marasmic kwashiorkor 62
Marasmus 61, 63, 63t
Micronutrient deficiencies 538
Microwave cooking 209
Mid-arm circumference measurement technique 461f
Mid-day meal program 485, 561
Milk
    and milk products 31, 608t
    and protein foods 290
    beverages 603
    hygiene 170
Minerals 268, 278, 289, 296, 299, 343, 398, 524
    elements 111
Minimal enteral nutrition 438
Moist heat methods 199
Monosaccharides 40
Muscle contraction and relaxation 116
Myocardial infarction 329

N

Nasogastric tube
    care 359f
    insertion 356
    measurement 357f
National Goiter Control Program 487, 567
National Nutritional Anemia Program 563
National Nutritional Policy 544
National Program for Prophylaxis Against Blindness 568
Nephrosis 321

Nerve impulse transmission 115
Niacin 95
    deficiency 110
Nicotinic acid 95
Night blindness 147
Non-alcoholic beverages 600
Nurse
    role 233
Nutrients 31t, 405t, 432t, 520t
    in therapeutic diet modification 232, 238
Nutrition
    concept 8
    education 581
        implications 583
        importance 582
        methods 584
        principles 585
    for sick child 470
    goals 433
    history 4
    in health
        importance 17
    in pregnancy 523
    program 484, 551, 554, 566
    Society of India 587
Nutritional
    assessment
        methods 458
    considerations in diarrhea 285
    deficiency 528
    problems of the child 478
    rehabilitation centers 455
    requirements 312, 431, 500, 508, 511, 520
    significance 599
    status
        assessment 457
        factors affecting 526
    stress 471

O

Obesity 148, 549
    assessment 550
Oligosaccharides 42
Oral rehydration
    salt 370
    therapy 370
Osteomalacia 81, 117
Osteoporosis 83, 117

P

Pantothenic acid 101
Parenteral
  access 475
  feeding 248, 475
  nutrition 437
Partial weaning 444
Pasteurization 217
Peer pressure 141
Pellagra 110
Peptic ulcer 290
Phosphorus 118, 321
Planning acid-ash diet 327
Planning
  alkaline-ash diet 327
  diets for adolescence 510
  low-oxalate diets 328
Polysaccharides 42
Potassium 128, 321, 323, 325
  modified diets 262
Precursors of nucleic acid 43
Pregnancy and breastfeeding 506
Premature infant 429
  feeding 427
Preparation of
  infant and environment 421
  milk formula for a day 414
Pressure cooking 202
Preterm nutrition
  importance 427
Preventing blood clots 272
Protein 49, 138, 268, 278, 289, 295, 298, 301, 309, 321, 323, 325, 332, 343, 523, 525
  allowance per day 60
  biological value 53
  complete 57
  diet
    low 240
  digestion 58
  energy malnutrition 528
  functions 55
  incomplete 58
  metabolism 59
  quality 57
  requirement
    factors affecting 56
  restricted diets 259
  sources 61t

sparing action 43
supplementary value 58
Provocative food tests 338
Pyridoxine 98

Q

Quetelet's index 32

R

Recurrent fever 277
Renal failure
  acute 322
Reproductive and Child Health Program 494
Retinol deficiency 109
Rheumatoid arthritis 315
Riboflavin 92
  deficiency 110
Rickets 80, 111, 146
Road-to-health chart 467, 468f

S

Scurvy 110, 147
Selenium 133
Skin and pressure ulcers 348
Sodium 127, 321, 323, 325, 332
  imbalance 128
  restricted diets 261, 332
Solar cooking 210
Specific nutritional deficiencies 146
Stress of illness 470
Strict elimination diets 339
Supplementary feeding
  program 453, 485
Syphon method 362

T

Tamil Nadu Integrated Nutrition Program 555
Tamil Nadu Integrated Nutrition Project 487
Thiamine 88
  deficiency 109
  role 90

Total parenteral nutrition
  infusion 475f
Trace elements 132
Triglycerides 65
Tube feeding 246, 359, 360, 477
Tuberculosis 343
Types of
  calculi 326
  drying 221
  insulin 308t
  special nutrition program 484
  surveys 457
  weaning 443
Typhoid fever 279

U

Unbalanced diets
  effects 145
Urinary calculi 326
Urolithiasis 326

V

Vertical nutrition program 552
Vision 590, 592, 594
Vitamin 72, 269, 278, 289, 296, 299,
  344, 398, 515t, 524
  A 73
    deficiency 109, 568
    prophylaxis program 486
  C 105, 272
    deficiency 110
  D 78
    deficiency 111
  deficiencies 109
  E 84
  K 86
    deficiency 111

W

Water
  functions 367
  importance 366
  soluble vitamins 88
Weaning
  foods 443, 446
    choosing 442
  importance 441
Wet beriberi 92
Wilson's disease 304
World Food Program 570, 571
Wounds
  healing 272

X

Xerophthalmia 109

Y

Yield energy 42
Youth clubs 489

Z

Zinc 123, 132
  deficiency 542